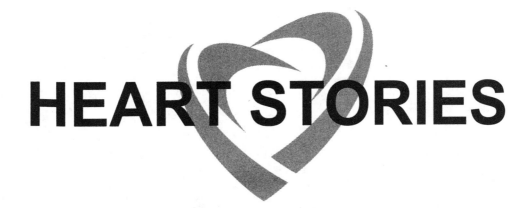

HEART STORIES

HEART STORIES

About Patients and the great Pioneers who saved them

Robert G. Hauser MD

ISBN-10: 0-692-81783-2
ISBN-13: 978-0-692-81783-4

GeorgiaMae Publishing LLC
Robert G. Hauser MD
1023 Barcarmil Way
Naples, FL 34110

rhauser747@gmail.com

Printed in Naples, Florida, USA

The logo on the front cover is published with permission of the
Minneapolis Heart Institute Foundation

This book is dedicated to my family—
Jennifer, Amy, Sarah, and particularly to my wife Sally—
for their love, support, and understanding.

"A physician can have no greater reward than the knowledge that he has been the means of bringing relief in a cruel disease, especially when this relief prevails over an agonizing symptom."

Sir Clifford Allbutt, 1915

ACKNOWLEDGEMENTS

I remember with deep gratitude the teachers and mentors who profoundly affected me as a physician and academic: Miss Marie Becker, Dr. Kip Weichert, Dean Richard Kiley, Dr. Edward Gall, Dr. Ormand Julian, and Dr. Joseph Messer. What they did for me at critical times in my career cannot be repaid with words; I can only hope that their efforts on my behalf were worth it.

I am indebted to Dr. Marshall Goldin for his critical review of my manuscript.

I was very fortunate to be a member of the Minneapolis Heart Institute (MHI) and the Minneapolis Heart Institute Foundation (MHIF). MHI was founded in 1982 by a group of cardiovascular specialists who were led by Drs. Robert Van Tassel, Richard Nelson, Fred Gobel, and Jim Daniel. MHIF is a separate non-profit organization dedicated to research and education and largely supported by the community and Abbott Northwestern Hospital. It was a great privilege to practice cardiology with my MHI colleagues, and to be a clinical investigator for MHIF.

I am grateful to Carol Pine for her guidance in preparing the manuscript, and to the staff of the Abbott Northwestern Hospital Library for their help in researching the materials for this book.

PROLOGUE

In Post-World War II America, members of the "Greatest Generation," who won the war and kept the country safe, returned home to peacetime life. They went back to school, married, had children, and built the largest economy the world had ever seen.

They also launched breathtaking advances in medicine. Penicillin killed the streptococcal bacteria that caused rheumatic fever. Vaccines virtually eliminated polio and other childhood diseases. Streptomycin and isoniazid cured tuberculosis and, in the process, emptied hundreds of sanatoriums. Surgical techniques that evolved in countless battlefield hospitals saved and rehabilitated peacetime victims of trauma and severe burns. Hospitals were no longer places where people died: they became sanctuaries for healing, birthing babies, and emergency care.

After 1945, the countries in Europe and Asia that were devastated by war recovered, albeit slowly, aided by the Marshall Plan. Their great academic institutions rebuilt their universities, restored their teaching faculties, and gradually resumed medical research.

Many countries introduced universal health care. Medical schools began graduating increasing numbers of physicians. Among them were some of the great scientists and technologists of the latter half of the 20th century. Moreover, a host of displaced persons and refugees attended universities in the west, providing a wealth of new talent and ambition. International scientific collaboration grew gradually at first but then accelerated rapidly, catalyzing discovery and innovation. Strong professional societies in the Americas, Europe, and Asia emerged to develop and promote excellence in cardiovascular care.

From 1945 to 1970, the most spectacular advances occurred in heart surgery. Millions of children and adults were suffering and dying from incurable cardiac conditions: blue babies, congenitally deformed hearts, and valves wrecked by rheumatic fever. After World War I a few courageous surgeons tried to repair them and failed. But the new generation of heart surgeons who emerged after 1945 were far more determined. Almost all of them had served in World War II and they possessed a bold "we-can-fix-it" attitude toward heart disease.

The clinical challenges before them were daunting: frail, purple children who were so weak they could not cry; women who could not breathe because their lungs were congested with the frothy, blood-tinged fluid of heart failure; men who dropped dead in the farm field or on the factory floor; and millions of adults who were debilitated by the yellow-white plaque clogging their arteries. By 1970, this new generation had established five pillars of cardiac surgery: the heart-lung machine, artificial heart valve replacement, coronary artery bypass, repair of complex congenital heart disease, and permanent pacemaker implantation

The next quarter century, from 1970 to 1995, was another period rich with discovery and invention. We saw advanced coronary care units, echocardiography, coronary angioplasty, nuclear imaging, and new treatments for peripheral vascular disease. Technology spawned a multi-billion-dollar medical device industry. This was an era when physicians born after 1930 drove many of the breakthrough innovations.

We learned that blood clots caused heart attacks and the faster we could remove them, the better chance our patients had to survive and resume productive lives. New and rediscovered drugs were evaluated in large randomized clinical trials, and many proved to be safe and effective: aspirin, statins, beta-blockers, ACE inhibitors, and thrombolytics (clot busters). Implantable defibrillators prevented sudden cardiac death in high-risk patients. Antirejection drugs dramatically improved survival after heart transplantation. Each discovery and clinical triumph emboldened us to go faster and climb higher.

The two decades after 1995 saw dramatic improvements in technology: drug-coated coronary stents, pacemakers for heart failure, durable tissue heart valves and valves that could be implanted without surgery. Techniques emerged to repair rather than replace the mitral valve. Artificial hearts morphed into a permanent solution for heart failure, rather than a bridge to transplantation. Novel blood thinners and cholesterol lowering drugs became available.

Many troublesome arrhythmias were cured with catheters that burned the heart tissue producing them, a technique called ablation. Imaging with high-resolution CT scanners and MRIs added new knowledge and improved our diagnostic and therapeutic capabilities. Research revealed significant gender differences in how heart disease manifests and responds to treatment in women. We applied systems of care to deliver better outcomes and developed guidelines to diagnose and treat heart disease based on the best available scientific data. Rather than practice in isolation, cardiologists, cardiac and vascular surgeons, and other caregivers formed integrated teams to deliver the highest quality and most appropriate care.

I wrote this book for everyone. I wrote it to educate readers and to show future generations what it took to throttle the epidemic of heart disease that exploded in the 20th century. It has been my privilege to practice cardiology during these extraordinary times. I graduated from the University of Cincinnati in 1968, and completed my cardiology training in 1973 at Rush Presbyterian-St. Luke's Medical Center in Chicago. During more than four decades, I have witnessed all of these advances in cardiac care.

When I graduated from medical school, a third of heart attack victims died at home or in the hospital. Heart rhythm disorders were killing or crippling hundreds of thousands of Americans every year. Severe heart failure was a death sentence. Preventive cardiology was practically unknown: the significance of high cholesterol was being debated, 50 percent of adults were smoking cigarettes, and high blood pressure was usually undetected and often poorly controlled. All of this changed for the better—much better—during the 47 years I practiced medicine and cardiology.

Patient stories are the centerpiece of this narrative. Their stories and the dialogues are fictionalized but they are based on actual patients, experiences, and my best recollections. With only a few exceptions, I knew and cared for all of them. Some patient stories are hybrids of several patients, and their histories have been further dramatized based on historical facts. The only exceptions to this are patients of historical interest whose health information is in the public domain.

I have interwoven these patient stories with the stories of the actual physicians, scientists, and engineers whose brilliance and determination brought my patients relief from pain and suffering. Some may think I glamorize the great pioneers, and ignored their human frailties and excesses. Such a sentiment may be justified, but it is what they did to improve the human condition that is central to this book.

From 1974 to 1986, I was a fulltime member of the Section of Cardiology at Rush University Medical Center in Chicago where I was Professor of Medicine. In 1987, I moved to Minnesota where I was Chairman and Chief Executive Officer of Cardiac Pacemakers, Inc., a division of Eli Lilly and Company, until 1992. In 1987 I also joined the Minneapolis Heart Institute, where I practiced clinical cardiology until October 2015.

During my clinical career I was fortunate to work with highly talented and dedicated physicians. Many of my partners and colleagues at Rush University Medical Center and the Minneapolis Heart Institute are included in this book. They are the men and women with whom I practiced for nearly five decades. Most of them participated in the care of my patients, and many of them were also research collaborators and personal friends.

This book is not intended to be a history of cardiology or heart surgery. It chronicles what I saw, experienced, and felt during this golden age of cardiovascular care. The stories begin with my first day as a doctor.

CHAPTER 1

At noon on Friday, June 28, 1968 I reported to the surgery office expecting to attend the interns' orientation, pick up my uniforms, and leave.

"You are on-call tonight, Doctor Hauser", the secretary said, smiling. It was the first time anyone except my family had called me "Doctor."

I replied, "I didn't know. The letter just said I should be here for orientation."

"This *is* your orientation. You are the intern on the cardiac surgery service. Here are your uniforms and pager. The head nurse wants you on the ninth floor."

"But…my wife and baby daughter are waiting for me in the car…we need to pay the movers…in Evanston."

She stopped smiling. "I don't know what to say. Your family will have to manage without you. You are needed on the ninth floor."

Twenty minutes later my wife Sally, seven month-old daughter Jenny, and two Pekingese were on Lake Shore Drive in our aging Buick, driving north to our new apartment in Evanston without me. They were on their own, and so was I, a newly graduated doctor who was about to spend an exhausting and anxiety-filled weekend as a new intern at Presbyterian-St. Luke's Hospital in downtown Chicago.

I stepped off the elevator onto the cardiac surgical unit. The head nurse was waiting for me. She wore an ankle-length starched white nurse's uniform and cap. "Are you Doctor Hauser?"

I nodded.

"Doctor, you have an emergency. The patient in 928 is very bradycardic [slow heart rate]."

I followed her. Looking over her shoulder she said, "I believe she is in heart block."

"Heart block…heart block," I muttered to myself.

"Would you like Isuprel®, Doctor?"

"Yes", I said hesitantly, not remembering the dose.

"A milligram in 250 of normal saline?" she asked.

Relieved, I replied, "Yes, yes please."

The patient in 928 was a young woman who had recently undergone repair of her mitral valve that had been damaged by rheumatic fever in childhood. The surgeon had opened the scarred valve through an incision in her chest the previous day. A rubber tube in her lung cavity drained bloody fluid into a clear glass bottle under the bed. She was pale and cool to the touch. Her pulse was slow and irregular. She looked up at me and smiled. Then her eyes closed.

My heart was racing and my mouth was dry. Panic extended its embrace. I was no longer a student. This dying woman was my first patient and I was her doctor.

The head nurse hung the bottle of Isuprel® on the pole at the head of the bed and connected the tubing to the intravenous catheter. She opened a thumbscrew on the plastic tubing and the solution began to drip rapidly. The medication should stimulate my patient's heart to beat faster. A minute passed. Nothing happened. The bedside monitor showed a heart rate of 22 beats a minute. Gradually her pulse increased…30…42…68…84 beats a minute. The drug was working.

Abruptly her heart rate rose to 120, then 150. Ugly extra beats appeared. "Slow it down." I ordered. The nurse turned the thumbscrew clockwise and the drips from the bottle decreased. After a few minutes, her heart rate steadied at 90 to100 beats per minute. The extra beats disappeared. She opened her eyes and whispered, "I'm so tired." I patted her shoulder.

"Should I call her cardiologist—Dr. Clark?" the nurse asked.

"Yes, please."

Another nurse entered. "Doctor Hauser, they need you in intensive care. Stat!"

I ran down three flights of stairs to the intensive care unit, taking two steps at a time. A patient who had open-heart surgery that day was bleeding bright red blood through large light brown rubber tubes in his chest. He was unconscious and on a ventilator.

Three nurses surrounded his bed. One was hanging a bag of blood, another was squeezing the chest tubes so the blood would drain faster, and the third was drawing up two large syringes of sodium bicarbonate. The third nurse—her nickname was "Smokey"—eyed me narrowly, placed both syringes in my hands, and said, "Here, Doctor, do something."

"Call the surgeon," I said, while injecting the contents of the first syringe into the intravenous tubing.

Smokey said, "He's in surgery. You're it."

"Let's get a hematocrit," I ordered.

A voice behind me said, "You don't need that. Give him two units of fresh frozen plasma. He's not clotting." I turned and faced an older man in light blue scrubs and a long white lab coat. "I'm Gene Delaney," he said, and we shook hands. Dr. Delaney was about 45 years old and graying. He had left his general surgical practice in downstate Illinois to train as a vascular surgeon. He would be my supervisor for the next 6 weeks

"I'll take over here," Delaney said. "You need to see patients on the ninth floor." He handed me a small black notebook containing about fifty pages. On each page in bold type were a patient's name, diagnosis, and procedures planned or completed. Also there were handwritten notes made by the previous intern who had gone off duty when I arrived. I shoved the notebook into my short white intern's coat pocket and headed for the elevator.

"Oh Hauser," Delaney called after me, "there's blood on your trousers. The chief doesn't like patients or families to see blood on anyone. Change them and meet me at five for afternoon rounds in the ICU conference room."

I changed my bloodstained trousers in the surgery locker room. Next door was a coffee vending machine but I did not have a dime. I needed caffeine but there was no time to go to the cafeteria. My pager beeped. I called the switchboard. "They want you in the catheterization laboratory. Dr. Clark is putting a temporary pacemaker in one of your patients."

Dr. Jim Clark was a young cardiologist who I met in my externship at Presbyterian-St. Luke's the previous summer. My patient with heart block from the ninth floor was lying on the X-ray table. Clark was in a surgical gown and mask. "Bob, thanks for taking care of this young lady," he said. "A temporary pacemaker should get her through the weekend. She may need a permanent pacemaker."

Clark inserted a thin plastic pacing catheter into a vein in her right arm at the elbow and guided the tip into the right side of her heart using X-ray fluoroscopy.

He asked the nurse to connect the pacing catheter to a black battery-powered electronic pacemaker and turn it on. The pacemaker stimulated her heart at 80 beats per minute.

My pager beeped. I pressed the button to stop the shrill high-pitched sound. It beeped again, and again. I called the switchboard, thinking the operator was impatient. "You have three pages, Doctor," the operator said briskly. I wrote down the numbers and called the one I knew to be the intensive care unit.

"Mr. Kane in 614 doesn't look good," the nurse said.

"Where is the medical intern?" I asked.

"He's here. He said to call you. He doesn't know what to do."

It was his first day too.

About half way to the ICU, the overhead paging system blared: "Doctor Hauser ICU, Doctor Hauser ICU, Doctor Hauser ICU." It was my first emergency page. There would be many more that weekend. Was it a cardiac arrest? I broke into a run.

The medical intern stood by the bed doing nothing. Mr. Kane was not breathing. I felt for a pulse—there was none—so I started chest compressions. He was recovering from open-heart surgery and the incision through his sternum (breastbone) was just beginning to heal. I clasped my hands and pushed downward on his chest. I could feel the edges of the freshly cut sternum sag under the force of my compressions. I prayed for the wire sutures to hold.

Meanwhile, a nurse wheeled the emergency cart into the room while another nurse connected him to an EKG machine. A respiratory therapist placed an airway in Mr. Kane's throat and began breathing for him with a facemask.

"Get the defibrillator," I said. I tried to stay calm, but my heart was pounding. I struggled to remember the precise sequence of what I needed to do. Soon it would become automatic.

I paused my compressions and looked at the EKG. Mr. Kane was in ventricular fibrillation, an ineffective, chaotic rhythm that portends death. He needed an electric shock to stop the fibrillation. The nurse spread a conductive gel on the defibrillator's two metal paddles and handed them to me. "Set it to 400," I said, as I placed the paddles on either side of his chest. I pressed the buttons on the paddles. The defibrillator's capacitors popped and a thousand volts drove millions of electrons through Mr. Kane's heart. He convulsed, as the powerful electrical energy made the muscles of his chest wall contract violently.

The shock was successful. Kane had a slow, regular rhythm. I could feel a strong pulse in his groin. His eyes fluttered. The respiratory therapist suctioned his mouth and throat. He gagged and grabbed the therapist's arm.

"Sir, you're okay! You're okay!" I shouted into his ear. "Just relax! Relax!" He groaned and let go of her arm.

The room was suddenly quiet. Everyone relaxed; the tide of adrenalin that gripped us receded. The emergency was over. Jim Clark arrived and I related what had happened. He ordered a chest X-ray and blood tests. I left to answer another page. It was 5 p.m., and I had yet to see even one of the two dozen or so patients on the 9th floor.

I was up most of the night reviewing charts and seeing hospital patients. I went through a pack of cigarettes and a pot of black coffee. Around 5 a.m., I went to one of the on-call rooms and managed to sleep for an hour and a half before my pager beeped. It was nearly shift change, and the night nurses were calling to update me on the sickest patients.

It was 7 a.m. Saturday morning and I had been on duty for 20 hours. I would go off duty in 11 hours at 6 p.m. My pager went off. It was Gene Delaney in the emergency room. "Hauser, I have a patient with a ruptured abdominal aortic aneurysm. He needs to go directly to the operating room. Javid is coming in. You and I will assist. We will do rounds later. Got it?"

"Got it," I replied, and headed for the surgery locker room.

Dr. Hushang Javid was putting on his scrubs when I arrived in the locker room. He was a refined, friendly man and a superb surgeon, completely unflappable no matter how desperate the situation.

"First day, doctor?" he asked. "Yes, sir," I replied. "I remember my first day," he said, sighing. He did not wait for a reply. "Do you know anything about this patient?" I told him that Gene Delaney had examined the patient in the emergency room. At that moment, Delaney entered the locker room.

"Hello Dr. Javid," Delaney said. "This patient is on warfarin for a DVT (deep venous thrombosis) and his prothrombin time (a measure of clotting) is quite long. I gave him vitamin K and ordered fresh frozen plasma. I'm afraid he's going to bleed, but I don't think we can wait."

"Let's go." Javid headed down the stairs to the operating room.

The three of us scrubbed at the sink. Through the window, we could see the anesthesiologist and two nurses positioning the patient on the operating table. Another nurse was unpacking the sterile instrument trays. A fourth nurse was hanging a bag of fresh frozen plasma.

The anesthesiologist stuck his head out the swinging door. "His pressure is 70, Dr. Javid. I think we should start Levophed."

Javid said, "Okay, but don't get his pressure too high. We're going to have enough trouble with bleeding."

One after another, we backed through the door into the operating room. Javid and Delaney gowned and gloved first. Javid stood on the patient's left, facing Delaney across the table. I stood next to Delaney near the head of the table.

"What's the pressure?" Javid asked the anesthesiologist.

"158," was the reply.

"That's too high, turn down the Levophed."

Javid made a long incision in the abdomen from just below the sternum and around the umbilicus. Delaney took a retractor, positioned it in the incision and motioned for me to hold it while he placed hemostats on bleeders and suctioned blood from the wound. The tissues seemed to fall away as Javid dissected through fascia and muscle. As he entered the abdominal cavity and retracted the bowel, the aortic aneurysm burst. A jet of bright red blood shot outward and splattered my cheek and neck.

Javid reached into the incision and placed a large clamp across the aorta. The bleeding stopped. The anesthesiologist had two bags of blood running. The scrub nurse handed me a second suction cannula and large cloth sponges to soak up the blood.

"Give him two more units of blood," Javid said to the anesthesiologist. "What's his protime? He seems to be clotting."

"The last protime was 16. We should be okay," the anesthesiologist replied.

Javid looked at me. "Are you okay, Bob?" he asked. I nodded.

So far, the patient had received seven units of blood. "What's his pressure?" Javid asked. The anesthesiologist pumped the blood pressure cuff and let it down slowly. "Ninety, ninety-five."

"That's good," Javid replied. "Let's go ahead."

The operation took two hours. Delaney assisted Javid as he cut the aorta and iliac arteries and inserted a synthetic woven Dacron® Y-graft. The longer, larger limb of the graft was connected to the aorta, while the two short limbs of the "Y" were connected to the common iliac arteries.

Afterward I showered and dressed into fresh white trousers, blue knit tie, white shirt, and short white coat. I called the switchboard and told the operator I was out of surgery. There were a dozen or more tasks to be done that morning but first I needed some food. I got a roll and coffee out of the vending machines. It was about 11 a.m.

Delaney told me to join the team making rounds on the ninth floor. The surgical residents were already there with Dr. James Hunter, a cardiac surgeon who worked in Javid's group. We saw 24 patients during the next three hours.

By 6 p.m., I was fading. "Get out of here, Hauser," Delaney ordered. "See you at 8 a.m. tomorrow." I had been on duty for 30 hours, but this would be one of the shorter shifts on this rotation.

Sally, Jenny, and the dogs—Gidget and Gerkerdee—were waiting for me in the faded bronze Buick at the front entrance of the hospital. I kissed Sally through the open window and she slid over to the passenger side as I settled behind the wheel. We drove north to Evanston on Lake Shore Drive. It was a beautiful evening, but all I wanted to do was have dinner and go to bed.

My first day as a doctor was over. I would remember it forever. Soon life outside the hospital would become a pit stop, a temporary reprieve from the incessant, grinding demands of acute patient care. As I drove along Lake Michigan with Sally and Jenny, I was relieved and reasonably satisfied with my performance. While panic had visited my doorstep, I had not let it in.

That night, lying next to Sally, I thought of the patients I had cared for during those 30 hours and asked myself what I could have done better. This would be my routine for decades to come.

CHAPTER 2

Early the following morning I drove down Lake Shore Drive to the hospital. The summer sun was already over Lake Michigan and joggers were running along the beach. One of them, a young woman, had a huge unleashed black Labrador retriever trotting at her side. The horizon blue water was tranquil and a few sailboats were slowly, silently cruising out of Belmont Harbor. In the distance I could see the John Hancock building looming over Water Tower Place. The view was exciting and seductive. I wondered what the next 36 hours would hold for me. It was a beautiful summer Sunday. Perhaps the hospital would be quiet.

I was wrong.

My pager beeped as I was parking my car in the lot across from Presbyterian St. Luke's Hospital, which is located on the Eisenhower Expressway just west of the Chicago Loop. Dr. Milton Weinberg wanted me in the ICU immediately. Weinberg was a cardiac surgeon who specialized in congenital heart disease—infants and children who were born with bad hearts.

Weinberg sat on the edge of Billy Samuel's bed. Billy had just arrived in the ICU from the operating room. He was unconscious, pale and shivering despite a mound of blankets. He had a breathing tube in his throat, and the green pediatric Bird respirator inflated his lungs every four seconds. The large black and white EKG monitor showed a regular rhythm. His heart rate was 100 beats a minute and the vertical spike of a pacemaker stimulus preceded each beat. I thought Billy must be nine or ten, but, in fact, he was fourteen.

"He was sent here from Moline in bad shape," Weinberg told me. "I operated on him early this morning and repaired a VSD (ventricular septal defect). We couldn't wait. He was on the heart-lung machine for 80 minutes. Now he has heart block. I have the temporary pacemaker set to a 100. He could need a permanent pacemaker, so I sewed on a permanent lead just in case. Can you watch him while I go to breakfast?"

Without waiting for my reply he continued, "I'm giving him a little Isuprel®. His blood pressure is okay but he's not making any urine. His mother is in the waiting room. I will speak to her on the way out." He thanked me and left.

I took Weinberg's place on the edge of the bed and felt Billy's legs. They were cool and dry. His nail beds were white. His shivers came in paroxysms and the nurse added another blanket. I touched his eyelids; they flickered -- a sign that the anesthetic was wearing off. The tiny drops of Isuprel® were emerging from the intravenous bottle at a rate of 10 drops a minute. A technician handed me a slip of paper with the results of Billy's last arterial blood gas. His oxygen saturation and carbon dioxide level were acceptable, but the acid in his blood was accumulating. I gave him half an ampule of sodium bicarbonate intravenously.

During the next 45 minutes, I reduced the dose of Isuprel® because it was causing numerous extra beats called premature ventricular contractions. His systolic blood pressure remained around 90. A rivulet of yellow urine appeared in the clear plastic tubing connected to the Foley catheter in his bladder. The shivering lessened and his skin felt warmer.

"How's he doing, doctor?" I turned to face a plump woman in a faded pink flower print dress carrying an olive green canvas handbag. "I'm Billy's mother." Her gray-streaked light brown hair was in a bun and she wore no make-up. She probably had not slept.

"A little better," I replied. "I'm Doctor Hauser, Mrs. Samuels."

Standing by the bed, she took her son's hand. "This is his second surgery," she said. "He was only three months old when he had the first one in Minnesota. The past year has been real hard on him. We kept him out of school most of the winter. Last week he came down with a chest cold and he just got worse. I sat up with him most nights. I know I should have brought him in sooner but we don't have any insurance…"

"You brought him to the right hospital," I said. "Dr. Weinberg is excellent. I think you should try to sleep. The nurses know where you are." She carefully placed her son's hand down on the bed and covered it with one of the blankets. "I'm very tired," she whispered, not wanting her son to hear how weary his mother was. "I'll go back to the waiting room now."

Weinberg returned from the cafeteria. He was about six feet in height, wore wire-rimmed glasses, and was polite and approachable. Later I would observe and occasionally be the object of his temper. I told him that Billy appeared to be improving and that his mother had returned to the waiting room. He thanked me, and I left to see patients on the ninth floor.

When I returned to the ICU later that day, Weinberg was still at Billy's bedside. The breathing tube was gone and the Isuprel® was no longer needed. Billy was waking up, breathing on his own. His eyes darted from Weinberg to me and then to the nurse. He moaned and closed his eyes.

"Well, Billy is doing better," Weinberg, said. "I was worried that the surgery was too late. In 1963 I spent time with Walt Lillehei at the University of Minnesota. He said never give up on young patients—no matter how sick they are. Kids have a way of bouncing back. I've always remembered that. If it weren't for Lillehei, we probably would not be doing this kind of surgery. Do you know anything about Walt Lillehei?"

I did.

In 1950 thousands of children died because they were born with all sorts of heart defects: holes that allowed blood to flow in the wrong direction, twisted arteries, incompetent valves, and missing parts. Surgeons could not repair them because no one had figured out how to open a heart, fix it, and keep the patient alive.

Many children died as infants. Others suffered recurrent lung infections, delayed physical development, and learning disabilities. The most common defect was a hole between the two main pumping chambers—the ventricles—called a ventricular septal defect or VSD. Patients with large VSDs rarely lived beyond age 20. During their foreshortened lives, they experienced fatigue and shortness of breath. Some of them turned blue as the pressure inside their lungs became higher than the pressure in their little bodies. There was no medical treatment, and no surgeon had successfully closed a VSD. Parents could only watch and grieve as their children struggled, deteriorated, and died.

But this dire outlook changed because a determined group of university surgeons in Minnesota figured out how to open the heart and repair VSDs and other lethal heart defects. In the process, they invented the first practical heart-lung machine and cardiac pacemaker. They were led by Dr. C. Walton "Walt" Lillehei.

Lillehei grew up in Edina, Minnesota, a fashionable suburb southwest of Minneapolis. His family had emigrated from Norway in 1885. Lillehei's father was a dentist who was serving in World War I when Walt was born on October 23, 1918. A bit of a loner, Walt spent his youth playing sports and tinkering with machines. He assembled a motorcycle from spare parts without a manual, and he modified a BB gun to shoot 22- caliber bullets. Nevertheless, he was an average student in high school. Then something clicked and in 1939 young Dr. Lillehei graduated with honors in the top 10 percent of his medical school class at the University of Minnesota. He interned at the Minneapolis General Hospital, later renamed Hennepin County Medical Center.

During World War II, Lillehei commanded a mobile army surgical hospital (MASH) unit in North Africa and Italy where he earned many commendations, including a Bronze Star and five battle stars. After returning home in 1945, he began his surgical training at the University of Minnesota under Dr. Owen Wangensteen.

A Minnesota farm boy of Norwegian descent, Owen Wangensteen wanted to be a farmer like his father. In 1914, when he was a junior in high school, his family's 50 sows were unable to deliver their piglets, and the local veterinarian said they should be sent to the slaughterhouse. Instead, Owen figured out how to help the sows deliver by using his hands. During the next three weeks he delivered 300 piglets. This success persuaded the elder Wangensteen that his son should study medicine. Owen graduated from the University of Minnesota Medical School in 1921 and received his surgical training at both the Mayo Clinic and the University where he received his Ph.D.

Owen Wangensteen became the chief of surgery at the University when he was just 32. He got the position, in part, because no one else wanted it. One candidate, a Harvard professor, declined the job and was heard muttering, "...there is nothing here and never will be." The medical school's leadership recognized Wangensteen's potential when he was only a surgical resident; they decided to groom him to be the next chief and sent him abroad to study in Europe.

Wangensteen spurned the financial benefits of a private practice so he could build a premiere academic program, setting high standards for his surgical staff and trainees. An innovator himself, Wangensteen developed a long nasogastric tube for decompressing the stomach and intestines that saved thousands of patients with life-threatening bowel obstructions. During World War II, so many wounded soldiers were treated with this tube that battlefield hospitals had units named "Wangensteen Wards."

In 1939, Wangensteen began to operate on patients who had a patent ductus arteriosus. The ductus arteriosus is a small vascular connection between the pulmonary artery and the aorta that normally closes shortly after birth. If the ductus arteriosus remains open, however, a variable volume of blood is shunted—diverted—from the aorta to the pulmonary artery and then to the lungs. This shunting means that the heart must work harder and, if a lot of blood is being shunted, patients eventually develop heart failure. In 1938 Dr. Robert Gross in Boston was the first to surgically close a ductus arteriosus. Wangensteen performed his first ductus arteriosus operation one year later, launching the great era of heart surgery at the University of Minnesota.

Owen Wangensteen was the perfect mentor for Walt Lillehei's restless intellect: he was open to almost any idea, but he insisted that any research conducted in his department be presented at national medical meetings and published in prominent surgical journals. The research had to be that good. He also demanded that his residents be thoroughly grounded in the basic sciences, especially physiology, and encouraged them to obtain their doctorates. Often he sent trainees to study under leading scientists at other universities. Wangensteen saw to it that Lillehei earned his Ph.D.

In 1951, something magical began to happen at the University of Minnesota. The Variety Club of the Northwest helped fund a 78-bed, $1.6 million heart hospital at the University that was devoted entirely to the medical and surgical treatment of heart disease. The idea of a heart hospital was born in 1944 when many children suffering from rheumatic heart disease waited months to see a specialist at the University Hospital.

The Variety Club, spurred by Al Steffers, a motion picture theater owner in Minneapolis, led the fund raising campaign. The Club enlisted the assistance of Warner Brothers in Hollywood to make a short film for moviegoers to view following the feature film. It starred Ronald Reagan, the future president of the United States, who exhorted the audience to join the battle against heart disease. Hundreds of theaters throughout the northwest featured the short film and the campaign raised a half million dollars, a sum matched by the University of Minnesota and the federal government.

In 1952, a year after the Variety Club Heart hospital opened, Dr. F. John Lewis, one of Wangensteen's talented young surgeons, performed the world's first successful open-heart surgery when he closed an atrial septal defect in the heart of a very sick five-year-old girl. An atrial septal defect is a hole between the two atria that results in shunting of blood, which overloads the heart. Lewis did this by lowering the youngster's body temperature to reduce the amount of oxygen that her brain, heart, and other vital organs needed. The technique, called whole body hypothermia, had been tested in animals.

After her was body cooled to 82° F, Lewis stopped the blood returning to the right side of her heart and cut open the right atrium. He could see the hole between the two atria, and he quickly closed the hole with stitches. Only five and a half minutes elapsed before normal blood flow was restored. The girl recovered, and Lewis repeated his landmark surgery on 32 additional patients with good results and very few deaths.

Lewis' technique was limited by the very brief period of time he could safely shut off blood flow and perform a repair. It would be difficult to fix more complex congenital defects, a reality that Lewis would encounter when he tried unsuccessfully to close ventricular septal defects.

Meanwhile Walt Lillehei was busy in his animal laboratory located in the attic of the University of Minnesota Medical School. Because he had no functional heart-lung machine, Lillehei and two of his residents—Drs. Morley Cohen and Herbert Warden—developed a procedure they called "cross-circulation" to experiment with open-heart techniques in dogs. One large dog supported the circulation of a second, smaller dog while Lillehei's team opened the little dog's heart. They connected the arteries and veins of the two dogs with plastic tubes and used a commercially available SigmaMotor finger pump to maintain blood flow between the two animals. It was elegantly simple and it worked. Originally, the

SigmaMotor pump propelled milk during processing for the dairy industry, and bars used the clear plastic tubes to connect beer kegs to taps.

Lillehei had an outrageous thought: Could this cross circulation technique work in humans? Could he use a healthy adult—the "donor"—to support the circulation of a child during open-heart surgery? Would the healthy donor suffer any ill effects and could this approach buy sufficient time to repair cardiac abnormalities that were more complex than an atrial septal defect?

To answer these questions, Lillehei and his team conducted more detailed studies in dogs. They operated on highly trained golden retrievers and found that the dogs performed their hunting duties as effectively after the surgery as they did before. The accumulated evidence suggested that cross-circulation was ready for clinical trial. With Wangensteen's support, Lillehei decided to move forward, even though cross-circulation risked the lives of two people—the patient and the donor. Someone observed that the procedure could have a 200 percent mortality rate.

Lillehei faced obstacles and principal among them was Dr. Cecil Watson, the University's chief of medicine. Watson was a nationally prominent internist and professor who specialized in liver disease. He had been involved in the atomic bomb program during World War II, and was instrumental in developing the American Board of Internal Medicine.

Watson and Wangensteen were powerful personalities, and the tension between them surfaced when Lillehei proposed using cross-circulation in order to repair a ventricular septal defect in 12-month-old Gregory Glidden from northern Minnesota. Watson could not prevent the surgery himself but he went to the head of the University Hospital, Ray Amberg, and exhorted him to stop Lillehei. The surgery, Watson said, was unethical and sheer madness.

Amberg, a former pharmacist, was in a difficult position. Recently, Dr. John Lewis had lost two patients in the University's operating room while attempting to close their ventricular septal defects using whole body hypothermia. For Gregory Glidden's operation, Lillehei planned to use his healthy father to support the circulation of his infant son. Lyman Glidden worked in the Mesabi Range mines and he was the only breadwinner for his wife, Frances, and their 11 children. If anything went wrong, both Lyman and his son could die. Along with the high human cost and public criticism, adverse publicity could negatively affect the legislature's willingness to increase funding for the University Hospital.

Gregory Glidden had been in the University's Variety Club heart hospital for several months and he celebrated his first birthday there. Lillehei and his team did everything possible to get Gregory in the best physical shape for surgery. The Gliddens had lost a 12-year-old daughter, Donna, to the ravages of a ventricular septal defect; she had died in her sleep in 1950. Unlike Donna who had a relatively normal childhood, Gregory had been sick almost from birth. Recurring "bronchitis" made him a frequent patient at the hospital in Hibbing, Minnesota. Eventually a physician heard a heart murmur and sent Gregory to the pediatric cardiologists at the University where a heart catheterization confirmed the presence of a large ventricular septal defect.

Lillehei met with Lyman and Frances Glidden and described how he proposed to repair Gregory's VSD. He explained that Lyman would have tubes connected to an artery and a vein in his leg, and his blood would be pumped back and forth to provide life-sustaining oxygen for his infant son. Lyman, who had the same blood type as his son, readily agreed.

The forty-year-old Ray Amberg listened to Cecil Watson's concerns, but he had great respect for Owen Wangensteen and knew of Gregory Glidden's desperate situation. He decided not to interfere.

Thus at eight-thirty a.m. on March 26, 1954, Gregory and Lyman Glidden were wheeled into Room II. The small green-walled operating room with no air-conditioning was devoid of the instrumentation that is standard today in all operating rooms. There was no reliable EKG or blood oxygen monitor, and respiratory assistance equipment for infants and children did not exist. Blood pH and electrolyte measurements took hours to process—even in emergencies. External pacemakers did not exist. If a patient developed heart block, the only treatment was intravenous epinephrine, an unreliable drug for managing very low heart rates in infants and children. No one had imagined or created an intensive care unit.

It was the wild west of cardiac care, an era when a patient's survival was in the hands of God and the doctors and nurses who spent long hours at a patient's bedside. They relied on their experience and senses—sight, sound, smell, and touch—because there were no digital displays, computers, or imaging machines to parse the myriad physiologic signals that foretold a patient's fate. Future generations of caregivers could only dream of acquiring the clinical intuition possessed by these mid-20th century practitioners.

Gregory and Lyman Glidden were anesthetized. Lillehei and his team inserted cannulas (tubes) into Lyman's femoral artery and saphenous vein. Then Lillehei opened Gregory's chest and placed tiny cannula's in his vena cava and subclavian artery. These cannulas were connected to Lyman's circulation by long clear plastic tubes that passed through a SigmaMotor pump. The pump moved Gregory's dark venous blood to Lyman where it traveled to his lungs for oxygenation and removal of carbon dioxide. Meanwhile, bright red oxygenated blood moved from Lyman's femoral artery to his son via the subclavian artery.

As Lillehei later observed, Lyman acted as a mother's placenta. Not only did Lyman's lungs provide a respiratory function, but his liver and kidneys also helped maintain Gregory's metabolic balance. This was particularly helpful at a time when the diagnostic instrumentation needed to monitor pH, electrolytes, and kidney function was not available.

Dr. Richard Varco, a short, stocky man with black hair and big hands, assisted Lillehei. A native of Montana and a University of Minnesota graduate, Dick Varco was a master surgeon, one of those highly gifted individuals who could visualize how to rearrange a patient's anatomy and then do it as God intended. Also in the room were Morley Cohen and Herbert Warden who had placed the cannulas in Lyman's blood vessels. Present too were Drs. Norman Shumway and Vincent Gott, both Wangensteen trainees, who in the years ahead would become world-famous heart surgeons.

Lillehei made a small incision in Gregory's tiny heart and saw the dime-sized VSD high up on the wall of the septum. The pre-operative diagnosis was correct. He proceeded to close the VSD with sutures while Varco expertly suctioned away a brisk flow of venous blood. All the while, Lyman's bright red blood kept Gregory's body fully oxygenated.

The surgery was complete in just 19 minutes. Cohen and Warden removed the cannulas from Lyman's artery and vein and closed the incisions. A few minutes later, Lyman awoke. The anesthesiologist had kept him "light," meaning he had limited the amount of anesthetic so it would not reach Gregory through his father's blood. Lillehei went to the waiting room to tell Frances that her husband and son had come through the surgery well.

At just 37, Walt Lillehei had accomplished a feat no surgeon before him had been able to do: close a ventricular septal defect and get the patient out of the operating room alive. The cross-circulation technique translated seamlessly from the research laboratory to clinical practice.

Gregory returned to the heart hospital with around-the-clock nurses and the following morning he took some nourishment. There was no evidence of brain or kidney damage. During the next few days, Gregory ate a poached egg and Cream of Wheat. All was going so well that Lyman, who had no ill effects from the surgery, and Frances returned home to Hibbing: there was work in the mine and, of course, the children.

For a week, Gregory did well, but then his breathing became labored and he started wheezing. Lillehei prescribed antibiotics. Lyman drove down to see his son, accompanied by Gregory's sister, Geraldine. By this time, Gregory was in an oxygen tent. Minutes after they arrived he began to suffocate. Lillehei took him to the operating room and performed an emergency tracheotomy (opening in the windpipe).

The child seemed to rally but his breathing problems continued. On April 6, Gregory's heart stopped. Every attempt to revive Gregory failed. He died at 9 a.m. His parents, alerted by the nursing staff that their son was not doing well, had driven down from Hibbing but they did not arrive until noon. Lillehei met with them and expressed sympathy and disappointment. The Gliddens consented to an autopsy, which showed that the repaired VSD was intact and the cause of his death was pneumonia.

Lillehei and his colleagues were convinced that cross-circulation was safe and would allow them to repair congenital defects that previously had been inoperable. With Owen Wangensteen's approval, Lillehei operated on two patients within weeks of Gregory's death. Both four year-old Pamela Schmidt and three year-old Bradley Mehrman had large VSDs and each operation was a complete success.

Lillehei announced his new surgical procedure at a press conference where he explained the cross-circulation technique using diagrams and photographs. He mentioned Gregory Glidden's death and concluded by bringing Pamela Schmidt on stage in a wheel chair. The story was published worldwide and, in today's vernacular, it went viral. Anxious parents, whose children were crippled by a variety of congenital heart defects, nearly overwhelmed Walt Lillehei and the University of Minnesota.

Would cross-circulation enable even more daring attempts to fix hearts? How long could you keep an adult "donor" connected to a young patient's circulatory system without doing harm? What would happen to these kids after their hearts were repaired? How long would they live? Would their lives be worth living? Lillehei and his team, with Owen Wangensteen's encouragement, would answer these questions by operating on increasingly complex congenital heart defects and conducting detailed follow-up studies.

Dozens of surgeons from the United States and Europe came to the University of Minnesota to observe the cross-circulation technique. Lillehei used cross-circulation to repair more VSDs and he tackled more difficult cases that became surgical firsts. Among them were *atrioventricular canal defect* (repair of openings between the atria and ventricles) and *tetralogy of Fallot* (VSD closure, removal of tissue obstructing flow from the right ventricle to the lungs, and repair of the pulmonary valve). Altogether, Lillehei and his team operated on 45 critically ill patients using cross-circulation, and 28 (62 percent) went home after surgery. Most impressive were the 22 patients who were still alive 30 years later. None of the cross-circulation "donors" died or sustained a long-term injury.

In 2013 I saw one of Lillehei's early cross-circulation VSD patients in a cardiology follow-up appointment at the Alexandria Clinic in Minnesota. He was a child when Lillehei operated on him and his father was the donor. Except for a long horizontal incisional scar across his chest, there was no sign that he had ever had life-threatening congenital heart disease.

Milton Weinberg was correct when he said that Billy Samuels was a direct beneficiary of Walt Lillehei's bold genius. However, there is much more to the University of Minnesota and Lillehei story than cross-circulation and the first successful VSD repairs. Weinberg had closed Billy's VSD using a heart-lung machine, a method for oxygenating and pumping blood through the body while the heart is shut down and its inner structures exposed for the surgeon to repair.

The development of the heart-lung machine began during the Depression when John Gibbon built a small oxygenator for animal experiments in Philadelphia. After World War II, IBM funded the development of a heart-lung machine that enabled Gibbon to successfully repair an atrial septal defect in an 18-year-old college student. This occurred in 1953. Unfortunately, Gibbon's next three patients died and he abandoned the technique. The 2000-pound Gibbon-IBM heart-lung machine was the key factor in the failures. It had too many moving parts and was just too complicated to use safely.

Dr. John Kirklin, a cardiac surgeon at the Mayo Clinic in Rochester, Minnesota, modified the Gibbon heart-lung machine and used it successfully beginning in 1955. But the Mayo-Gibbon model was both complicated and expensive to operate, requiring a cadre of technicians and physicians in addition to the surgical team. No other heart center had the financial or technical expertise to reproduce the Mayo-Gibbon experience.

Walt Lillehei recognized that cross-circulation did not offer a long-term, practical way to operate on tens of thousands of patients, including adults, who needed open-heart surgery. The world needed a heart-lung machine that did not require costly investment and legions of technicians, so Lillehei asked one of his young residents, Dr. Richard DeWall, to work on it.

DeWall grew up in Morris, Minnesota, an agricultural town 150 miles west of Minneapolis. After serving in the Navy during World War II, he graduated from the University of Minnesota Medical School in 1953. During his internship at Staten Island Hospital in New York City he cared for a teenage Portuguese sailor who was dying of heart failure due to a leaking mitral valve caused by rheumatic fever. This experience inspired DeWall to design a mechanical mitral valve and he created a crude prototype. After returning to Minnesota, he visited his former teacher, Richard Varco, at the University's heart hospital. Varco was impressed by DeWall's passion and creativity and introduced him to Walt Lillehei who gave DeWall a job in the animal laboratory. Soon DeWall was deep into cross-circulation research, and the mitral valve project was shelved.

The young Dr. DeWall, who would be recognized for his mechanical genius, became very skilled at operating the SigmaMotor pump and tubing used for cross-circulation. Lillehei brought him into the operating room where DeWall became what today is called a perfusionist -- an individual who operates equipment to support a patient's circulation during open-heart surgery. One day, after a successful cross-circulation case, Lillehei bemoaned the limitations of the technique. For starters it could not be used to operate on adults. Lillehei told DeWall: "What we need is a simple, reliable heart-lung machine. If it interests you, that would be a good project to work on in the lab."

Years later DeWall would recall: "He gave it to me as an option. That was Walt's generosity. He didn't force anything on anybody, and neither did Dr. Wangensteen." Lillehei admonished DeWall not to go to the library and do literature searches: "Don't be prejudiced by the mistakes of others."

The oxygenator was the major barrier in developing a safe and effective heart-lung machine. In the lab, DeWall experimented with a variety of approaches, including hyperbaric oxygenation that forced oxygen into plasma. However, when the high pressure was lowered, bubbles formed and bubbles could cause strokes, heart attacks, and death if they entered human circulation.

Using long polyvinyl tubing shaped in a helix, DeWall found that he could trap the bubbles so they would not enter the blood stream. This innovation prompted him to abandon hyperbaric oxygenation and do what everyone said *not* to do: oxygenate blood with bubbles. By figuring out how to keep the bubbles from escaping into a patient's circulation, DeWall had found a profoundly simple and safe way to oxygenate blood during heart-lung bypass.

DeWall tested the bubble oxygenator on 10 dogs in the laboratory. Years later DeWall wrote, "Every dog survived and none had any physical disability. They all looked good." Lillehei came down to the lab, took the dogs out of their cages, and walked them around in a grassy field next to the research laboratory. There were no apparent ill effects. Lillehei asked DeWall if the oxygenator could support a 25-pound patient. To do so the oxygenator would have to be upsized, which DeWall managed to do by employing larger polyvinyl tubing. He got the tubing from a company in Hopkins, Minnesota, that manufactured it for making mayonnaise. After more testing, they were ready for the first patient.

On May 13, 1955, Lillehei repaired a VSD using DeWall's bubble oxygenator. The oxygenator did exactly what DeWall had designed it to do, and the operation was a success. Subsequently, surgical teams at the University of Minnesota repaired VSDs, tetralogy of Fallot, atrial septal defects, and other complex congenital defects for patients ranging in age from 16 weeks to 21 years using the DeWall-Lillehei bubble oxygenator.

For the second time in two years heart surgeons from around the world flocked to Minnesota. Prominent among them was Dr. Denton Cooley from Texas. In February 1955, Lillehei had presented his cross-circulation results at the prestigious Society of Thoracic Surgeons in Houston. In the audience was his friend Cooley, who was impressed with Lillehei's data and enthralled by his movie depicting an operation on a child.

Four months later, Cooley visited Lillehei to observe a cross-circulation operation. As Cooley recalled in his memoir—*100, 000 Hearts*—Lillehei treated him and a colleague to a delicious steak dinner the night before the surgery. After the meal and several double martinis, they finally got to bed around 1 a.m. Both men were a bit shaky the next morning but Cooley recalled, "Walt and his team performed the operation superbly and successfully."

Cooley was impressed with DeWall's uncomplicated and inexpensive bubble oxygenator. That afternoon he drove 90 miles south to Rochester, Minnesota, where he spent the night at the home of Dr. John Kirklin, head of heart surgery at the Mayo Clinic. After a thimbleful of sherry and early dinner, they all retired at 9 p.m. The following morning Cooley observed Kirklin successfully close a ventricular septal defect using the elaborate and baffling Mayo-Gibbon heart-lung machine. Cooley returned to Houston where eventually he adopted the DeWall-Lillehei bubble oxygenator.

The DeWall-Lillehei bubble oxygenator was an instant success because it was easy to use, efficient, inexpensive, heat sterilizable, and had no moving parts. The materials were cheap, so the oxygenator was disposable. Open-heart operations performed routinely only in Minnesota at the University and the Mayo Clinic soon became possible at dozens of hospitals around the world. Cooley remarked that DeWall's oxygenator was the "can opener" that enabled the expansion of heart surgery. It was the first of many disruptive technologies that would shape cardiac care during the decades ahead.

Five days after his surgery in June 1968, Billy Samuels was up walking the halls of the pediatric surgery floor. He pushed an iv pole holding the temporary pacemaker that continued to stimulate his heart 100 times a minute.

Billy's appetite was insatiable; he ate everything the dietician placed on his tray, and asked for more. His mother brought in all sorts of food—pizza, ice cream, and chocolate cake. Every day I turned down the rate of the temporary pacemaker to see if Billy's own natural rhythm was coming back. But the heart block persisted. Without the pacemaker, his pulse was in the low thirties.

Billy's heart block occurred during surgery when the conduction system that carries impulses from the atria to the ventricles was injured. The conduction system is located close to the region of the VSD that Weinberg had repaired. Often the injured tissue recovers and normal conduction and heart rates resume, but recovery may take days or weeks.

Neither temporary nor permanent pacemakers existed when Walt Lillehei began repairing VSDs in 1955. Ten percent of his patients—one in 10 infants, children and young adults—were dying after surgery due to heart block. Later Lillehei said, "We began a very intensive crash program in our experimental laboratory to find a better treatment." He and his co-workers, including Vincent Gott, found that they could cause the heart to beat by attaching insulated conductive wires of their own design to the surface of the right ventricle and delivering small electrical pulses from a Grass™ stimulator. In 1935, Albert and Ellen Grass developed this stimulator to study the brain in the Harvard physiology department. Subsequently they formed a company and built stimulators for multiple research applications. Fortunately, Dr. Maurice Visscher, chairman of the physiology department at the University of Minnesota, had purchased one.

Shortly after his team discovered they could pace the heart with the Grass™ stimulator, Lillehei operated on a patient with a very large VSD. Complete heart block occurred while the patient was still in the operating room; the heart rate was less than 20 beats a minute. Lillehei asked Dr. Vincent Gott to bring the Grass™ stimulator over from the research laboratory.

When it arrived, Lillehei attached one Teflon insulated stainless steel wire to the heart, and a second wire to the patient's skin. Both wires were connected to the Grass™ stimulator. The patient's heart rate increased to 100 beats a minute, driven by the small electrical pulses from the stimulator. At last there was a reliable way to manage patients with heart block during and soon after surgery.

There was one major logistical problem: the bulky black Grass™ stimulator operated on AC current. To move a patient to the bathroom or X-ray department required a long extension cord or a nimble doctor or nurse who had to dash between electrical outlets to keep the patient's heart beating. A power outage could be catastrophic. In fact, during the summer of 1957 a thunderstorm shut off the hospital's electricity for six hours. The heart rates of patients paced by line-powered Grass™ stimulators dropped precipitously. No one died as a result but Lillehei realized that the solution was a *wearable battery-operated* pacemaker that would reliably stimulate the heart 24 hours a day, without fail.

"I began talking with a young man who we hired to help with our operating room equipment," Lillehei said. "The hospital electricians would not come into the operating room because it wasn't in their contract, so we hired this fellow, Earl Bakken, to be there during heart operations to keep all of our equipment running well—the electrocardiogram and Sanborn pressure monitors. One day I told Bakken that the Grass™ pulse generator was working pretty well but it runs on regular wall current." Lillehei asked Bakken, "We need a wearable battery-driven unit…Can you do that?"

Bakken replied simply, "Yes."

Earl Bakken grew up in a blue-collar neighborhood in northeast Minneapolis. As a kid, he built all sorts of machines in the basement of his home. His parents, Osvald and Florence, encouraged their son's interest in electronics and he had a workshop crowded with vacuum tubes, copper wire, and multiple copies of *Popular Electronics*.

After serving as a radar technician in World War II Bakken returned to the University of Minnesota where he studied electrical engineering and married Connie Olson, a medical technologist at Northwestern Hospital in south Minneapolis. Earl often found himself hanging around the hospital waiting for Connie to get off work. He helped the hospital staff fix equipment, such as EKG machines and centrifuges. Soon he and his brother-in-law, Palmer Hermundslie, started a company to repair medical instruments. They named it Medtronic—short for "medical" and "electronics." Bakken left graduate school and began working out of a garage. During its first month, Medtronic made eight dollars fixing a centrifuge. It was hardly an auspicious beginning.

After he agreed to build Lillehei a battery-operated pacemaker, Bakken returned to his garage and found an article in *Popular Electronics* describing a circuit for an electronic metronome. It was perfect because its cadence could mimic the rate of the human heart. Bakken purchased some electronic components, including transistors that were just becoming available for home projects. Within a few weeks he built the first external heart pacemaker based on the *Popular Electronics* metronome design. After Vincent Gott tested Bakken's pacemaker in the animal laboratory, Lillehei began using it to treat patients with heart block.

The Bakken-designed external pacemaker was an unqualified success. In a short time, Medtronic was building external pacemakers and pacing leads (wires) for hospitals around the country and in Europe. Bakken's chance encounter with Lillehei was the true beginning of the modern pacemaker industry.

Billy Samuel's nurse paged me a week after his surgery. Billy's pulse was irregular and he was complaining of "thumping" in his chest. I went to his room. Billy seemed fine, but his mother was understandably anxious. Except for heart block, Billy had breezed through his surgery and was ready to go home to Moline, a scenic city on a bluff overlooking the Mississippi River.

I listened to Billy's heart and lungs with my stethoscope: his rhythm was irregular but I heard nothing else unusual. The nurse brought in the EKG machine. I began to smile as the signals made by the pacemaker and Billy's own heartbeats appeared on the EKG paper.

"What is it," his mother exclaimed. "Is something wrong?"

"No, not at all", I said, "Billy's own rhythm is back. The heart block is gone. The pacemaker just doesn't know that its pacing pulses are competing with Billy's own heart beats." I turned the pacemaker off and repeated the EKG. Billy now had a beautiful sinus rhythm—all his own—and he would not need a permanent pacemaker. He and his mother returned home to Moline the following morning.

The Lillehei era was remarkable for its breakthroughs: repair of "inoperable" congenital heart defects, development of the first practical blood oxygenator, and creation of the first battery-powered external pacemaker. These lifesaving innovations were foundational: they were platforms for expanding the treatment of heart disease in its many forms.

Lillehei literally opened the door to the heart's interior structures and made them accessible for repair, replacement, and reconstruction. In addition to congenital defects, he operated directly on the aortic and mitral valves. These were crude and largely ineffective attempts to restore valve function by modern standards, but they expanded cardiac surgery's horizons.

In 1986, Lillehei published two studies detailing the long-term results of the heart surgeries he had performed from 1954 to 1960. Among 106 patients with tetralogy of Fallot, a very complex congenital heart disease, 84 patients were still living, 34 had graduated from college, two had received Ph.D. degrees, two were physicians, and one was a lawyer. These outcomes far exceeded the expectations of almost everyone—except Walt Lillehei. Some of his peers thought he was rash. Rash he may have been, but 30 years later there was an impressive group of grateful patients.

Looking back, it is compelling to wonder: What were the special ingredients that enabled Lillehei and his Minnesota team to accomplish so much in such a short time? Certainly there was Lillehei himself, a passionate man who was devoted to his patients, and was not afraid to take risks when they were justified and backed by research. He refused to accept suffering and death as inevitable.

Then too there was Owen Wangensteen, a master teacher and mentor. In 1979, Lillehei, reflecting on Wangensteen, said: "He had an unusual knack of spotting talent in people who didn't even know they had talent at all. Many of those people that he selected as residents were rejects from other places because they did not fit the conventional mold of a surgical fellow. But, in Dr. Wangensteen's eyes, they had some particular thing that he thought was very favorable to surgery."

Wangensteen did not care about a resident's color, religion, or ancestry; he included everyone, and exposed them to a unique training program that emphasized science and innovation. Years after he trained under Wangensteen, the foremost cardiac transplant surgeon of his era, Dr. Norman Shumway, wrote:

> *"One of Wangensteen's greatest attributes was that he had a total lack of envy. When I first arrived in Minneapolis as an intern, people were coming from all over the world to watch Dr. Wangensteen operate. When open-heart surgery got started there in 1952, they were not coming to see Wangensteen anymore. They were coming to watch Lillehei, Lewis, and Varco. Did this bother Wangensteen? Not a bit. He was so proud of what was going on with these young men that he just basked in the reflected glory of their contributions, and helped to advance and develop them…. He always referred to himself as the regimental water carrier, and his job was to be sure that the troops had enough support."*

The Lillehei era at the University of Minnesota era came to an end in 1966, when the medical school decided to replace the retiring Wangensteen with an outsider, Dr. John Najarian. Organ transplantation was a rapidly evolving field and University leaders believed their school was falling behind. Najarian was a prominent transplant surgeon and immunologist, and he arrived in the summer of 1967 to lead the department of surgery.

Walt Lillehei left the University to become Chairman of Surgery at Cornell University in New York. It was not a happy experience. He returned to Minnesota in 1975 to serve as a clinical professor of surgery and medical director of St. Jude Medical, a heart valve company. Dr. C. Walton Lillehei died on July 5, 1999, at 80. The Lillehei Heart Institute is now the center for cardiovascular research and education at the University of Minnesota.

CHAPTER 3

John Young was assigned to my clinic in 1972 when I was a cardiology fellow at Presbyterian-St. Luke's Hospital in Chicago. He was 58 but looked 80 and had long-standing severe mitral regurgitation (leaky valve).

Every few months, acute heart failure and shortness of breath brought John to the emergency room. Both of his ventricles—pumps—were huge: we did not have echocardiography in those days, but the chest X-ray revealed that his enlarged heart occupied most of his chest cavity. Surgery to replace the valve would have killed him. Toward the end of his life John became so exhausted by the least amount of activity that I visited his apartment weekly in north Chicago to give him intravenous diuretics.

On a cold, rainy day in early March I found John sitting with a blanket covering his swollen legs. He was gaunt, his eyes sunken. His neck veins were engorged. Each breath was labored. I could hear his wheezes without a stethoscope. His heart murmur was not as loud as it had been, a sign that the pressure and blood flow in his heart were trending in the wrong direction.

John was a widower. One of the neighbors walked John's dog, Taffy, a Heinz 57, several times a day because he could no longer climb three flights of stairs to his one-bedroom apartment. John's daughter lived in west Chicago and visited him on the weekends. She had her own struggles: three kids, a fulltime job, and a chronically unemployed husband. Yet she cared about her father, and brought him groceries and did his laundry.

I finished giving John his diuretic and asked if he needed anything. "Yes, let's end this," John said. His statement was so matter-of-fact that, at first, I missed his intent.

He looked at me with kind eyes and a weak smile. "Doctor Hauser, I don't want you to come back here anymore, and I don't want to go to the hospital again. I think we should just stop. It's not worth all the trouble."

"John," I said, "this is no trouble at all—it's on my way home..."

"Doc," John interrupted, "I'm so tired. You are just not helping me. I know that no one can help me. These drugs are keeping me alive when I don't want to live anymore."

This was defeat, utter helplessness. I put the syringe and vial back in my black bag and we sat in his living room for a few minutes, looking into each other's eyes and not speaking. The silence symbolized our shared futility.

Eventually I reminded John that he had my phone numbers and left.

I do not know exactly when John died. It must have been shortly after that last visit. I can still see his face as he gently dismissed me from his care.

The medical treatment of severe, symptomatic heart valve disease in the mid-20th Century was largely ineffective, as it is today. Short-term relief with digitalis and diuretics was helpful. But most patients, like John, did not survive five years, and during those years they often were unable to perform the most basic tasks of daily living. Toward the end of their lives, they had shortness of breath, even at rest, unable to lie down, legs swollen, bellies full of fluid, and coughing blood as the tiny capillaries in their lungs burst under the pressure of unrelenting congestion. Eventually overwhelming fatigue and organ failure triumphed: death was a blessed relief, and mercifully not to be delayed. This was the fate of tens of thousands of patients every year in every country on earth.

In 1960, a young heart surgeon and a wealthy middle-aged engineer in Oregon were about to change the management of valvular heart disease. In the process, they would offer hope to the multitude of patients praying for relief from their suffering. One of these patients was Rose Fisher.

Rose was born in 1928 and grew up on a farm west of Kankakee, Illinois. Her father raised cows, hogs and planted corn and beans on 160 acres of fertile prairie while Rose and her sister took care of the chickens and goats.

In the middle of the Great Depression, when the Fisher family struggled to keep their farm, Rose contracted scarlet fever after a bad strep throat. First she developed a fever, and then the telltale scarlet rash appeared on her cheeks and neck. Her tongue looked like a giant strawberry. She hallucinated, and her limbs twitched. The doctor came to the farmhouse and made the diagnosis. He gave her aspirin because in 1936 that was all he had to offer.

The county health department placed a sign on the front door: QUARANTINE – SCARLET FEVER – CONTAGIOUS – NO ENTRY – By Order of the Health Commissioner. A week later Rose was better but she could not return to school until the quarantine was lifted. Instead, her teacher sent schoolbooks and assignments to her home. Each Friday for the next three weeks, her mother gave her tests in reading and arithmetic. Eventually the schoolbooks were burned because they may have been contaminated. After 21 days, the health department allowed Rose to return to school.

Scarlet fever was the result of infection by the Group A streptococcal bacterium that caused Rose's sore throat. The same infection also caused rheumatic heart disease, an inflammation of the heart muscle and valves. She and her parents did not know it at the time but the rheumatic process attacked every cell and tissue in Rose's heart.

The two leaflets of her mitral valve became swollen and boggy with a mixture of water, white blood cells, and protein. The mitral leaflets became permanently deformed, swollen, and partially fused. Initially the valve opened and closed normally, allowing blood to flow freely without leaking. Rose had no symptoms, no shortness of breath or fluid retention. Yet the scarred valve began a slow, relentless devolution from its virgin state to a knurled, calcified structure that leaked and obstructed blood flow from her lungs to the left ventricle (main pumping chamber). This disease activity would go on slowly, mutely, for years.

During World War II Rose attended high school and worked every morning and evening on the farm. She was the class valedictorian and won a scholarship to the University of Illinois. After graduating with a business degree in 1949, Rose joined an architectural firm in Chicago. There she met and married Al Fisher, a U.S. Army combat veteran, who had received his civil engineering degree from Purdue University.

Rose and Al formed their own construction company and bought a home in Rogers Park, four blocks west of Lake Michigan. Fisher Construction prospered, buoyed by suburban growth and the need for a robust highway system. The company specialized in building the bridges that spanned the new interstate freeways. They borrowed money to purchase trucks and cranes and hired veteran crews. Al supervised the projects while Rose managed the finances. She was adept at winning contracts with low bids that yielded a decent profit by keeping costs down.

In 1960, at the age of 32, Rose found herself pregnant for the first time. Her obstetrician told Rose she had a heart murmur and asked if she had had rheumatic fever. Rose told him of her bout with scarlet fever. The doctor said she had the classic murmur of mitral stenosis but, because she had no symptoms, he expected the pregnancy to go well. Eight months later Rose delivered a healthy boy without difficulty. They named him John, after her father, who had been killed the previous year when he was struck by lightning during the fall harvest.

By the spring of 1968, young John was in school and Fisher Construction was debt free and growing. The Fisher family moved six miles north to Kenilworth where John would attend Joseph Sears primary school. Once a month they spent the weekend with Rose's mother who was still living on the farm in Kankakee. John and his father fished in a pond near the house and Rose relaxed on the screened porch, reading books that her father had left her.

They were visiting the farm on Easter Sunday when Rose first felt her heart racing. The episode lasted about an hour but she did not mention it to anyone. Then at home on a particularly humid night in July, Rose suddenly became very short of breath; her heart pounded and seized like a faulty engine. She felt faint and could not stand. Al called an ambulance. It was a converted Cadillac but it was equipped with oxygen that helped Rose's breathing.

The ambulance ride from Kenilworth to Evanston Hospital was brief. In the emergency room, she was found to be in atrial fibrillation, a rapid, irregular rhythm originating in the top chambers of the heart (atria). Her lungs were full of watery edema and she was wheezing.

Rose received oxygen, morphine, and an injection of diuretic that acted on her kidneys to remove salt and water. She was also given digitalis to slow her heart rate. Over the next two hours Rose produced more than a liter of urine; her breathing was less labored and her heart rate slowed. She was admitted to the small intensive care unit and a cardiologist was consulted. He listened to her heart and told Rose that she had heart failure caused by mitral stenosis and atrial fibrillation. She needed a heart catheterization and might require heart surgery.

One surgical treatment was mitral valve commissurotomy, a repair that splits the scarred commissures between the two leaflets of the valve so they could open more freely. The procedure had been developed after World War II. Because there was no heart-lung machine at the time, this surgery was performed on the beating heart through an incision in the left chest. The surgeon entered the heart with his finger via the left atrium and opened the scarred mitral valve with a tiny scalpel or metal dilator.

Mitral commissurotomy worked well for many patients but it was ineffective and even dangerous for those whose mitral valves were also leaking or regurgitant: the surgery could make the leakage worse and result in death. Rose was one such patient: she had both mitral stenosis and mitral regurgitation, a valve that was narrow and did not close. When her heart contracted, some of the blood that managed to get through the valve to the ventricle regurgitated back into the left atrium toward the lungs. It was a toxic combination, made more lethal by rapid atrial fibrillation.

"Good morning, Mrs. Fisher," I said as I entered her private room on the ninth floor of Presbyterian-St. Luke's Hospital. "I'm Dr. Hauser." Rose looked at me but did not reply. She was leaning forward in bed, grasping the handrails with both hands. Her breathing was labored. She was using every chest muscle to move air into and out of her lungs. Her long dark brown hair was moist and matted and converged on her forehead in a sharp widow's peak. Rose's high cheekbones were flushed and her dark eyes were sunken beneath well-groomed eyebrows. The oxygen tube in her left nostril was taped to the bridge of her nose. The valve on the oxygen tank by the bed was wide open.

Rose raised her head to bring her eyes level to mine. After clearing her throat, she whispered, "I thought I was going to see Dr. Muenster?"

"You are, Mrs. Fisher," I replied. "I'm the intern. Dr. Julian asked Dr. Muenster to be your cardiologist. He will see you sometime this morning." She nodded, dropping her head, exhausted after whispering a few words.

I ordered more diuretics and digitalis. Rose was breathing easier by the time Muenster arrived. I had met him the previous summer when I was still a medical student. He was a brusque, big man with silver white hair and he chain-smoked. By reputation Muenster was a solid, pragmatic cardiologist who was particularly skilled in the catheterization laboratory. Patients liked him for his sense of humor and ability to put them at ease.

Thirty minutes later Muenster came out of Rose's room and sat down in the doctor's charting area next to the nurse's station. He looked over at me and growled, "Mrs. Fisher is still in heart failure. We can't do the catheterization if she can't lie flat on the table." I told him the drugs I had ordered and he told me to double the diuretic doses. "Be more aggressive," he said. "I want to do the catheterization this Thursday."

"Dr. Julian has her on the surgery schedule for a valve replacement Friday morning," I said.

Muenster stood, lighted a cigarette, and said, "We'll see. Go over her head to toe. She's been healthy but we don't want to miss anything before taking her to surgery."

Over the next two days the diuretics removed nine pounds of water from Rose. Thanks to digitalis her heart rate was in the 70s as long as she was resting. Her appetite improved and she could sleep without awakening breathless and coughing.

Heart surgery may be risky, so it is vital to determine the correct diagnosis and assess the severity of the disease before taking patients to the operating room. Unnecessary surgical deaths have occurred because the pre-operative diagnosis was wrong, or the severity of the disease had been misjudged. Diagnostic catheterization would assure more precision.

On Thursday, Rose was brought to the catheterization laboratory on the tenth floor of the Jelke Building of Presbyterian-St. Luke's Hospital. She was lifted onto the X-ray table, and a technician placed adhesive EKG electrodes on her arms and legs. Positioned over her chest was a fluoroscopy tube that Muenster would use to guide the catheters into precisely the right location. Heart catheters are long, thin, hollow tubes made with a variety of plastic materials.

After anesthetizing the tissue in her right arm, Muenster inserted catheters into her brachial artery and vein at the elbow. Using fluoroscopy, he positioned the catheters into the right and left sides of her heart. He measured the pressures in her pulmonary artery and left ventricle. The pressure in the pulmonary artery was much higher than in the ventricle, and this difference in pressures was consistent with severe mitral stenosis. Because of her chronic rheumatic inflammation, Rose's valve opening was very small and it restricted blood flow from her lungs to her body. When rapid atrial fibrillation occurred, there was little time for blood to flow through the diseased mitral valve.

Muenster drew samples of blood for calculating the quantity of blood her heart was pumping each minute. It showed that her heart was pumping about half the amount of blood that would be normal for a woman her size. Later, Muenster would use the pressure and blood flow data to compute the area (opening) of Rose's mitral valve; this would show that her valve opening was only a small fraction of its normal size.

Lastly, Muenster injected dye into the left ventricle and recorded an X-ray movie called a ventriculogram. The movie showed dye being pumped out through the aortic valve from the ventricle, which is normal, but dye also flowed briskly backward through the mitral valve, filling the left atrium. This reverse jet was distinctly abnormal and confirmed that Rose's mitral valve was also leaking—regurgitant. Her mitral valve's opening was both narrow (stenotic) and did not close properly (regurgitant).

Later that day I was in Rose's room when Muenster explained the results of the heart catheterization. Al Fisher listened silently; his face was pasty and he looked like a condemned man who had accepted his fate. Muenster said Rose needed her mitral valve replaced. It was scheduled for the following morning. Rose asked a number of good, practical questions. She looked at her husband. "Do you have any questions, honey?" she asked. Al stood and took his wife's hand. "Not right now," he replied. "Maybe when the surgeon comes in."

Around 6 p.m. Dr. Ormand Julian and one of the surgical residents came to her room. Julian was the chief of cardiovascular surgery and renowned as an innovator, teacher, and leader in the surgical community. He had an engaging smile in a round, inquisitive face. His horn-rimmed glasses reinforced his professorial manner. A decade later, one of his associates, Dr. Marshall Goldin, would say, "I did my best to pattern myself after him. I`m sure everyone he trained felt the same way. He treated every individual he met as though that person was the single most important person around."

"Hello, Mrs. Fisher," Julian said. He introduced himself and the resident. "I would like to talk to you about the surgery. Then you can decide if you want it. I discussed the results of your catheterization with Dr. Muenster. He told me you need your mitral valve replaced." Julian paused and reached into the side pocket of his white lab coat. "This is the Starr-Edwards valve we will use tomorrow—if you agree," Julian explained. "It's an excellent valve. In fact, I know Dr. Starr, one of the inventors, quite well."

Albert Starr was born in 1926 in New York City where he attended public school. He was a bright young man who advanced rapidly and graduated from high school two years early. After flirting with physics and economics, he settled on medicine and entered Columbia Medical School in 1945. The school was on a wartime schedule and the students attended year-around. Starr excelled; he was elected to Alpha Omega Alpha, the honor medical society, in his third year. He applied for a surgical internship at Massachusetts General Hospital in Boston and Johns Hopkins in Baltimore. Hopkins accepted him but Starr had his eye on Boston and he did not reply immediately to Hopkins' offer.

Then he received a call from Dr. Alfred Blalock at Johns Hopkins. Blalock was a world famous heart surgeon, having performed the first "blue baby" operation in 1944. "Starr," Blalock exclaimed in his southern drawl, "we have never had anybody who turned down a surgical internship at Johns Hopkins. What are you waiting for? You have to tell me now if you're coming to Hopkins or not."

Starr accepted. Hopkins was his second choice but it turned out to be the best choice because Alfred Blalock was one of the great teachers of his generation. Born in rural Georgia, Blalock gained fame for research into the causes and treatment of shock. In 1944, he performed the first Blalock-Taussig shunt on a dying girl with dark blue lips and purple fingernails. With the help of his talented research assistant, Dr. Vivien Thomas, a brilliant African-American man, Blalock sutured the girl's subclavian artery to the pulmonary artery. This delivered additional oxygenated blood to her lungs. Immediately the girl's color improved—she turned pink—and survived. Blalock and Dr. Helen Taussig, a pediatric cardiologist who suggested the surgical technique, were celebrated widely for their achievement.

Starr assisted Blalock during heart surgery and learned the meticulous surgical techniques pioneered by Dr. William Halsted, the first surgeon-in-chief at Johns Hopkins. Starr's chief resident was young Dr. Denton Cooley. In 1950 Starr was drafted and spent 18 months as a battle surgeon in Korea. He returned to New York where he completed his general and thoracic surgery residencies at Presbyterian Hospital.

In 1956, open-heart surgery was just beginning in New York and Starr was part of it, assisting senior surgeons in closing atrial septal defects—a surgery pioneered by F. John Lewis at the University of Minnesota. Initially the mortality rate was high because the surgical techniques were evolving with each patient. In time, however, the methods were fine-tuned, and the DeWall-Lillehei bubble oxygenator made the heart-lung machine a more reliable and practical method for supporting a patient during open-heart surgery.

Toward the end of his thoracic surgery residency, Starr was recruited to start an open-heart program at the University of Oregon. He was barely thirty and he looked more like twenty. On his way to Oregon, he stopped at the Cleveland Clinic, the University of Minnesota, and the Mayo Clinic to acquaint himself with the latest techniques. In 1957, he arrived in Oregon and performed his first open-heart operation—a successful VSD repair—in 1958.

Shortly after Starr arrived in Oregon he was visited by a retired electrical engineer, Lowell Edwards, who had become wealthy by designing a fuel injection pump for World War II fighter planes. The semi-retired Edwards was graying, a bit rickety, and he had a tremor. He was a Quaker and was bothered by the fact that his pumps were used in military aircraft. For this reason, Edwards wanted to invent something that would help people, and he had an idea for an artificial heart. Dr. Herbert Griswold, the chief of cardiology at the University, was a personal friend and he arranged for Edwards to meet the newly arrived Albert Starr. While the artificial heart was an interesting concept, Starr said they first needed to create an artificial mitral valve. No one else was doing it, so together Starr and Edwards decided to develop one.

Later, Starr wrote: "We didn't have to invent a new type of valve—there were many designs employed by hydraulic engineers—we simply had to select the best one for us. We did a lot of brainstorming. I met with Edwards at least once a week and we spent hours talking about the valve. We thought it should be fully assembled, so that all the surgeon needed to do was sew it in."

The Edwards family had a summer home on Sandy River, 40 miles east of Portland and a winter home in Santa Ana, California. Edwards had labs in both locations. His wife, Margaret, remembered awakening in the middle of the night and seeing light from her husband's laboratory reflecting off the trees: she knew he was out there trying out a new idea for the mitral valve. After a year's work, he had a prototype valve ready for animal implants.

The first Edwards designed experimental valve had two Silastic™ rubber leaflets that opened and closed on themselves, much like the natural mitral valve. It clotted when they tried it in dogs, so Edwards built a valve with a Silastic™ ball that moved up and down in a cage made of Lucite™. It functioned like the ball valve in a bottle stopper. When the left atrium contracted, the ball moved down, allowing blood to flow into the left ventricle (main pumping chamber). When the left ventricle contracted, the ball moved up, preventing blood from leaking back into the atrium.

Researchers at the Mayo Clinic had tried the ball valve design but it had clotted in animals and they abandoned the project. Starr had a solution to this. He asked Edwards to build a special valve for dogs because they were more prone to clotting than humans. The dog version had a Silastic™ shield on the sewing ring that prevented clotting. It worked, and soon Starr and Edwards had a group of healthy dogs with valve implants that became long-term survivors. They refined the design, implanted it in more dogs, and performed heart catheterizations to document the valve's performance.

Starr was a careful investigator and sought to devise the very best valve possible before proceeding to patients. He wanted to implant the valve in more dogs and follow them longer. But the chiefs of cardiology and surgery demurred. They had patients in the hospital who were near death, and whose only chance for survival was the Starr-Edwards™ valve.

Starr relented, and went ahead with the first implant on August 25, 1960, at the University of Oregon in Portland. The patient was a 33-year-old woman whose mitral valve was severely damaged by rheumatic fever. Two attempts to repair the valve had failed. She had severe mitral regurgitation—leaky valve—and had been hospitalized for many weeks with repeated bouts of acute heart failure. She was rapidly approaching the end of her life. The woman survived the operation but she died suddenly the next day of a massive air embolism when she sat up for a portable chest X-ray. Starr had failed to appreciate how critical it would be to remove all of the air from her heart and pulmonary veins before closing the incision.

The first successful surgery occurred a month later when a 52-year-old man, Philip Amundson, had his mitral valve replaced with a Starr-Edwards™ valve on September 21, 1960. He had had two prior surgeries on his mitral valve, and he was dying in the hospital. His mitral valve was heavily calcified and almost completely destroyed by scar tissue. Even so, the surgery was successful. Amundson returned to work, and lived another 15 years; he died after falling from a ladder.

Starr and Edwards could rapidly modify their valve and refine their surgical techniques without the regulatory restrictions and delays we experience today. The U.S. Food and Drug Administration did not regulate medical devices until 1976. Consequently, the inventors were able to rapidly implement improvements. One major enhancement was replacement of the thermoplastic Lucite™ cage with a more durable cage made of Stellite™, a cobalt-chromium metal alloy.

Starr presented the results of his first eight mitral valve surgeries in 1961: six patients had survived the surgery. This was a landmark event because they were the first long-term survivors of mitral valve replacement anywhere. Starr and Edwards learned to use the anticoagulant warfarin (Coumadin®) to prevent blood clots from forming on the valve and they addressed the danger of infection on the valve by insisting on meticulous sterile techniques and the use of antibiotics before and after surgery.

The Starr-Edwards™ prosthetic mitral valve marked a turning point in valve surgery. When they created a model for the aortic valve, Starr soon reported successful cases of combined mitral and aortic valve replacement. Other centers adopted the valve, and eventually centers like the Mayo Clinic were reporting single-digit mortality rates, a remarkable achievement because these patients were so ill.

In 1963, Albert Starr showed an X-ray movie of his first triple valve replacement at the American Association of Thoracic Surgery: the patient, who had severe rheumatic valve disease, had her aortic, mitral, and tricuspid valves replaced with Starr-Edwards™ prostheses. At the end of the movie, Starr received an unprecedented standing ovation. Dr. Ormand Julian was in the audience.

Rose took the Starr-Edwards™ mitral valve from Dr. Julian and held it in her hand. "Will I be able to hear it?" she asked Julian, handing the valve to her husband.

"Good question," Julian replied. "The answer is yes, but most patients get used to it in time."

"How risky is this surgery?" she asked.

"There is a ten percent risk of a serious complication," Julian replied. "We are concerned about infection, and we will give you an antibiotic, beginning tonight. We also worry about pneumonia after surgery, so the nurses will make sure you cough and take deep breaths even though the incision may make it painful to do so."

"Where do you make the incision?" Rose asked.

Julian pointed to his breastbone and motioned up and down. "Right here," he said. "It's a good incision—if there is such a thing. The breastbone doesn't move much during breathing, so the pain is less than an incision between the ribs." He paused and smiled. "Anything else?"

Rose and her husband looked at each other for a moment. Then Rose said, "Okay, Dr. Julian, thank you. I guess I need it. I won't get better without it." She looked at him, eyebrows raised. "Is that true?"

"That's quite true, Mrs. Fisher."

"I just want to see my son grow up." Rose whispered, her voice dropping an octave.

Julian nodded and smiled. "I understand."

Meanwhile a new patient had been admitted to the room next to Rose. John Leonard was a 68-year-old semi-retired insurance salesman who had been rejected from military service because of a heart murmur. He was good-humored with curly hair that was dyed black. He had shortness of breath with activity for at least a year and he had begun suffering chest pressure when he carried groceries or climbed stairs to his office. Recently, he had blacked-out while carrying a heavy suitcase at the train station. These were the classic symptoms of severe aortic stenosis, in which the valve's leaflets scar and become fused so that the opening through the valve is a tiny fraction of its original size.

I examined John in his hospital room across the hall from the nurse's station. His murmur was harsh and the sound normally made by the aortic valve was absent because the scarred and calcified leaflets barely moved. The murmur was transmitted upward to the carotid arteries in his neck. All of his pulses were sluggish because too little blood was being pumped through the damaged valve.

"What do you think, doc?" John asked when I finished

"The valve leading out of your heart is called the aortic valve," I replied. "It is scarred. Your catheterization tomorrow will tell us how serious it is."

"Do you think I will need surgery?"

"That will be up to Dr. Muenster, your cardiologist," I hedged. "But it's definitely a possibility."

"Okay, what's next then?"

"Chest X-rays and blood tests. Then you can relax with the family. Dr. Muenster should meet with you this afternoon." I turned to leave.

"Hey," John said, reaching for his wallet on the bedside table. "When I'm done here, let's have lunch and talk about your life insurance." He handed me his business card.

"Okay, sounds good," I agreed, smiling. I liked this kind of guy.

Muenster performed John Leonard's catheterization on the same day as Rose Fisher's procedure. The measurements confirmed the presence of severe aortic stenosis. John Leonard needed open-heart surgery. Like Rose, his surgery would be on Friday and he too would receive a Starr-Edwards™ valve.

The following day, I served as second assistant during John Leonard's aortic valve replacement. In the operating room I inserted a central venous catheter through a vein in John's left arm and another catheter into the ulnar artery at his wrist. I did both through small skin incisions and connected the catheters to transducers that would display his blood pressures on a monitor.

Howard Peacock was in charge of the heart-lung machine. He was an extremely gifted, personable African-American perfusionist who was an acknowledged pioneer in his field. Indeed, he had built some of the early blood oxygenators. Howard prepared the heart-lung machine's disc oxygenator and roller pumps that would sustain John Leonard while his heart was stopped and his aortic valve replaced.

Dr. Hassan Najafi entered the operating room, holding his wet hands and forearms up until the scrub nurse gave him a sterile towel. He was an elegant, extremely polite, serious man who always looked like he had just stepped out of an Armani advertisement. Najafi had grown up and studied in Iran and came to Chicago where he trained under Dr. Julian. His first assistant was Dr. Bill Ostermiller, the senior cardiac fellow who would complete his training at the end of the year and begin a successful cardiac surgery practice in southern California.

I waited while Najafi and Ostermiller draped Mr. Leonard who was comfortably asleep with a breathing tube in his throat. The anesthesiologist sat at the head of the table taking notes and graphing John's vital signs. Chopin played softly in the background. Howard Peacock sat on a stainless steel bench behind the heart-lung machine watching the discs in the oxygenator slowly rotate in Ringers lactate, a special electrolyte solution he used to prime the pump. I stood next to Ostermiller and across from Najafi. Above us was a glass observation dome; three visiting surgeons watched.

Najafi made an incision down the middle of the sternum from just below the sternal notch to the xiphoid process. Ostermiller followed along with an electric cautery to stop bleeding from tiny veins and arteries. Najafi took an oscillating saw from the scrub nurse and cut through the sternum. He placed a self-retaining retractor in the incision and spread it, exposing the heart that was enclosed in a shiny sac (the pericardium) that he opened delicately with the cautery.

Ostermiller made an incision in John's right groin and dissected out the femoral artery and femoral vein. Next he placed thin cloth tapes around each vessel to serve as tourniquets to control any bleeding. Then he made an incision in both vessels and inserted long plastic cannulas into the artery and vein. Each cannula was connected to clear plastic tubing that was handed off to Peacock who attached them to the heart-lung machine. Meanwhile Najafi inserted a cannula into the right atrium and connected it to the tubes draining blood from the femoral vein.

The circuit between John Leonard and the heart-lung machine was complete: dark unoxygenated venous blood moved from the femoral vein and right atrium to the heart-lung machine where it was oxygenated and pumped back into John's body via his femoral artery. The heart-lung machine kept the blood warmed to body temperature.

John's heart and lungs, therefore, were "bypassed". Najafi slipped two flat electrodes behind his heart and induced ventricular fibrillation with a small battery-powered pulse generator that delivered a high frequency current. The fibrillating heart could no longer pump blood. John Leonard's life was totally dependent on the heart-lung machine.

Najafi clamped the aorta above his heart and opened it with a short horizontal incision. I stood next to Ostermiller and suctioned small puddles of blood as they accumulated in John's chest. I watched as Najafi inserted two small tubes into the openings of the left and right coronary arteries just above the aortic valve. These cannulas delivered a flow of oxygenated blood from the heart-lung machine to the arteries that perfused his heart muscle.

Najafi removed the diseased valve. The calcified scar tissue was so tough that he had to use a rongeur—a sharp pliers-like instrument—to excise the valve, in pieces, being careful not to tear the heart's fibrous skeleton or leave fragments that later could travel to the brain and cause a stroke. Next, the scrub nurse handed Najafi the Starr-Edwards™ valve mounted on a circular frame suspended on a white plastic rod.

I held the rod while Najafi placed sutures through the tissue around the opening where the aortic valve had been. Each stitch was then passed through the sewing ring of the Starr-Edwards™ valve. This was repeated until sutures had been placed in a 360-degree circle through the tissue and around the new valve. At this juncture, Najafi positioned the valve within the space previously occupied by the diseased aortic valve. He had Ostermiller tie each suture, making sure the prosthetic ball moved freely within the Stellite metal cage.

Najafi closed the incision in the aorta with multiple sutures. He asked the anesthesiologist to lower the head of the table and inserted a large bore needle into the aorta just above the valve. Blood tinged bubbles came through the needle until all residual air was removed. Any air bubbles left behind could cause a stroke or heart attack.

Najafi released the aortic clamp. The electrical current that was fibrillating the heart was turned off. Ostermiller placed two defibrillator paddles on either side of John's heart. The circulating nurse pressed a button on the external defibrillator beside the operating table and a shock was delivered to his ventricles.

John Leonard's heart should have begun to beat, but it did not move. His heart was paralyzed, except for random twitches. The EKG monitor showed the irregular electrical wavelets of ventricular fibrillation, rather than the sharp, regular spikes of a normal rhythm. Najafi applied another shock and another: ventricular fibrillation was replaced by asystole—a flat line on the EKG. Now his heart was both electrically and mechanically silent.

The heart-lung machine continued to circulate oxygenated blood. Najafi injected an ampule of calcium chloride and a milligram of epinephrine into the left ventricle. Nothing happened, the heart did not move. He tried massaging the heart. "It's as hard as a rock," Najafi said, looking at John's heart in his hands. He administered more drugs to no avail. We stood there, watching, silent. He tried two or three more electrical shocks. The heart was in contracture, a sustained spasm without relaxation. Blood could not get into or out of John's heart.

Was it possible that the new valve was malfunctioning? Perhaps the ball had become stuck in the metal cage. Desperate, Najafi opened the aorta and inspected the valve. All of the sutures were in place and the ball moved freely. Najafi again closed the incision in the aorta.

The room was quiet except for soft music and the whirring of the heart-lung machine. An hour passed. The visiting surgeons who watched us from the observation dome left. Najafi paged Muenster and asked him to come to the operating room. When he arrived Najafi explained the situation. Muenster stood at the head of the table and looked down on John Leonard's inert heart. "I've seen this a couple of times," he said, "I have never seen the heart recover."

Najafi sighed. "I'm going to talk to Mrs. Leonard," he whispered. He stepped back and removed his gloves and surgical gown; his blue-gray scrub shirt was dark with perspiration. Twenty minutes later Najafi returned to the operating room. He spoke quietly to the anesthesiologist and told Howard Peacock to stop the heart-lung machine. It was 2:25 p.m. John's life had ended.

The room was silent. The whirring of the heart-lung machine and sounds from the ventilator were suddenly absent. No one spoke. All of us had been in this operating room when John had been wheeled in seven hours ago. He had been joking with the orderlies, telling them that they needed life insurance and he would be delighted to sell it to them.

This was the first death of one of my patients. I had encouraged John Leonard to have the surgery. I felt responsible. It would not always be this difficult, but I would never be indifferent.

The scrub nurse began to remove the instruments from her tray, placing them in a stainless steel container for cleaning and sterilization. The anesthesiologist finished his charting and left. Two orderlies appeared with a white enameled cart and a body bag from the pathology department. Najafi asked Mrs. Leonard for permission to do an autopsy and she had agreed. We needed to understand what had happened.

I left the operating room and checked in with the page operator. She told me to call Dr. Julian in his office right away. Instead of calling I walked down the hall and entered his office. The secretary was on the phone but she motioned for me to go in.

Julian looked up from his desk and said, "Mrs. Fisher's surgery went well but she was on the heart-lung machine for nearly 90 minutes. You're on call tonight?" I nodded. "Good. Keep a close eye on her. I've spoken to Bill Ostermiller, too." Then he gestured for me to close the door to the outer office. "Do you have a cigarette? My secretary has taken mine again." I gave him a Parliament. We sat there smoking.

I told Julian about John Leonard. "We have no clues why this happens," Julian sighed. "This is the ninth or tenth case we have had like this. I hope we can learn from his autopsy."

Julian glanced toward the outer office where his secretary had her desk. "She'll know we're smoking in here," he said. "We're both in trouble." I was not aware at the time but Julian was already suffering from coronary artery disease.

I took the stairs down to the ICU. Rose Fisher was just being wheeled into the intensive care unit from the operating room. The anesthesiologist and three nurses surrounded the cart. I helped them lift her onto the bed. She was cool and beginning to shiver. Her eyes were closed. The anesthesiologist connected her endotracheal tube to a Mörch piston-operated respirator under the bed. The EKG electrodes were attached to a black and white monitor. There were two intravenous lines delivering blood and Ringer's lactate, a crystalloid solution containing glucose and electrolytes. The arterial and central venous catheters were connected to pressure transducers.

It was 4 p.m. Rose had been in the operating room for eight hours. When the nurses were finished they allowed her husband to visit for a few minutes. Al Fisher took his wife's hand and massaged it gently. "She's cold," he said softly. He turned to me. "Why is she so cold?" he asked. I said it was common after heart surgery and explained that the blood vessels were constricted but they would eventually relax as the anesthetics wore off.

Rose had two tubes coming out of her chest; they were draining rivulets of blood into a plastic container. The container was marked in cubic centimeters (ccs) so that the nurse could chart the amount of drainage per hour. A Foley™ catheter in her bladder was draining urine into a plastic bag hanging on the bed; it too was calibrated in ccs. Rose's progress would be mapped in measurements of blood and urine out, fluid and blood in, arterial and central venous pressure, oxygen saturation, heart rate and rhythm, and a host of blood chemistries including pH (acidity), potassium ions, and urea nitrogen. These were the data available in 1968, and none of them directly addressed the function of Rose's new valve or the two most important chambers in her heart—the left and right ventricles. This technology would not appear for another decade.

John Leonard's death weighed on me, but I had a night on call ahead and there was little time for reflection. Three new patients were admitted on the ninth floor and I took care of them before 10 p.m. when a late meal, consisting of coleslaw and cheeseburgers, was available to the house staff in the cafeteria. After that, it was coffee and cigarettes until breakfast. Around midnight, Bill Ostermiller called to say he was going into the operating room to repair a ruptured aneurysm and he wanted me to keep an eye on Rose Fisher in the surgical intensive care unit.

I learned to use my stethoscope because it was the only tool I had. In 1968, we relied almost exclusively on our senses to assess and manage patients. Intensive care units were "intensive" because the nurses were experienced veterans. They were assigned to care for one or two patients at a time. I soon learned that doctors admitted patients to the ICU, but it took great nursing care to get them out alive.

ICU technology was primitive. The heart rhythm monitor was a portable black and white television with a "bouncing ball" that faintly traced the patient's EKG on a 16-inch screen. Rhythms were not stored or recorded. Abnormal rhythms that could be harbingers of an impending disaster were often missed unless a knowledgeable person happened to be watching the monitor. Automated drug infusion pumps did not exist. Critical medications and fluids were delivered directly from the intravenous bottle and measured in drops per minute. There were big drops and little drops, depending on the medication, and either a nurse or a doctor had to count the drops as they emerged from the iv bottle.

The lights had been turned down in Rose's room even though she had yet to open her eyes. Her skin remained cool. I pressed on one of her fingernails and watched the blood refill the capillaries in her nail bed: the flow was sluggish. There was scant urine in the bag. Her blood pressure was 100 over 80 and her heart rate—she was in a regular rhythm—was 100-110 beats per minute.

"Dr. Ostermiller ordered a unit of blood before he left for the operating room," the nurse said. I listened to Rose's lungs. Her breath sounds were clear on both sides. Her central venous pressure was low. "Good, and give her digoxin," I said. "I'll be in the on-call room."

At 2:30 a.m., Rose's nurse shook me awake. "Fisher's heart rate is 180! We can't get a blood pressure!"

The lights were on in Rose's room and the head nurse was there. "We called Dr. Ostermiller but he can't leave the operating room." She looked at me, waiting for orders. Rose had no pulse. The EKG monitor showed a very rapid, irregular rhythm called atrial fibrillation. Her heart was beating so fast that the ball in her new artificial valve did not have time to open or close: it was floating, suspended in the valve's Stellite™ cage. We did not have much time.

"Get the defibrillator," I barked. "We need to get her out of this rhythm." Everyone moved quickly. One nurse disconnected Rose from the respirator and started ventilating her with an Ambu bag. Another nurse wheeled in the defibrillator. I applied the EKG electrodes to her chest so we could synchronize the shock to her heartbeat. Then I placed the two defibrillator paddles on Rose's chest and delivered a 200-joule shock.

The electrical energy jolted Rose's body and disrupted the signal on the EKG monitor. I felt for a pulse in Rose's groin. It was strong. In seconds, the EKG signal came back and was visible on the monitor. Rose was in a normal rhythm at 80 to 90 beats a minute. The Starr-Edwards valve was opening and closing, allowing blood to be pumped forward, providing oxygen and nutrients to Rose's starved brain and body. The crisis had passed.

The nurses removed the defibrillator electrodes from Rose's body and covered her with a blanket. I turned to leave and found Al Fisher standing in the hall. He had been sleeping in the waiting room when the flurry of activity woke him. I explained what had happened and said his wife was stable and that both of us should get some sleep. He nodded and, without a word, walked back to the waiting room.

All of us were weary, sapped by anxiety and serial emergencies and the knowledge that another catastrophe was brewing somewhere to someone who would need our help. I went to the on-call room and slept for two precious hours.

The sun was shining through the large window in Rose's room. It was 6:30 a.m. Ostermiller was still in the operating room. He was assisting Julian's longtime partner, Dr. Sam Dye. They were struggling to save the life of a truck driver from

Wisconsin. I wanted to check on Rose before going to 7 a.m. rounds with the senior surgeons.

The night nurse was going off duty. "She's waking up, Dr. Hauser. Putting out good amounts of urine, too. Still in sinus rhythm." All of this was good news. Later, I would ask Muenster if I could give her quinidine sulfate to keep her in sinus rhythm. On the way to rounds, I stopped by the waiting room. Al Fisher was asleep on the couch. I did not wake him. Perhaps this would be a better day.

Rose Fisher recovered from her surgery and lived 13 years. She died of a stroke in 1981, two months after John, her only child, graduated from Notre Dame. Starr-Edwards™ valves underwent several modifications, but the model Rose received performed well in tens of thousands of patients for many years. A number of these patients lived more than 30 years. Very few valves failed mechanically, a tribute to Lowell Edwards and his engineers. The major problem with the Starr-Edwards™ and other mechanical valves continued to be blood clots that formed on the valve. The clots dislodged and traveled to the brain or other organs. For this reason, patients took daily warfarin (Coumadin®), a blood thinner. Some of them suffered severe bleeding, usually in the gut, but also in the brain.

If Rose had been treated medically, she would have had a 50 percent chance of dying within 5 years, and during that time she would have been progressively disabled by congestive heart failure. With the Starr-Edwards valve, her longevity more than tripled, and she continued to manage Fisher Construction with her husband until the day she died. Rose saw her son grow-up, as she had wished.

Albert Starr remained in Portland and practiced surgery at both the University of Oregon and Providence St. Vincent Hospital. Lowell Edwards built Edwards Laboratories in Santa Ana to manufacture the valves. Eventually Edwards Laboratories manufactured a pacemaker and I worked with Starr to develop a sophisticated microprocessor-based model. Lowell Edwards died in 1982 at 84. He and his wife gave generously to the University of Oregon.

Starr-Edwards™ valves were implanted in more than 175,000 patients before other mechanical and tissue heart valves replaced them. Edwards Laboratories went on to develop many novel cardiovascular devices including the first successful aortic valve to be implanted using a catheter without open-heart surgery. In 2016, the renamed Edwards Lifesciences Inc. was valued at $20 billion.

John Leonard died from a condition that in 1972 Denton Cooley named the "stone heart syndrome." It was an extreme manifestation of reduced blood flow to the heart muscle during open-heart surgery. Over many years, John Leonard's heart muscle had hypertrophied (thickened) because it had to squeeze harder to pump blood through the small opening in his aortic valve. When deprived of oxygen during surgery, the mass of his heart muscle rebelled and went into irreversible spasm, like a Charley horse that never went away.

At autopsy, the inner third of John Leonard's heart was red with ruptured blood vessels that flooded the tissue with red blood cells and serum, immobilizing the muscle bundles, starving the cells of oxygen and glucose, and ultimately causing his death. The pathologist called it a "hemorrhagic subendocardial myocardial infarction" and it was a phenomenon he had seen only in patients who died during open-heart surgery. The "stone heart" was its manifestation.

This and other heart muscle problems that occurred during heart-lung bypass prompted much basic and clinical research. After John Leonard's death, Hassan Najafi's inspired research found that cooling the heart during surgery with topical ice slush could mitigate the damage. He was among the first to employ techniques that keep heart muscle healthy and functioning during open-heart surgery. Thanks to Najafi and others, deaths like John Leonard's are now rare.

CHAPTER 4

Atherosclerosis has been killing people for millennia. It has been found in the arteries of Egyptian mummies, and it spares no race, gender, or age. Fatty streaks in the lining of an artery are usually the first sign that a man or woman is developing atherosclerosis. These cholesterol rich, fat-laden plaques can be found in children and young adults, and they signal the beginning of a decades-long process that can ultimately compromise blood flow to any organ.

The atherosclerotic plaques invade every layer of the arteries that supply blood to the heart, brain, kidneys, and legs. Plaques are not uniform; rather, they are quite diverse, even in the same artery, and they may be solid and stable, or frail and brittle. Plaques may aggregate, forming discrete blockages, or they may be dispersed along the entire length of an artery.

Plaque is composed of scar tissue, muscle cells, and lipids. This milieu is stirred by inflammation and noxious chemicals that create pools of fat and erode the lining of the artery. Tiny clots form when the thin fibrous lining cracks. These clots become scarred, adding another layer to the plaque. The process repeats itself until layer upon layer accumulates, expanding the plaque, and distorting and narrowing the channel where blood must flow. Sometimes a plaque ruptures, and bleeds, forming a clot large enough to completely obstruct blood flow. Acute clot formation can be a seismic thrombotic condition that precipitates heart attacks, strokes, and or the loss of a limb or loop of bowel.

Although atherosclerosis descended on the world centuries ago, its full impact was not felt until the 20th century when the average life expectancy crept past 50 and 60 years. Previously, most people died of infection, childbirth, war, and malnutrition. Aging in the modern era meant that people lived long enough to develop severe atherosclerosis with all of its manifestations, primarily angina (heart pain), myocardial infarction (heart attack), and congestive heart failure. Cigarette smoking was a notable catalyst, triggering plaques to rupture and bleed. Other risk factors were high blood pressure and diabetes.

Many people never develop atherosclerosis, even at an older age and with multiple risk factors. They are the likely beneficiaries of a favorable genetic makeup that protects them from the disease. At the other end of the spectrum are patients like Harold Swanson, whom I met for the first time in 1969. His family had a striking history of coronary artery disease that affected its men before they were 55 years of age. It would take almost every major advance in the treatment of coronary artery disease that I witnessed during my career to keep Harold alive and well.

Harold Swanson was third generation Swedish-American. The first of his family's immigrants changed their name from Svensson to Swanson when they landed at Ellis Island in 1892. There were three brothers: William, Nils and Bjorn. Two of them became farmers in Wisconsin and Minnesota. Harold's grandfather, Bjorn, was recruited in Sweden to work on the Lake Forest estate of a wealthy meatpacking family.

Bjorn Swanson married Lucy Nevers in 1897. Lucy was the daughter of Marion and Louis Nevers who owned a clothing store in Highland Park, a bustling lakeshore community south of Lake Forest. Lucy had thick auburn hair and milk-white skin and she was a graduate of Lake Forest College with a liberal arts degree.

Lucy gave birth to Richard in 1898 and Amanda in 1900. After completing his contractual obligation to the meatpacking family, Bjorn and Lucy opened the first Swanson's Restaurant in their home in downtown Highland Park. Lucy cooked and Bjorn did everything else, including waiting tables and washing dishes.

For years, Bjorn and Lucy never took a day off or considered a vacation. Then Bjorn received a letter from his oldest brother, William, who had married a St. Paul girl and settled on a farm near Olivia in western Minnesota. William had heart failure and could no longer work the farm; he was 42 and suffered increasing fatigue and shortness of breath. Shoes could not accommodate his swollen feet and legs, so he wore thick socks and rubber boots. The neighbors helped out, but they had their own farms to work. William's letter was a plea for help.

Bjorn quickly boarded a train from Chicago to St. Paul and he sent a telegram to his brother Nils in Lacrosse, asking him to meet him. They spent the night at a boarding house and then set out for Olivia in Nils' Model T Ford. Two days later, they arrived in Olivia to learn that their brother had died during the night. William left a wife, Lorna, and three sons. Bjorn and Nils offered to take them in but Lorna said she was going to keep the farm for her boys—this was William's last wish.

During the return trip to St. Paul, Nils told his brother that he was taking pills to relieve chest discomfort that he experienced when performing heavy work. Nils' squeezing chest tightness was classic angina pectoris—an ominous sign for a 39 year-old relying on physical labor to support his family. The cause of his angina was coronary artery disease, and Nils was one of millions of Americans who would suffer its ravages.

The new Swanson's Restaurant prospered during World War I when Highland Park, like other north shore communities, welcomed sailors from the Great Lakes Naval Station and soldiers from Fort Sheridan. When Richard joined the army, Amanda took a leave from her studies at Northwestern University to help in the restaurant.

On a bitterly cold, windy evening in December 1918, Bjorn Swanson, 46, collapsed and died behind the restaurant. He had been setting out the garbage cans for collection when his heart fibrillated and he fell forward into a snow bank. Amanda found him face down: her father was not breathing and she could not feel a pulse. The doctor said Bjorn had died of a coronary thrombosis -- blockage of blood flow to his heart caused by a clot in his coronary artery.

The previous week, Richard was discharged from the Army and he took over running the restaurant. Lucy continued to work in the kitchen, devising new entrees and desserts. They had a loyal clientele. Prohibition was in effect and customers often had dinner at Swanson's and spent the rest of the evening in one of the local speakeasies.

In September 1929 Richard married Edith Merrill, a nurse at Highland Park Hospital, who frequently dined with her parents at the restaurant. She was tall, blonde, narrow at the waist, and had striking oval green eyes. The stock market crashed a month after their wedding. A year later, the Great Depression took hold. Highland Park was not spared. Unemployment became the norm. Some families endured winters in tents and tarpaper shacks on the edge of town and in vacant lots. Every day a dozen people came to the back door of Swanson's Restaurant begging for food and a job. Richard fed many but he could employ only a few.

On a warm summer night in July 1930, Edith gave birth to a son. Harold Swanson was the first of his family to be born in a hospital. It was no longer necessary or fashionable to give birth on the kitchen table or in the bedroom. Edith stayed in the hospital for five days. When she returned home, Edith found that Richard had hired a young woman, Doris Hart, to help with baby Harold. She was one of the many who had asked him for a job at the restaurant. Despite being gaunt and disheveled, Richard sensed something special about her. At first, Edith was not pleased but Doris proved to be not only a loving and caring nanny for Harold but also a bright and energetic helper in the restaurant.

Harold had red hair and fair skin, a throwback to his Irish ancestors on the Nevers side of the family. The Depression years were difficult for everyone and Swanson's Restaurant operated on a thin edge. There was no money for anything but the absolute necessities. Their savings, accumulated during the good years, dwindled. Fortunately, Prohibition ended in 1933, and with the last of their savings, Richard built a bar at the front of the restaurant. Beer and liquor resuscitated their finances.

In 1939, Hitler invaded Poland. France and Great Britain declared war on Germany. The United States would become, as President Franklin Roosevelt declared, the "arsenal of democracy". The economy recovered as the country once again mass-produced the implements of modern warfare. The draft brought recruits to the Great Lakes naval station. By 1941, most people in northern Illinois had jobs.

World War II came to America on December 7, 1941, when Japan attacked Pearl Harbor. The country mobilized its people and vast industry. Together with its allies, the United States defeated Germany and Japan in less than four years. By September 1945, the world was at peace, at least for a while, and America was untouched by the devastation of war.

Swanson's Restaurant had been caught up in the war wave and prospered as people with money in their pockets packed the bar and dining rooms at all hours. Most of the factories were operating three shifts and so did Swanson's. The restaurant opened at 5 a.m. and closed at midnight. Richard found it difficult to find enough good help, so Edith and young Harold pitched in during odd hours and Doris Hart became Lucy's indispensable second in command in the kitchen.

The war had taxed the physical and emotional reserves of the Swanson family. In 1946, Lucy reluctantly retired and handed over the kitchen to Doris. But it was Richard who had aged most of all. Like his father and uncles, Richard developed coronary artery disease at 48 when he was stricken with angina pectoris. Richard did not smoke and he had no symptoms or signs of high blood pressure or diabetes mellitus. His cholesterol levels were unknown because such measurements were done only for research purposes. Unbeknownst to Richard, his total blood cholesterol was over 500, nearly three times what is now considered normal. Even if he did know it, there was no treatment except diet. Most physicians were unaware or unconvinced of cholesterol's role in the genesis of coronary artery disease.

In 1952, Richard sought help at the Mayo Clinic in Rochester, Minnesota. His angina kept him from working in his restaurant; he took a nitroglycerin tablet before eating or bathing. Occasionally he was awakened a night with a squeezing, burning sensation in the middle of his chest. To gain relief he placed two or more nitroglycerin tablets under his tongue and let them dissolve. Richard had consulted with specialists in Chicago but his condition failed to improve despite multiple medications, including morphine.

The Mayo doctors tried several new drugs. One after another seemed to help, but the angina always returned. Disappointed and dispirited, Richard returned home and turned the restaurant over to Harold who had recently received his degree in business administration from Loyola University in Chicago.

Swanson's Restaurant had thrived during and after the war, but tastes had changed. Double decker hamburgers, steaks, roast beef, fries, chili, and pie alamode reflected America's gastronomic rebound from the deprivations of the Depression and the food rationing of World War II. Fried fat and sugar went well with beer and bourbon. Lucy's delicate entrees of fish, pasta, fruits, and vegetables appealed to a dwindling niche of health-conscious patrons. Moreover, major highways bypassed downtown Highland Park and future interstates would shunt more traffic away from the north shore communities. Harold was convinced that change was vital if the restaurant was to survive.

With his father's reluctant consent, Harold made two critical strategic decisions: Swanson's would move west to U.S 41 and revamp its menu. The old restaurant was demolished and the land sold to a bank. The new Swanson's Restaurant was an attractive red brick building with white columns at the entrance. The interior was three times larger and the expansive bar area included a dance floor. Patrons loved it, and the restaurant quickly became the most popular eatery on the north shore of Lake Michigan.

Richard died in 1957 of congestive heart failure. Lucy, who had been declining for years, lived long enough to bury her son. At the age of 27 Harold was the only male Swanson left. Coronary artery disease had taken the lives of Bjorn, Nils, William, and Richard, all before 60. Harold, the last Swanson male, would not be spared.

I saw Harold Swanson for the first time in the spring of 1969 when he was admitted to Presbyterian-St. Luke's Hospital for coronary angiography. He had green eyes and short straight dark red hair surrounding a balding pate. An older woman was in the room.

"I'm Doris Hart," she said, extending her hand. I am Mr. Swanson's assistant." She wore a white lace-trimmed bib-style shirt and gold wool slacks; her only jewelry was a modest diamond set in a thin gold ring on her right hand.

"I'm Doctor Hauser, the intern on this floor. I believe you are being admitted by Dr. Muenster for a coronary angiogram."

Harold nodded, and Miss Hart said, "That's correct, doctor. Do you know when Dr. Muenster will be in?" I replied, "No idea. But I have a few questions."

For the next 25 minutes, I learned the details of Harold's history. Like his father and grandfather, he had developed symptoms of coronary artery disease at a young age—37 years. His angina had begun a year and a half before; it predictably came on with physical activity after eating.

Recently the pattern had changed: the burning discomfort was accompanied by aching in his armpits and nausea. Heavy cigarette or cigar smoke could trigger an attack, so he avoided the bar area at his restaurant. Harold had hypertension but a new medication—methyldopa—had brought his blood pressure under control.

His family doctor had measured Harold's cholesterol and found it to be very high; he prescribed a rice diet. By the 1960s a growing number of doctors believed there was a link between dietary cholesterol and coronary artery disease.

Isosorbide dinitrate, a nitroglycerin type drug, moderated Harold's angina but it caused distracting, gnawing headaches. He avoided using sublingual nitroglycerin for the same reason. Propranolol was the only drug that truly helped: he could at least take a walk after dinner without pain or a throbbing headache. Propranolol was a relatively new drug that Sir James Black discovered in 1964. It was the first of a class of drugs known as beta-blockers. Propranolol worked by lowering the heart rate and blood pressure, thus reducing the amount of oxygen the heart needed to pump blood.

As Harold's angina worsened, his doctor increased the dose of propranolol to control his symptoms. Side effects appeared, including fatigue and impotence: neither was acceptable to a 38-year-old man. Then Harold read a *Chicago Tribune* article about Dr. Rene Favaloro's new surgical technique at the Cleveland Clinic. It seemed promising. He wanted to know if it would allow him to get off the damn drugs.

In 1923, a boy was born to a carpenter and dressmaker of Sicilian decent in La Plata, a university city fifty miles south of Buenos Aires. His name was Rene Favaloro and he inherited his parents' talent for sewing and delicate woodworking. Years later, he reflected: "My parents taught me both ethics and hard work: nothing can be gained without effort." His uncle was a doctor and Rene often went with him to see patients in their homes. Later, Rene said, "I thought my uncle had a wonderful job."

Favaloro's dark hair and brown eyes were set in a square, serious face. He attended six years of elementary school, and six years of secondary school. "My parents aspired to a university education for their sons," he wrote, "and my mother took on additional work as a dressmaker, often laboring late at night over a pedal-driven Singer sewing machine…and my father did not know what it was to take a rest, working even Saturdays and Sundays until late at night."

As a result of their parents' labors, Rene and his brother, Juan José, attended medical school in La Plata. "We had first-class teachers in the humanities, mathematics, and engineering," Favaloro recalled. "Some of them had very strong humanistic and altruistic ideas, and we were all greatly influenced by them." Indeed, Favaloro's humanism and selflessness would shape his career.

In 1948, Dr. Favaloro graduated first in his medical school class. He interned in the old Hospital Policinico of La Plata where he received excellent training in general surgery. Favaloro was offered a position in the advanced surgical training program, but only if he signed a paper pledging his loyalty to the Peronist party and the National System. Argentina's president was Juan Peron who, together with his wife Eva ("Evita"), espoused a vague ideology—Peronism—that appealed to the working classes and unions. Peron was viewed by many of his countrymen to be a fascist and a demagogue with dictatorial tendencies. Favaloro refused to sign the pledge, foregoing an opportunity to study thoracic surgery.

Instead, Rene became a rural doctor in Jacinto Aráuz, a small town west of the Provence of La Pampa, a fertile plain southwest of Buenos Aires. "This internal exile," he said, "was provoked by various motives, among them my love and respect for liberty, which at that time was curtailed by the policies of the government in office. It signified an end to my first steps in thoracic surgery…"

Shortly thereafter, his brother graduated from medical school and joined him. Together they built a 23-bed clinic and operating room in Jacinto Aráuz where there was no hospital. During the next 12 years, they performed more than 10,000 surgical procedures in their clinic.

The brothers also provided primary care and practiced public health. Still, Favaloro could not help but think to himself: "This is not the place for you, it never was: you are capable of bigger things and you are wasting your time." He had always wanted to be a thoracic surgeon and his surgical role models were Dr. Clarence Crafoord, a prominent thoracic surgeon in Sweden, and Dr. Enrique Finochietto of Buenos Aires. He read too of the emerging field of cardiovascular surgery and the work done by Blalock, Lillehei, and Kirklin in the United States. During his infrequent visits to La Plata, he told one of his former professors, Dr. José Maria Mainetti, that he was determined to leave his practice in Aráuz and train in cardiothoracic surgery.

"Apply to the Cleveland Clinic because the staff is skilled and forward-looking," Mainetti told him. "I have seen the work of Dr. Mason Sones and his colleagues in the catheterization laboratory and they are undoubtedly years ahead of any other cardiology center in the United States," he said, "and then there is Dr. William Kolff who is working on an artificial heart…and Dr. Donald Effler who seems to be an excellent surgeon. I believe it is the ideal place for you."

On Favaloro's behalf, Mainetti wrote twice to the chief of surgery at the Cleveland Clinic, Dr. George Crile Jr., but never received a reply. After three months of waiting, Favaloro took matters into his own hands. He said good-bye to his family—he would forever remember the pain in his mother's eyes—and flew to Cleveland with his wife, Toni. It was the first time either one had been in an airplane. Neither was fluent in English, although Rene had taken English lessons from an Australian tutor.

> *"[During the flight] I slept fitfully," Favaloro wrote. "Had I done right? I had cut short my career as a country doctor, which had given me so many happy moments…Would I have the aptitude to enter the field of thoracic and cardiovascular surgery? Would I be accepted in the Cleveland Clinic? Perhaps I would be back home sooner than expected…Without doubt at the age of 39 I would be faced once more with a great challenge. Would it be too late? I did not think so, for the years spent in Aráuz had made me strong and given me an extraordinary power of resistance."*

Arriving in Cleveland, Rene went directly to George Crile's office and presented the letter of introduction from Professor Mainetti. Crile was the son of a founder of the Cleveland Clinic and a prominent surgeon and author. After Favaloro explained the purpose of his visit, Crile called Donald Effler, the chief of thoracic and cardiovascular surgery. Minutes later, Rene was sitting in Effler's office on the ninth floor of the Clinic.

Effler was a big man with an athletic build, wide face, and penetrating eyes. He said Favaloro could not be a trainee at the Clinic because he had not taken the examination required of foreign medical graduates. Instead, Effler told Favaloro that he could be an observer but would not receive a salary or support of any kind. Favaloro leaped at the opportunity. He promised to work with "dedication and responsibility." Effler instructed him to report to the education department to register as an official observer.

Favaloro met with the head of the education department, a notoriously fussy bureaucrat. When he learned that Favaloro was from Argentina, he said, "You are from a wild county. I don't know what sort of education you have." The man continued with insults directed at Argentina. Exasperated and angry, Favaloro said he would not tolerate further abuse of his country. He left, thinking that he would return soon to Jacinto Aráuz. Favaloro told Effler what happened. "Forget it," Effler said. "Officially registered or not, you will present yourself on my service tomorrow at eight o'clock on the dot."

The Favaloros had about $10,000 to last them until Rene passed the foreign medical graduate exam and hopefully became a resident trainee at the Clinic. They moved into a cheap hotel occupied by low-income elderly couples. It had a kitchenette where they subsisted on Campbell's soup, rice, and chicken. Eventually Effler arranged for them to move into an apartment in an old building near the Clinic.

Favaloro became a jack-of-all-trades: transporting patients, inserting urinary catheters, and cleaning the heart-lung machine. He also served as a surgical assistant and observed Effler during lung and heart surgery. At night, he studied for the foreign medical graduate examination. "Those first days gave me a global idea of the complexity of the work being carried out in the Clinic," he wrote, "and of the enormous responsibility which I would have to confront if I wished to qualify in this specialty."

After passing the foreign medical graduate examination Favaloro became a junior surgical resident at the Clinic. In 1964, he was appointed chief resident, and Effler arranged for him to visit Dr. Denton Cooley in Houston. Effler was interested in the DeWall-Lillehei bubble oxygenator because it was easier to use than the time-consuming heart-lung machine employed at the Clinic. Favaloro assisted Cooley during surgery, and studied the bubble oxygenator. Cooley was impressed with Favaloro's capacity for work and wrote Effler that his chief resident was very skilled in the operating room.

Favaloro would always remember how Effler praised those who performed well. Like many great teachers, Effler gave his colleagues the credit they deserved. One afternoon a patient, who was a prominent Cleveland businessman, was not doing well in the operating room. Effler and Favaloro had replaced his aortic valve, but they could not get the heart to stop fibrillating. Effler left the operating room to tell the relatives the bad news. While he was gone, Favaloro tried a new solution containing high concentrations of potassium, glucose, and insulin that he had learned about from Dr. Sodi-Pollares, a cardiologist in Mexico City.

Favaloro injected the mixture directly into the patient's aorta near the openings of the two coronary arteries. He waited a few minutes and shocked the heart again. It began to contract, slowly at first but then faster, pumping in a regular rhythm. The patient's blood pressure rose. The heart-lung machine was no longer needed. Effler was surprised and pleased. He returned to the waiting room and told the family that Favaloro had saved their loved one—taking no credit for himself.

When Favaloro completed his training in 1966, Effler offered him a staff position at the Clinic. However, Favaloro declined and instead returned to Argentina hoping to create a heart surgery program. He spent months trying to garner support from the Argentine medical establishment. After receiving no encouragement, he returned to Cleveland and began his pursuit of a surgical treatment for coronary artery disease.

Early on, Favaloro met Dr. F. Mason Sones who was revolutionizing cardiology with diagnostic coronary angiography. The son of a mechanic, Sones was born in Noxapater, Mississippi, in 1918 and graduated from the University of Maryland Medical School in 1943. After serving in the Air Force, he trained at Henry Ford Hospital in Detroit where he learned cardiac catheterization. In 1950, the Cleveland Clinic recruited him to start a catheterization laboratory, and by 1956 Sones had built a state-of-the-art facility. The advanced X-ray imaging equipment was so large that it was housed in a pit excavated in the basement of the Clinic at the then-exorbitant cost of $150,000.

Sones had performed the first selective coronary angiogram by accident in 1958 when a catheter he had placed in the aorta of a 26-year-old man slipped unseen into the right coronary artery. At the time, it was widely believed that injecting X-ray dye directly into a coronary artery would cause a heart attack or ventricular fibrillation. Sones, to his horror, watched as a large volume of dye coursed down the artery.

Expecting the heart to fibrillate, Sones grabbed a scalpel and was about to open the patient's chest to perform cardiac massage when he noticed that his patient was awake. The heart monitor showed a slow rhythm. On impulse, Sones shouted for the patient to cough, which he did, and within minutes, a normal rhythm returned. The patient survived the large dye injection without any ill effects. (Coughing helped to clear the dye from the young man's heart; today, "Cough! Cough!" is heard often in every catheterization laboratory after dye is injected into a coronary artery).

Most physicians would have thanked God that a tragedy had been averted, but Sones had one of those seminal moments in history: he realized that it could be safe to insert a catheter directly into the coronary artery, selectively inject a small quantity of diluted X-ray dye, and take a movie as it filled the coronary artery with dark contrast.

Coronary angiography was born on that day. In a few years, it would transform the diagnosis and treatment of coronary artery disease. Up to this time, doctors diagnosed coronary artery disease based on a patient's symptoms, the electrocardiogram (EKG), and intuition. The margin of diagnostic error was large because, unlike Harold Swanson, many patients with significant coronary artery disease had no typical symptoms. Coronary angiography not only improved diagnostic accuracy, but it also revealed the location and severity of the plaque that was blocking blood flow.

This new diagnostic test identified new diseases, including coronary artery spasm and spontaneous coronary dissection—a tear in the artery. It unlocked new frontiers for cardiologists and cardiac surgeons. For the first time they were able to see, in great detail, the cholesterol and fat-laden plaque that blocked blood flow to the heart's muscle. Such knowledge would prove vital as new therapeutic interventions were conceived, applied, and evaluated. This momentous advance was a potential lifesaver for millions of people, including young Harold Swanson.

Sones was an innovator who abhorred writing scientific papers. He rarely published his work, preferring instead to present his results at medical meetings and to cardiologists who visited his laboratory at the Cleveland Clinic. In October, 1959, he attempted to dissolve a clot by infusing streptokinase into the right coronary artery of a 43-year-old patient suffering an acute heart attack. Five years later, in 1964, he tried to dilate (angioplasty) an artery in a 45-year-old man. He even collaborated with Lowell Edwards to create a "roto-rooter" catheter to drill through arteries that were totally blocked by calcified plaque. Decades later, other physicians would convert Sones' prescient impulses into successful therapies.

Rene Favaloro was fascinated and inspired by Sones' coronary angiograms. Often at night, he would study the films in his apartment and review them with Sones the next day. The two of them worked with Dr. William Proudfit, the chief of cardiology, to understand the correlation between what was seen on the angiogram and the symptoms that patients experienced. Plaque that occupied more than 70 percent of the diameter of the lumen (channel) of a major coronary artery was often associated with angina or shortness of breath, particularly during physical activity or emotional stress. But some patients had no symptoms, even when a major artery was completely blocked.

Sones and Favaloro and became close friends, despite being opposites in personality and behavior. Favaloro was tall, focused, and humble. Sones was short, hypercritical, and often bombastic. At one point, Sones was banned from making rounds in the hospital because he was so disruptive to the medical staff. Nurses feared him and tried to hide when he was around. Together, however, Sones and Favaloro were a symphony, and their harmonious collaboration opened new vistas in the treatment of coronary artery disease.

Favaloro studied hundreds of Sones' coronary angiograms. He observed that the most serious coronary artery obstructions were usually close to the point where the coronary arteries originated at the aorta. This fact would prove vital to the success of coronary artery surgery.

In 1994 Favaloro wrote:

"At the beginning of 1967, I began to think about the possibility of using the saphenous vein from the leg in coronary surgery. The Cleveland Clinic had accumulated a lot of experience using the saphenous vein in patients with occlusion of the circulation in the lower limbs [legs] and renal [kidney] arteries. I asked myself: why not the coronaries?"

Favaloro and Effler experimented with a variety of techniques to surgically repair coronary arteries using the saphenous vein. One method involved cutting out the plaque and repairing the artery with a patch of saphenous vein. Another technique excised the diseased section and interposed a vein graft by suturing either end directly to the artery. The results were mixed. Many of the repaired coronary arteries developed clots, causing heart attacks. Some patients died during or shortly after surgery.

Favaloro and his team agonized over these deaths and complications. Attempts to remove the plaque, called endarterectomy, also yielded disappointing results. Attacking the plaque with surgical instruments often caused more harm than good. Coronary artery surgery was about to join the growing list of promising treatments that ultimately proved ineffective or unsafe.

At this point, Favaloro could have thrown in the towel, but he was not that kind of person. Instead of operating directly on the diseased coronary artery, Favaloro decided to leave the fragile plaque alone because touching it with a scalpel or scissors often triggered an uncontrollable inflammatory response and blood clots. It was a critical decision. He would use the saphenous vein as a conduit—a kind of flexible pipe—and simply shunt blood around the blockage. One end of the saphenous vein would be sutured directly to the aorta just above the aortic valve and the other end to the coronary artery beyond the blockage. The fat-laden and calcified yellow sludge clogging the artery would thus be bypassed, like traffic redirected around a congested city. This surgical procedure would become known as aorto-coronary bypass, or coronary artery bypass grafting (CABG).

"My first paper reported a patient with a saphenous vein bypass to the right coronary artery," Favaloro recalled. "The evolution from patch graft to bypass graft took place in just a few months." Soon he and his colleagues were doing aorto-saphenous vein bypass grafts to the left coronary artery and combining bypass surgery with valve replacement.

In December 1968, Favaloro published the results of 171 coronary artery bypass procedures in the *Journal of Thoracic and Cardiovascular Surgery*. It was the largest experience published up to that time. The mortality rate was so low (4 percent) that several prominent cardiologists challenged the report's credibility. Favaloro invited these skeptics to Cleveland where they examined the records and confirmed that the results Favaloro reported were indeed accurate.

Favaloro's work created a sensation in the medical community. Hundreds of patients with severe, symptomatic coronary artery disease were treated at the Clinic with bypass surgery. The surgery list grew so much that some patients had to wait two to three months for their operation.

Auditoriums were standing room only wherever Favaloro spoke at medical meetings. On one memorable occasion, in London, the usually well-behaved specialists crashed through the closed doors of a completely full lecture hall, interrupting the morning presentations by Favaloro and a group of prominent cardiovascular specialists, including Dr. Paul Dudley White of Harvard and the Massachusetts General Hospital. The session chairman eventually regained control by promising to repeat Favaloro's lecture that afternoon.

This unassuming general practitioner from rural Argentina had become an international celebrity because of his pioneering innovation. Favaloro could have basked in his fame and become a very wealthy man, but these were not his priorities. When asked by several of his countrymen to return to Argentina to become chairman of the cardiovascular department in Buenos Aires, he wrote a letter to Donald Effler. In it he said:

> "...*as you know there is no real cardiovascular surgery in Buenos Aires. Patients are going every day to San Pablo and the United States. Some of them are rich enough to afford the trip but some are coming under great financial strain (one patient sold his home in order to be able to make the trip). Some of them cannot even afford to think about coming. They die slowly but surely without the proper treatment...*

"Destiny has put on my shoulders once more a difficult task. I am going to dedicate the last one-third of my life to build a thoracic and cardiovascular center in Buenos Aires. At this particular time, the circumstances indicate that I am the only one with the possibility of doing it...I know I am taking the difficult road...If I do not do this my conscience would constantly be telling me: 'You chose the easy way'".

Effler read Favaloro's letter and replied:

"Your letter does not come as a surprise but nevertheless it comes as a great disappointment to me...Your professional work and your tremendous drive has made an impact on the Cleveland Clinic Foundation, and more than that, upon the specialty of thoracic and cardiovascular surgery, itself. Needless to say I am very proud...I think you are doing the right thing."

Rene Favaloro returned to Argentina and, largely with money he donated and raised, created the Favaloro Foundation, a center for patient care, education, and research that was based on the Cleveland Clinic model. A surgeon establishing and personally financing a basic research department was unprecedented. The Favaloro Foundation evolved into an institute for cardiology, cardiothoracic surgery, and organ transplantation. It elevated the level of medical education all over Latin America.

The morning after Harold Swanson entered Presbyterian-St. Luke's Hospital in 1969, Joe Muenster performed a coronary angiogram. It was less than one year after Rene Favaloro had published the results of his pioneering work in coronary bypass surgery.

The angiogram showed that Harold's right coronary artery was totally blocked just beyond its origin from the aorta. The artery beyond the blockage received some blood via small branches from the left coronary artery, known as collaterals, and appeared to be free of any plaque. The left coronary artery had some plaque build-up, but none of it was severe enough to compromise blood flow.

By the standards of the time, Harold was a candidate for coronary artery bypass. Acceptable medical therapy had failed to control his symptoms. His bypass would be one of the first performed in Chicago, and Dr. Hassan Najafi would do it.

At 9 a.m. the following day, Harold was wheeled into the operating room, anesthetized, and covered with sterile cloth drapes. Through a long incision, Najafi removed a length of saphenous vein from Harold's left leg; he wrapped the section of vein in a saline soaked sterile dressing and handed it to the scrub nurse. Next, he and Bill Ostermiller opened Harold's chest through a sternotomy incision and placed Harold on the heart-lung machine. Najafi inspected the right coronary artery and identified where the bypass would be anastomosed (connected) to the artery. This would be well beyond the total blockage as seen on the angiogram.

By this time, four additional people entered the operating room to observe this landmark surgery. Principal among them were Drs. Ormand Julian and John Graettinger, the chief of cardiology. Also present were Joe Muenster and a photographer. All were properly garbed in scrub suits and masks. Julian stood next to the anesthesiologist at the head of the table so he could look directly down onto Harold's exposed heart and confer with Najafi.

"Dr. Julian," Najafi said, pointing to the right coronary artery, "I think this is where the distal anastomosis should go."

"How does the artery feel?" Julian asked.

"It is soft here where I want to attach the vein. I can feel the hard plaque where the angiogram showed it would be."

"Good. I would go ahead then," Julian said.

Najafi took the section of saphenous vein from the scrub nurse and cut it to a length that would allow the vein to extend from the aorta to the coronary artery without stretching (too tight) or kinking (too loose). At each end of the vein, he made a small incision to enlarge the opening and tapered it to a 45-degree angle. Then he made a small incision in the coronary artery and attached one end of the vein graft to the artery with individual sutures.

Najafi placed a small clamp on the lower portion of the ascending aorta to isolate a small section of the wall. He then cut a triangular hole in the aorta and anastomosed the other end of the vein graft. The clamp was released allowing blood to flow through the vein graft and around the blockage. It was an elegantly simple surgical procedure.

Harold Swanson left the hospital six days after his bypass surgery. He convalesced at home for five weeks and returned to work. The sternotomy incision caused occasional discomfort but he rarely needed a pain pill. Best of all, he was taking no drugs because his once-crippling angina was completely gone.

The dread that Harold had once felt as each day unfolded also disappeared. No longer did he avoid the simple tasks of living: dressing, eating, shopping for groceries, and loving. Harold was liberated. The optimism that had deserted him two years earlier now returned with renewed vigor.

Swanson's Restaurant was no longer the center of his universe. Though it had been in his family since 1900, he sold the restaurant to Doris Hart for $350,000 cash and a promissory note for an identical amount payable to him in five years with interest.

Four months later, Harold decided to visit his cousins in Wisconsin and Minnesota. He bought a new dark blue Volvo station wagon, filled it with clothing sufficient to last a month and headed northwest. Harold's first stop was LaCrosse where his grandfather's brother, Nils, had farmed until his premature death due to coronary artery disease.

Nils' widow, Harriet, raised their two sons. Gerald, the oldest boy, became a naval fighter pilot, and was killed in 1944 when his shot-up plane crashed as he attempted a carrier landing during the Battle of the Philippine Sea. The second son, Morgan, inherited the farm from his mother and expanded it to more than five thousand acres. At 72, Morgan Swanson was a successful farmer and businessman, active in local politics, and a fervid Green Bay Packers football fan.

After three days at Morgan's farm south of LaCrosse, Harold drove through St. Paul and Minneapolis and headed west on highway 212 to Olivia, the "Corn Capital of the World." The sons of his great uncle, William, were farming the same land south of Olivia that their grandfather had purchased in 1901. William's widow, Lorna, had rented out the land until the boys were old enough to work the fields themselves. Lorna was still alive at 90. Two of her grandsons had attended agricultural college at the University of Minnesota and the third grandson was finishing his medicine residency at Hennepin County Hospital and soon would open a practice in Renville County.

Harold occupied the guest bedroom on the third floor of the expansive farmhouse. The evening before Harold's planned departure for the drive back to Illinois, Lorna and her two daughters-in-law invited the neighbors to dinner. The Larson, Novak, and Schultz families were large and filled every room on the first floor. The children ranged from newborns and toddlers to polite, muscled farm boys and sturdy, cheerful farm girls.

The men congregated around the fireplace in the living room, while the women gathered in the kitchen and dining room. Harold moved among them. He had already met a few during trips to town or visits to their farms. Standing with the men in the living room was a solitary woman. She spoke to them of sugar beets and tractors, new pest-resistant seeds, and Ford trucks.

Harold had to move around the circle of men to see who had gained the attention of this all-male group. The woman had short, curly brown hair, hazel eyes, high forehead, dimples, and full lips; she was about Harold's height. She spoke with authority and her hands were in constant motion. Her name was Jean Novak and she was the oldest daughter of Jim and Sally Novak who owned 240 acres south of the Swanson farm on US 71.

Harold managed to sit across from Jean at dinner. "I understand you are returning home tomorrow," Jean said matter-of-factly above the clatter of silverware. She did not wait for a reply, "I have always wanted to visit Chicago. Where do you live?"

Harold described Highland Park and his recently sold restaurant. He liked this woman. Jean was thirty, unmarried, and very different. She had forsaken the traditional role of the farmwoman: namely babies, homemaking, and community service. To his credit, Jean's father had permitted and encouraged his daughter to work alongside her brothers and learn the finer points of crop management. She was a decent mechanic, good businesswoman, and tireless during the harvest. Jean got them into sugar beets and she figured out how to get the beets to the processing plant on time. All of this had left little opportunity for dating, much less courting, and now Jean was well past the age when most women married.

After dinner, Jean and Harold sat on the screened porch. Harold told her about his surgery and desire to do something other than running a restaurant. Then, on impulse or instinct, he said, "Drive back with me to Chicago. I'll show you around, visit the museums, and go to a concert in Grant Park. You can take the train home or I will drive you. At the most you'll be gone 10 to 12 days".

Jean looked at this 41-year-old balding redhead with Irish green eyes and crooked smile. He was attractive in an odd way and the last thing she wanted to say to him was that she was too busy with the farm. Except it was the truth, and there was no possibility she could leave with the sugar beet harvest coming up.

"I'd like to go," she said, leaning toward him on the wicker couch. "But we are in the middle of …"

"I'll wait 'til you're done," Harold interrupted. "And you don't have to worry about anything. I'm not one of those guys."

"I'm not worried, not at all." Jean extended her hand. "It's agreed, then."

In September of 1970 Harold Swanson and Jean Novak arrived at his home west of Highland Park. They dined at Swanson's Restaurant where Jean met Doris Hart. For the next seven days, they visited all the sights Harold had described: The Art Institute of Chicago, the Museum of Science and Industry, and the Shedd Aquarium. They went to a Cubs game (the Cubs lost), attended a concert in Grant Park, and spent an evening on Rush Street.

Harold proposed on the day prior to Jean's planned departure home. They were huddled together on the Highland Park beach where a cool northwest wind was signaling summer's end. Harold said, "I don't expect an answer right away. Take your time." Jean kissed him on the cheek and took his hand. "I don't need to. My answer is 'Yes.'"

Two weeks later Harold and Jean arrived in Olivia, and announced that they would marry after the harvest.

In 1985, Favaloro and his wife returned to Cleveland. Mason Sones was dying of lung cancer and he wanted to see his Argentine friend one more time. The two of them sat alone on the last day of their visit. Favaloro wrote: "We looked at each other in silence and our view became crowded by the tears we both shed. I managed to say: 'Well, let's not act like this. After all we will be seeing each other again one day in Heaven. 'Sones replied: 'You believe that, Rene? I have my doubts.'" They shared a long embrace, crying disconsolately. Sones died on August 29, 1985.

By 2000, the Favaloro Foundation faced severe financial problems. In the midst of a deep recession, it was $75 million in debt and close to bankruptcy at the hands of the government. Favaloro appealed to the government, to his friends in the United States, and to President Fernando de la Rua for financial assistance.

After receiving no reply from the government or de la Rua, Rene Favaloro wrote a final letter, saying he was "tired of being a beggar". Then he pointed a pistol at his chest and shot himself in the heart. He was found dead in his home on July 29, 2000.

A week later, the *New York Times* reported:

> *"It has been more than a week since Rene G. Favaloro, Argentina's most esteemed surgeon and a pioneer in the heart bypass operation, committed suicide. But the outpouring of grief seems to be compounding day-by-day, opening a channel of despair so profound that Argentines are raising the deepest of questions about themselves and their country.*
>
> *As wreaths of flowers pile up in front of Dr. Favaloro's research foundation, newspapers are publishing extra columns of letters to the editor in a deluge of long, sorrowful and often bitter diatribes blaming the entire society for the suicide. Dr. Favaloro's photograph is on covers of magazines filled with details of the suicide and theorizing by Argentine writers about what Dr. Favaloro's death means."*

Coronary artery bypass graft surgery became the most frequently performed heart operation. By 2000, more than half a million patients a year were undergoing this procedure in hundreds of hospitals on every continent except Antarctica. Several major improvements were introduced, primarily the use of the internal mammary artery rather than the saphenous vein as the conduit for bypassing the left anterior descending coronary artery.

Yet the basic principles discovered and evolved by Rene Favaloro remained unchanged. While Favaloro did not perform the very first coronary bypass operation, he and his colleagues at the Cleveland Clinic embraced the procedure, made it work, reported their results, and taught other surgeons how to do it well and safely. Today the Favaloro Foundation is thriving, offering multispecialty patient care at The University Hospital in Buenos Aires, and education and research at Favaloro University.

The vein bypass graft to Harold Swanson's right coronary artery continued to supply oxygenated blood to his heart. But inside Harold's left anterior descending coronary artery, a soft atherosclerotic plaque was slowly accumulating more fat. Within the plaque were puffy cells called macrophages that replicated and gulped bad cholesterol. Occasionally inflammatory chemicals caused the surface of the plaque to erode, fracture, and bleed. Miniscule clots formed. Fibrin strands in the clots trapped cells from the blood stream and formed fragile tissue, adding thin microscopic layers to the soft plaque. Calcium molecules penetrated the plaque and hardened the fibrous tissue. The pathologic process was fitful; it would lay dormant for months or years until something noxious triggered a reawakening.

At that time, there were no statins—cholesterol lowering drugs—and the benefit of aspirin in coronary artery disease was uncertain. Meanwhile Harold felt nothing as the stealthy disease lurched forward, fueled by lipids, stress, and the Swanson genome. The left anterior descending coronary artery and the blood flowing through it were in jeopardy and so was the mass of muscle comprising his main pumping chamber. This looming plaque could make Jean Swanson a widow.

CHAPTER 5

In July of 1969, I climbed the stairs to ward K-3 of Cincinnati General Hospital on a typically muggy summer morning. I was now a junior medicine resident and would be in charge of this ward for the next six weeks. My starched white pants were already wilting in the heat and humidity.

General Hospital occupied the same buildings where my cousins had trained during the 1930s. Indeed, I had been a medical student on ward K-3 where I had learned the basics of the physical examination from a very distinguished African-American internist, taken my first night calls, and learned how to perform minor surgical procedures and spinal taps.

The ward had a wide and long, high ceiling room that accommodated 24 to 30 patients. Large windows on either side provided sunlight and ventilation. At the end of the ward was a room for six to eight patients who were less ill. The sickest patients were at the front of the ward near the nurses' desk. Two private rooms were reserved for isolating patients with infectious diseases like tuberculosis. At night when the overhead lights were off, we used gooseneck lamps to examine patients, draw blood, and insert catheters.

Patients were transported in old wood and wicker wheelchairs. The hand-cranked steel beds were relics of another era. There were no heart monitors. When a patient was admitted with a heart attack, we connected him or her to the single American Optical™ defibrillator that had a small orange-tinted glass oscilloscope monitor displaying one lead of the electrocardiogram. The defibrillator's eight-inch round monitor was visible to the nurse provided she was sitting at her desk and there was no glare from the sun or fluorescent lights. Because there was no audible alarm, a life-threatening rhythm could go undetected. If a second heart attack victim was admitted, we had to decide which patient was most likely to survive: this patient would be triaged to the monitor.

Waiting for me were two interns who were as green as I had been only 12 months before. The chief medical resident was already there. He was irritatingly officious but seemed competent. During the next hour and a half, we assessed each of the 32 patients on the ward. The majority were African-Americans who suffered from a variety of common disorders. Most had chronic obstructive pulmonary disease or heart failure due to cigarette smoking, long-standing and untreated hypertension, or poorly controlled diabetes. Several young women were being treated for pelvic inflammatory disease due to gonorrhea. Eloise, 19, a University of Cincinnati undergraduate, was in one of the isolation rooms recovering from near-fatal meningococcal meningitis. In the other isolation room was a medical resident with tuberculous pericarditis, an infection involving the sac around his heart.

At 10 a.m. Dr. Richard Vilter, the director of the Department of Medicine, arrived on the ward to welcome us to his training program. I knew Vilter from my medical school rotations. He was 57-years-old and a renowned internist, hematologist-oncologist, and master clinician. Like Owen Wangensteen at the University of Minnesota, Vilter was devoted to teaching and research and he closely supervised an outstanding department of medicine. The medical community would remember the "Vilter era" from 1956 to 1978 as the years when the Cincinnati Medical Center emerged as a premiere teaching hospital.

That afternoon we admitted Tom McClellan, a 53-year-old construction worker, who had a heart attack while pushing a wheelbarrow filled with wet cement. He was a heavy smoker but otherwise healthy. We connected him to the ward's only American Optical™ monitor. Thirty minutes later Tom's heart went into ventricular fibrillation. Instead of regular coordinated contractions, the muscle of his ventricles shimmied, producing random polymorphous waves of useless mechanical energy. Blood coming back to the heart from his body and lungs pooled and stagnated, forcing the four chambers of his stricken heart to stretch and dilate. Tom's vast circulatory engine stalled. Death was imminent.

Tom could have died quietly and unnoticed because the American Optical monitor had no alarm, but a patient in the next bed saw him slump over and shouted for the nurse. An intern rushed to his bedside and placed defibrillator paddles on Tom's chest. The shock sent electrical current through Tom's heart, causing his muscle cells to contract simultaneously, extinguishing the ventricular fibrillation and allowing his biologic pacemaker—the sinus node—to stimulate his heart and restore effective blood flow.

Tom started breathing on his own. He struggled to sit up but a nurse gently laid him back and took his blood pressure; it was normal—116 over 64—and his heart rate was 92 beats per minute. I listened to his heart and lungs. There were no signs of congestion. Tom's condition had not changed except for the circular red burn marks on his chest from the high voltage defibrillation shock. Prompt defibrillation saved his life and prevented heart damage.

Using electricity to stop life-threatening heart rhythms began in 1947. Dr. Claude Beck operated on the heart of a 14-year-old boy in Cleveland when the youngster's heart went into ventricular fibrillation. Beck massaged the boy's heart for 45 minutes but the fibrillation persisted. He knew of research by his colleague, Dr. Carl Wiggers, a physician and physiologist at Case Western Reserve. Wiggers was using an experimental alternating current defibrillator in the animal lab to defibrillate dogs. In a desperate attempt to save the boy's life, Beck called for the experimental defibrillator to be brought into the operating room.

Beck massaged the boy's heart while he waited. It took some time before the machine finally arrived. Beck placed the metal electrodes directly on the boy's heart and delivered a high voltage shock. The heart continued to fibrillate. Beck injected procainamide—an antiarrhythmic drug—directly into the left ventricle and again shocked the heart. This time, the boy's heart stopped fibrillating, a normal rhythm took over, and he survived. Claude Beck had performed the world's first successful human defibrillation.

Subsequently, surgeons who participated in a training course sponsored by the Cleveland Area Heart Society reported that they had successfully defibrillated more than 20 patients using Beck's technique. One patient, in particular, was quite remarkable.

In June 1955, Dr. Albert Ransone, who practiced at the University Hospital in Cleveland, developed indigestion and some chest discomfort. He was 65 years old and otherwise healthy. An EKG revealed mild, non-specific abnormalities. As he left the hospital, however, Ransone collapsed and fell to the floor unconscious.

In the emergency room, he was blue and had no pulse. Doctors gave him oxygen via a facemask and injected a solution of epinephrine directly into his heart, all to no avail.

Cardiopulmonary resuscitation with closed chest massage was unknown in the 1950s. Within five minutes Claude Beck opened Dr. Ransone's chest through an incision between the fourth and fifth ribs and massaged his heart, squeezing it rhythmically so that blood began to flow. Beck could see that Ransone's heart was fibrillating. He called for an experimental defibrillator, similar to the one he used on the 14-year-old boy in 1947.

Meanwhile, Beck placed a tube in Ransone's trachea and ventilated him with an anesthesia bag. His skin color improved and he intermittently took breaths on his own. Beck opened the pericardium, the sac around the heart. A few minutes later, the defibrillator arrived and Beck wrapped the electrodes in sterile gauze sponges, applying them to Ransone's heart. But several shocks were unsuccessful. Beck realized that the dry sponges insulated the electrodes so that no current could flow to Ransone's heart. He soaked the dressings in saline, a salt solution, and repeated the shock. It worked: the shock defibrillated the heart and it began to beat on its own, restoring blood flow.

Ransone awoke the following morning, but understandably remained confused and disoriented for several days. Then he became more like himself—cheerful and talkative; he could recall nothing that happened during the 36 hours after he collapsed. A week later, he left the hospital and he eventually resumed his medical practice.

Remarkably, Dr. Ransone lived another 28 years, dying in 1984 at 93. He had retired to Florida and remained active. He slipped away quietly one morning sitting in a chair in his home, while his housekeeper read to him. His case illustrates the value of prompt electrical defibrillation—and God's beneficence.

During my high school summer vacations in 1956 and 1957 I served as an orderly at Mercy Hospital in Hamilton, Ohio. There I observed open chest heart massage. But unlike Beck's success with Dr. Ransone, I never saw a patient survive. The drawbacks to open chest resuscitation were obvious: only a surgeon could do it and the instruments had to be available. If more victims of cardiac arrest were to survive, someone had to invent a method to restore blood flow anytime, anywhere, and without opening the chest.

William Bennett Kouwenhoven was nicknamed "Wild Bill" by his friends and colleagues. His Dutch ancestors came to America in 1623 and settled on the western edge of Long Island, now Brooklyn, where Bill was born in 1886. He graduated from the Brooklyn Polytechnic Institute with degrees in electrical and mechanical engineering and in 1913 obtained a doctorate from the prestigious Karlsruhe Institute of Technology in Germany. In 1914, he was an Instructor in Electrical Engineering at Johns Hopkins University. Eventually he became the dean and chair of the department.

Electricity was novel in the early 20th century and doctors knew little about its effects on the human body, including the heart. In 1925, Consolidated Edison of New York (ConEd) had become so concerned with the unexplained deaths of its lineman that it commissioned a study at Johns Hopkins to explain these tragedies and to find solutions.

Kouwenhoven joined the Hopkins research team. They found that even brief contact with the AC current in power lines could cause ventricular fibrillation and sudden death. The obvious preventive measures were safety procedures that diminished accidental exposure to "hot wires." But ConEd and other utility companies around the country wanted a way to treat, i.e. stop, ventricular fibrillation on the scene. The Hopkins team found that properly timed AC current also could defibrillate the heart. This observation led to Wiggers' development of the AC defibrillator that Beck used successfully in 1947.

Beck's approach to defibrillation required an open chest and placement of electrodes directly on the heart. This was not feasible or practical for the vast majority of patients. So during the 1950s Bill Kouwenhoven at Johns Hopkins and Dr. Paul Zoll at Beth Israel in Boston each developed external defibrillators with electrodes that were placed on the patient's chest to deliver shocks to the heart through the skin.

The Zoll™ defibrillator delivered AC shocks of 240 to 720 volts and Kouwenhoven's defibrillator delivered shocks of 440 volts (it also weighed 200 pounds). Both were successful inventions. In 1956, Zoll reported four patients he treated successfully with an external defibrillator; and, in 1957, the Kouwenhoven defibrillator was used for the first time to save a 42-year-old patient.

Like so many advances in medicine the next major step forward in resuscitation occurred by a combination of serendipity and astute observation. Guy Knickerbocker was a doctoral student in electrical engineering who worked in Kouwenhoven's laboratory on closed chest defibrillation. One day in 1958, Knickerbocker noticed that placing the heavy defibrillating paddles on the chest of a dog in ventricular fibrillation would produce a pulse on the blood pressure monitor. Simply pressing on the dog's chest produced a pulse. He pushed again and again, creating a series of pulses that resulted in blood flowing to the animal's body even though the dog's heart was fibrillating. Knickerbocker's observation marked the beginning of closed-chest cardiac massage.

Kouwenhoven, Knickerbocker and surgeon Dr. James Jude, embarked on extensive laboratory studies to define the best method for performing this technique. They found that optimum blood flow resulted when clenched hands were pressed downward on the sternum, compressing the heart against the spine. With this method, they could keep an animal in ventricular fibrillation alive for 30 minutes and then successfully defibrillate it with an electric shock. They called it cardiopulmonary resuscitation or CPR.

By 1960, Kouwenhoven's team reported their findings, and their article in the *Journal of the American Medical Association* remains a classic. Their first patient was a 34-year-old woman who came to the emergency room with a gallbladder attack. She was taken to surgery where her heart stopped during the operation. Within two minutes of closed-chest massage, her pulse returned without defibrillation. Another patient was a 45-year-old man who had a heart attack and collapsed in ventricular fibrillation. After 20 minutes of closed-chest massage, an external defibrillator restored a normal heart rhythm.

An estimated 100,000 to 200,000 lives are saved *every year* with CPR. And while some minor modifications have been made, the method described by Kouwenhoven and colleagues remains in use. Fittingly, Johns Hopkins granted Dr. William Kouwenhoven its very first honorary medical degree in 1969.

The two key elements of successful resuscitation—closed-chest massage and external defibrillation—were firmly established by the early 1960s. Subsequently defibrillation improved with the introduction of the American Optical direct current defibrillator, similar to the one we used to defibrillate Tom McClellan at Cincinnati General Hospital. Direct current, delivered by a particular type of capacitor, causes less heart muscle damage and arrhythmias than alternating current.

Still, most cardiac arrest patients, especially victims of a heart attack, were dying of ventricular fibrillation outside the hospital. This fact inspired Dr. Frank Pantridge in Belfast, Northern Ireland, to create the first mobile coronary care unit, a forerunner of modern emergency medical teams (EMTs), known as paramedics.

Pantridge had barely survived five years of imprisonment after the Japanese captured Singapore in World War II. After the War, he became a cardiologist. In 1964, Pantridge was practicing at the Royal Victoria Hospital in Belfast, Northern Ireland, when a man collapsed from a heart attack outside his hospital. He pushed a heavy defibrillator on a cart to the scene. Using a long extension cord for power, Pantridge successfully defibrillated the man. Afterward he was told that many retired military men died outside the hospital due to ventricular fibrillation caused by heart attacks. Pantridge responded, "Well, if that's so, we had better go out there and pick 'em up, hadn't we?"

There were two problems: defibrillators weighed 155 lbs. and they required AC current. Undeterred, Pantridge and his colleagues wired together two 12-volt car batteries to power the heavy defibrillators. Soon emergency medical teams lugged massive "portable" defibrillators into homes and bedrooms to perform out-of-hospital defibrillation. Eventually smaller battery-powered defibrillators became available, and one was used to treat former President Lyndon Johnson when he suffered a heart attack in 1972 while visiting his daughter in Virginia.

Modern mobile coronary care began in 1980 when Dr. Leonard Cobb at the University of Washington in Seattle showed that many lives could be saved by training emergency medical technicians (EMTs) to perform defibrillation as well as CPR on victims of cardiac arrest outside the hospital. Cobb, a graduate of the University of Minnesota Medical School, was inspired by Pantridge's work. Cobb's "Seattle system" was widely adopted by emergency medical services throughout the United States.

Tom McClellan was the last patient treated for a heart attack in Cincinnati General Hospital, which was built in 1915. The new General Hospital was completed in the summer of 1969. We placed our patients on carts and into wheelchairs, and moved them from the old K-3 pavilion to the new hospital next door. It had 417 beds, five intensive care units, and a separate 6-bed coronary care unit (CCU). For the patients and for us the new hospital was like a different planet, a world that was a century ahead of the one we had just left.

The CCU was a relatively new concept in 1969. It had been pioneered by Dr. Hughes Day in Kansas City and Dr. Desmond Julian in Sydney, Australia. The idea was to place heart attack victims in a special unit that was staffed by highly trained nurses and equipped with the instruments that were necessary to resuscitate a patient quickly. The critical therapies were external defibrillation and CPR and it was clear that patients had to be treated within minutes of a cardiac arrest. Many CCUs cut hospital heart attack mortalities in half, a stunning achievement in an era when the most we could do for heart attack patients was put them to bed and hope for the best.

Dr. Eugene Braunwald, the pre-eminent cardiologist of the 20th Century, proclaimed that the CCU was the single most important advance in the treatment of acute heart attacks. This statement would hold true for the remainder of the century until, in the new millennium, major innovations in patient care from Denmark and Minnesota spread around the globe.

CHAPTER 6

Hattie Williams gave birth to her daughter in 1898 and she named her Blanche after a favorite aunt. Both Bill and Hattie Williams were children of plantation slaves who had become landowners in Mississippi after the Civil War. In 1892, however, the state legislature passed a new constitution that disenfranchised African-Americans. The Williams lost their farm and they became tenants on the land they had once owned in Leflore County.

Blanche was the youngest of five Williams children. Her parents raised them in conditions of abject poverty and in constant fear of the Ku Klux Klan. When she was 16, Blanche left home with her two older brothers. They were part of the Great Migration when nearly a half million African-Americans left Mississippi in the early 20th century to seek a better life in the north and west.

It took them more than a month, but eventually they arrived in the south side of Chicago. However, they found themselves in a cauldron stirred by unemployment, disease, and discrimination. In many ways Blanche and her brothers were worse off in Chicago than their family back in Mississippi. Her brothers decided to return home, but Blanche found work as a servant in a home on Astor Place in downtown Chicago. She would not retreat.

Blanche met James "Jimmy" Simpson at the Pilgrim Baptist Church when, by happenstance, they sat next to each other at a Sunday service. During the service, the Reverend told the congregation to stand and "take the hand of your neighbor" and Jimmy reached out to Blanche. "When I took her hand," Jimmy said later, "I decided to hold on, and she didn't resist!" Three months later, they were married and moved into an apartment near Michael Reese Hospital where Jimmy worked as an orderly. When the country entered World War I, Jimmy volunteered and served as a medic in the all-black 92nd Infantry—the Buffalo soldiers. Before he left for France, Blanche delivered their first child, a boy, James Jr.

Shrapnel from an artillery shell hit Jimmy on the last day of the war at Pont-a-Mousson while he applied a tourniquet to a wounded soldier's leg. Most of the shrapnel remained in Jimmy's body for the rest of his life. He was awarded a Silver Star for gallantry under fire and a Purple Heart for the multiple wounds he sustained.

Jimmy was discharged in the spring of 1919 and returned home to Blanche and his young namesake. Over the next seven years, Blanche and Jimmy had three more children. In 1922, Jimmy secured a good job at the new Hines Veterans Administration Hospital and they gladly moved the family out of South Chicago to a home near his new workplace in Maywood, Illinois. Blanche, who had continued to work full time during the war, became a full-time homemaker.

The first time Blanche Simpson blacked-out, she was sitting alone in her kitchen shelling string beans. "I woke up with my face in the bowl of beans," she said. "It was 1958. Jimmy was upstairs taking a nap. I didn't bother to tell him. I thought it was a fluke."

A month later, it happened again and this time she was with Jimmy. They were walking home from church when she abruptly dropped face down on the concrete sidewalk. Blanche was unconscious for a few minutes; her nose was broken and bleeding, and there were abrasions on her chin and forehead. Jimmy felt for her pulse; it was slow but strong. "You're okay, honey," he whispered. "I'll get you to the hospital."

Blanche objected: "I'm not going to the hospital. This is Sunday and the boys are coming over for dinner." Jimmy ignored her and carried Blanche to his car. He drove to West Suburban Hospital where he knew the doctors in the emergency room. The EKG showed that Blanche had partial heart block: every other beat from the top of her heart (atria) was being conducted to the ventricles. The doctor thought Blanche had blacked out when the partial heart block briefly advanced to complete heart block and she had no heart beat at all. They tended to Blanche's broken nose and abrasions and admitted her to the hospital for observation.

Blanche remained in the hospital for five days and had no further spells. Jimmy made an appointment to see a cardiologist in downtown Chicago. The specialist said her heart block was serious and that she could expect more attacks.

He prescribed isoproterenol tablets that she could place under her tongue when she felt symptoms coming on; if she was unconscious Jimmy could administer the tablets. The isoproterenol would stimulate her heart to beat; it was the only therapy available. Blanche could not leave her home alone and she certainly could not drive: "I might just as well be dead!" she exclaimed.

Two more attacks occurred over the next year and they became more frequent. Blanche's medication dosage changed to a long-acting tablet that she took every day. Jimmy never left her alone. He retired from the VA hospital. Their life devolved into a constant state of anxiety and fear that her heart would stop forever. "I seriously considered stopping the medicine," Blanche said later to a friend, "but it would have devastated my husband. He was so considerate and devoted, I could not have done it to him."

The isoproterenol kept Blanche's heart beating, but it also kept her bowels in constant turmoil. She could not leave the house. Jimmy insisted she wear a football helmet during the day because she had fallen so often. By 1959, Blanche had far outlived the normal life expectancy of a patient with her condition, but she felt like a prisoner confined to home. Only Jimmy's constant surveillance kept her alive.

On a Monday morning in December 1960, Jimmy received a call from a doctor at the VA Hospital. He knew of Blanche's situation and told Jimmy that a small Minnesota company named Medtronic had developed a portable electronic device that could keep her heart beating. The doctor described how the wire was attached to the heart through an incision in the chest and connected to a device called an external pacemaker. A patient could wear the Medtronic device on a belt. Dozens of patients of all ages were walking around with this "portable pacemaker," the doctor said, and one of his VA patients was even playing golf.

Two weeks later, Jimmy drove Blanche northwest to the University of Minnesota where children and young adults who had open-heart surgery were kept stable with Medtronic pacemakers. Blanche refused to wear the helmet to her appointment with the world-famous heart surgeon, Dr. C. Walton Lillehei. He said Blanche was a candidate for the procedure but there was a waiting list. The wait could be three or four months. Disappointed, but hopeful, Blanche and Jimmy returned to Chicago to wait.

Three months later, in March 1961, the minister of their church gave them a clipping from the *Saturday Evening Post* entitled "Making Hearts Behave." The article described the fully implantable pacemaker invented by an upstate New York engineer, Wilson Greatbatch, with cardiothoracic surgeon, Dr. William Chardack. The revolutionary device manufactured by Medtronic was expensive, $375, but Jimmy was determined that Blanche would have one.

Wilson Greatbatch was born in 1919 and grew up on the south side of Buffalo. His father had emigrated from England where he was a union organizer and unable to get a job. He met Wilson's American mother at a singing club in Buffalo. Wilson attended West Seneca High School, sailed with the Sea Scouts on the Niagara River, and built a radio transmitter with his high school friends. In 1938, he joined the Naval Reserve as a radioman and he went on active duty in 1940. During World War II, Greatbatch specialized in repairing radar equipment, and served as an enlisted gunner with a dive-bomber squadron on the carrier Monterey.

After the war, Greatbatch married Eleanor Wright, his childhood sweetheart. He worked for a year, and entered Cornell University to study electrical engineering under the GI Bill. Years later Greatbatch said, "Cornell made it possible for undergraduate students to participate in very high levels of research as a part of our education. We appreciated that."

Greatbatch was interested in radar, but he got a job in Cornell's psychology department making various electronic instruments for medical research. There he met two surgeons who told him about complete heart block. Just like Blanche Williams, the hearts of such patients often stop—do not pump blood—and they black out. These patients had a life expectancy of about one year. The condition was considered untreatable and terminal. Heart block was killing thousands of people every year.

"When I heard about this disease I knew we could fix it," Greatbatch said years later. But transistors did not exist in 1950 and it was impossible to build an implantable device with vacuum tubes. "There were external pacemakers at that time", Greatbatch said. "Paul Zoll in Boston was building big TV-sized boxes that were plugged into the wall with the end of the wires running over to the patient.

That patient's world was the length of an extension cord. A friend of mine in Minneapolis, Earl Bakken, was building pacemakers that could be worn on a belt. They had wires going right through the skin. That was only marginally satisfactory, although some people lived a long time."

One evening in 1958, Greatbatch arrived home and announced to Eleanor that he was quitting his several jobs. He was going to use $2,000 in savings to support the family for two years while he built a fully implantable heart pacemaker in the barn behind their home. Earlier he had accidentally built a pacemaker circuit when he placed the wrong transistor in a heart sound recorder for a local cardiologist. The "wrong" transistor caused the circuit to produce electrical pulses at 60 times a minute, the same frequency needed for a heart pacemaker.

When Greatbatch showed his pacemakers to Buffalo cardiologists, they expressed very little interest. "Fine idea," one doctor observed, "but these patients all die in a year or so…Work on something else."

Then in the spring of 1958, Greatbatch visited Dr. William Chardack, Chief of Surgery at the VA Medical Center. "He wanted me to help him with a blood oximeter problem," Greatbatch recalled. "I couldn't help him much. But I broached my pacemaker idea. He walked up and down the laboratory several times, looked at me strangely, and said 'If you can do that, you can save ten thousand lives a year.' Three weeks later we implanted our first model in a dog."

During the next two years, Greatbatch and Chardack solved multiple design and technical problems. The pacemaker needed a battery. They chose ten small mercury batteries just like the ones used in the famous "Walkie-Talkie" portable radios built during World War II. Next they found a way to hold the electronic circuit and batteries together in a single unit by placing the components in an oval metal mold and pouring in liquid epoxy. When the epoxy hardened, it was removed from the mold and coated with white Dow Corning silicone. Finally, they needed a wire lead to connect the pacemaker to the heart. After trying numerous metals and configurations they decided to use the Hunter-Roth pacemaker lead manufactured by Medtronic in Minnesota.

They tested the pacemaker and wires in the animal laboratory. Years later, recalling their first successful experiment, Greatbatch wrote, "I seriously doubt if anything I will ever do will give me the elation I felt that day when a two-cubic-inch electronic device of my own design controlled a living heart." This pacemaker was the first of many Greatbatch inventions that helped tens of thousands of patients. A deeply religious man, he said that his good work was the "Lord working through me."

The surgery to implant this first pacemaker was performed in two stages, about 6 weeks apart. During the first stage, Chardack opened the chest of a 77-year-old patient who had heart block. Chardack sutured the Hunter-Roth™ lead to the surface of his right ventricle. Next he closed the incision and brought the lead out through the skin where it was connected to a Medtronic external pacemaker that the patient wore on the belt of his trousers for a month.

On June 6, 1960, the patient returned to the operating room. The external end of lead, which was outside his chest, was soldered to the pacemaker's electronic circuitry. Immediately the pacemaker began stimulating the heart at 55 beats a minute. In order to sterilize the pacemaker and lead, Chardack and his associate, Dr. Andrew Gage, placed them in a plastic bag containing ethylene oxide. Some minutes later they removed everything from the bag and implanted the pacemaker under the skin in the patient's abdomen. It was a moment of pure exhilaration. The Chardack-Greatbatch pacemaker was doing exactly what it was designed to do: restore a normal heart rate.

Greatbatch and Chardack entered into a 10-year agreement with Earl Bakken. Medtronic would manufacture their pacemaker under a licensing agreement that would give Bill Greatbatch engineering design control over all Medtronic pacemakers during the 1960s.

Blanche Simpson had a Medtronic Chardack-Greatbatch™ pacemaker implanted in the summer of 1961 at the Mayo Clinic in Rochester, Minnesota. Surgeons opened her chest through a small incision under her left breast and sewed the Hunter-Roth lead onto her heart. They tunneled the lead under her skin to just below her waist where they created a pocket of tissue to hold the pacemaker.

Immediately, Blanche had a regular heart rate of 70 beats per minute. The additional blood flow created by a normal pulse was invigorating and liberating. Her fatigue vanished and she no longer blacked out. The dreaded Isuprel® tablets were no longer needed. She was free to be alone and to go wherever she wished. Jimmy no longer felt obligated to stand watch at all hours of the day and night. Best of all Blanche could throw out the football helmet. It was a miracle: her life had been resurrected.

I met Blanche and Jimmy Simpson a decade later in 1972 when she arrived by ambulance at the Presbyterian St. Luke's Hospital emergency room. She had blacked out at home and fallen down the stairs, sustaining multiple cuts and contusions but no broken bones.

When I examined her she was conscious, lying on a gurney. Despite her pain she smiled when I introduced myself.

"I'm Dr. Hauser, the cardiology fellow", I said. Blanche extended her hand and I took it in mine and held it for a moment.

"Doctor Hauser, this is my husband, Jimmy." Blanche had golden brown skin and freckles. Silver strands streaked her hair. She was lovely.

I smiled and shook Jimmy's hand. He was my height, dark, balding, with short gray hair and a mustache. He wore metal frame glasses on a long straight nose. Jimmy jiggled the fedora in his hands as he spoke. "Doctor, the pacemaker has been a blessing. Don't get me wrong. But it has been one thing after another. What's happening now?"

I nodded my head in agreement and said, "I understand. We will find out what went wrong. I'm sorry this has happened." Jimmy did not relax.

The EKG showed that Blanche's heart rate was 30-35 beats per minute and there were regular pacemaker spikes at 70 beats per minute which were not capturing—pacing—her heart.

"Mrs. Simpson, your pacemaker is not working," I said, looking back and forth between them. "We need to do some tests to see why, but first we are going to put in a temporary pacemaker. It's precautionary, in case your heart stops again"

"When will you do this?" Jimmy asked.

"Right now," I replied.

The nurse handed me a chest X-ray that had been taken when Blanche arrived. I held it up to the fluorescent light. I could see the pacing wire where it was attached to her heart. I traced it with my finger to the point where it was connected to the pacemaker. The wire was broken—fractured—near the pocket of tissue in her abdomen that enclosed the pacemaker.

"What do you see?" Jimmy asked.

"The wire is broken," I replied.

"Will I need more surgery?" Blanche asked. "I've already had five operations."

In fact, Blanche had six operations since her first pacemaker had been implanted at Minnesota's Mayo Clinic in 1961; depleted pacemaker batteries were the reason for the first five procedures and the sixth involved repair of a broken pacing wire. These six pacemaker failures were all heralded by symptoms—some severe—that were related to an extremely slow heart rate. But this was the first time that Blanche suffered cuts and bruises. Luckily, she had not been seriously injured.

"You will need another pacemaker operation, Mrs. Simpson," I said. "Dr. Clark will have to decide what kind of surgery."

I asked Jimmy to carry the X-ray while I pushed the gurney to the elevator. Jim Clark was already in the catheterization laboratory. I slipped on a lead apron and scrubbed and put on a sterile gown and gloves. After anesthetizing the tissue around the femoral vein in her groin I inserted a small plastic temporary pacing catheter and guided it into Blanche's right ventricle using fluoroscopy. Clark connected the lead to the external pacemaker and set it to 70 beats per minute.

Blanche needed a completely new pacemaker system. During the last 11 years, there were many pacemaker improvements and the most important was development of a lead that could be inserted into the heart through a vein below the collarbone. It was no longer necessary to open a patient's chest. Because the surgery only required local anesthesia, the risk of permanent pacemaker implantation had decreased substantially. These advances were primarily the result of inspired efforts by two surgeons, Dr. Seymour Furman in the Bronx, a borough of New York City, and Dr. Victor Parsonnet in Newark, New Jersey.

Dr. Clark explained the procedure to Blanche and Jimmy. "Your pacemaker wire has broken twice now," he said. "It's time to put in a new one." He explained how the new lead would be inserted and that the new pacemaker would be located below her right collarbone.

It was 1972 and this would be my first permanent pacemaker implant. Jim

Clark would supervise. I entered the operating room where Dr. Marshall Goldin had already draped Blanche with sterile sheets. Goldin made a two-inch incision below Blanche's right collarbone. Next, he isolated the cephalic vein, which ran in a groove of tissue that also contained an artery and nerve. He used a small curved iris scissors to cut an opening in the vein. Goldin took the slim silicone-insulated pacemaker lead from the scrub nurse and inserted it into the opening in the vein. He stepped aside and I took his place at the table.

I asked the technician to move the X-ray's C-arm over Blanche's heart. The video screen was directly across from me. I advanced the lead from the cephalic vein to the superior vena cava. Clark told me to remove the metal stylet and bend it an inch from the tip at a 30-degree angle. I replaced the stylet. The tip of the lead now looked like a hockey stick. I advanced it into the right atrium toward the tricuspid valve. With a beginner's luck, the lead crossed the tricuspid valve and dropped into the tip of the right ventricle.

"Good. Stop. Perfect," Clark said. "Let's test thresholds".

Only one milliampere of current was needed to stimulate Blanche's heart through the metal electrode at the tip of the pacing lead. I asked Blanche to cough and take a deep breath. The lead was stable. I connected it to a Cordis pacemaker powered by mercury-zinc batteries. Goldin placed it in the pocket of tissue he fashioned under her skin and closed the incision with sutures. The procedure took slightly more than 30 minutes. This was my first pacemaker implant, but it was one of the easiest of the hundreds I would do during my career.

In 1973, I led a National Institutes of Health-sponsored project testing two nuclear battery models for implantable pacemakers. Patients like Blanche Simpson had to undergo frequent surgeries because mercury-zinc batteries lasted only two to three years. The frequent surgery was inconvenient for patients, and each operation risked infection and other wound complications.

The quest for a longer-lived battery led to several types of nuclear batteries and a rechargeable battery. The rechargeable battery would eventually be available, but it was not a commercial success. Patients had to charge their pacemakers every week for an hour.

Four companies, including Medtronic and Cordis in Miami, Florida, produced nuclear pacemakers, but they were heavily regulated. Hospitals were required to track patients and submit endless forms to the Nuclear Regulatory Commission. Consequently, nuclear pacemakers were impractical, so few physicians used them.

I implanted one nuclear pacemaker, and it occurred after I joined the fulltime cardiology staff under Dr. Joseph Messer at Rush Presbyterian-St. Luke's Hospital in 1974. Messer grew up in Watertown, South Dakota, and attended Harvard where he received his medical degree in 1956. Prior to coming to Rush, Messer had been the Chief of Cardiology at Boston City Hospital. He was, and is, an astute clinician, gifted teacher, and leader with integrity.

Libby Palmer was a 16-year-old girl who had undergone surgery for a ventricular septal defect as a child. Like many such patients, the surgery produced complete heart block and Libby had a permanent pacemaker. In time, as Libby grew, the pacemaker wires attached to the surface of her heart fractured and her heart rate dropped to 20 beats a minute. Connecting new wires required another open-chest surgery. The skin and tissue around her pacemaker became infected and the wires had to be surgically removed while the infection was treated with antibiotics. After a long hospital stay, she was given a new pacemaker.

More pacemaker and lead complications occurred. The large pacemakers eroded through her skin. Leads broke. Batteries failed prematurely. She had 13 pacemaker operations during her young life.

One afternoon in 1976 I was standing in the hall of our clinic when Libby stepped off the elevator. Her pacing lead had fractured and she was being paced intermittently. Her heart would not beat for many seconds and she blacked out twice at home. Libby started to walk toward me when she collapsed, falling to the floor, unconscious. We rushed her to the catheterization laboratory and inserted a temporary pacemaker.

Her parents were frantic and I can still remember the anguish on her father's face. Pacemakers had been implanted under the skin of Libby's chest and abdomen. The scars embarrassed her, and they signified the inadequacies of pacemaker technology during that era. Now she was a teenager and a year behind in school because she had spent so much time in the hospital. Her closest friends were the nurses and technicians in our clinic. The situation called for a new approach: we needed to get creative and think "outside the box."

I thought back to our nuclear battery studies. I had implanted 30 nuclear pacemakers in German shepherds. We had to keep the dogs from chewing at the pacemakers under their skin. Mike Haklin, a superb surgical technician, and I conceived of placing the pacemaker in a polyethylene Dacron® pouch and suturing it inside the animal's chest. We used large Teflon® sutures to suspend the pacemaker from the dog's ribs in a tightly sealed pocket. It worked well: in two years, none of the dogs developed wound complications.

Would this approach work for Libby? The nuclear battery could produce sufficient energy to power Libby's pacemaker for the rest of her life. Radiation was not an issue; multiple studies proved that the lifelong radiation dose from a nuclear battery was safe. The real concern was the durability of the pacemaker leads and the electronics: how long would they last?

I spoke with Libby and her father and told them what I had in mind. Libby was desperate for a chance at a normal life. Her father had many good questions. I conferred with Marshall Goldin and asked him to meet with Libby and her family. By the end of the afternoon, everyone agreed to go ahead with this novel operation.

It took several days to secure the nuclear pacemaker from the Cordis Corporation. I filled out multiple forms for the Nuclear Regulatory Commission and met with the hospital's radiation officer who was required to be in the operating room with a radiation tester. On a Friday morning, Libby entered the operating room. The radiation officer did his tests and detected no radiation from the pacemaker. Silly as they seemed, the regulations could not be ignored.

Goldin made a short incision between Libby's two ribs and dissected the pleura (lining of the chest cavity) away from the inside of her chest wall. He placed the Cordis™ nuclear pacemaker with the Dacron® pouch inside Libby's chest beneath her ribs and secured it with wire sutures. The old lead was connected to the pacemaker. Before closing the incision, we watched the monitor for many minutes to be certain that the pacemaker was working correctly.

Our clinic followed Libby's progress for a year or two until she left Chicago. A decade later, one of our clinic staff saw Libby in a grocery store in Illinois. She was married, had a child, and was doing well.

Libby had the nuclear pacemaker for 28 years, with no other surgeries needed, until 2004 when her cardiologist in Florida decided she needed a more sophisticated model. Libby's story is unique because an uncommon device and a novel surgical technique came together this one time to help a truly desperate patient. Other patients in the United States and Europe have also had their nuclear pacemakers for many decades. However, in the 1970s we sorely needed a long-lived, non-nuclear pacemaker battery that could last 10 years.

In the early 1970s, I met Wilson Greatbatch at a medical meeting in downtown Chicago. He introduced himself as "Bill" and that is how I always addressed him. Bill could have been a professor or Oxford Don. His dark hair was combed straight back and he had a mustache below a broad nose and framed glasses. He was a born teacher and one of the most unassuming men I have ever known.

At that meeting, Greatbatch spoke to our group—mostly cardiologists—on the reliability of pacemakers and their component electronic parts. Then he described a new battery he had developed; it was made of lithium iodide and he predicted it would last 10-20 years. Lithium batteries had a tendency to explode, but Greatbatch had solved that problem with a proprietary manufacturing process. Of course we were skeptical, but Bill Greatbatch was the inventor of the implantable pacemaker and spoke knowledgably and convincingly about the lithium iodide battery's potential to be a reliable energy source.

A few weeks later, a meticulously dressed man in a business suit dropped by my office. He introduced himself as Manny Villafana. He was tall, balding, with a soothing smile, and soft voice. "Dr. Hauser, I'm the president of Cardiac Pacemakers," Villafana said. "We have a pacemaker that we think will last 10 years." He removed a shiny rectangular metal pacemaker from his suit pocket and handed it to me. "The lithium battery and electronics are hermetically sealed inside to keep moisture out. We just implanted the first one in Milwaukee a few months ago. We call it the Maxilith™." The Maxilith™ was powered by Greatbatch's battery.

I learned years later that Medtronic had rejected Greatbatch's lithium battery in 1971. Instead, Earl Bakken, Medtronic's founder and president, decided to stay with a "new and improved" mercury-zinc battery. By rejecting Greatbatch's lithium battery, Medtronic had inadvertently opened the door to the pacemaker market that it had created and dominated for more than a decade. Villafana eagerly stepped in and, with several former Medtronic employees, he launched Cardiac Pacemakers Inc. (CPI) in St. Paul, Minnesota in 1972.

CPI built the first lithium battery pacemakers, and quickly gained market share. Meanwhile, Medtronic suffered a major product problem when its mercury-zinc Xytron™ pacemakers failed by the thousands due to moisture entering the improperly sealed metal can that housed the integrated-circuit electronics. The moisture caused the electronics to short circuit, resulting in abrupt pacemaker failure. Without pacing, a few patients died while others suffered blackouts or heart failure. We replaced dozens of the Xytron™ pacemakers with models from other manufacturers, including CPI.

In a short time, Medtronic's share of the pacemaker market plummeted from 80 percent to below 40 percent. Other pacemaker companies also had a variety of product problems, which provided impetus for passage of the Medical Devices Amendments of 1976 that gave the FDA broad powers to regulate the medical device industry. FDA regulation was welcomed by many physicians, including myself, but in the years ahead we would become disillusioned with the FDA's inability to protect our patients from defective products.

The Cordis pacemaker that we implanted in Blanche Simpson in 1972 was powered by mercury-zinc batteries. These batteries lasted just 26 months and Blanche was back for another replacement surgery in 1975. This time she received a CPI Maxilith™ pacemaker. It would be the last surgery she would ever need. The lithium battery pacemaker functioned perfectly for 12 years, until her death in 1986 at 88. Blanche's devoted Jimmy died a year earlier of prostate cancer. Most patients like Blanche would have been dead within two years of her first blackout spell in 1958. Pacemakers—and Jimmy—had given Blanche 28 years that she would not have enjoyed without them.

Greatbatch's company became the major battery supplier for the pacemaker industry and it grew into a billion-dollar medical device manufacturer. His company manufactured many components for a variety of implantable medical devices. Bill Greatbatch, who died at 92, was elected to the National Inventors Hall of Fame, a fitting tribute to a man who held more than 300 patents.

In 1979 Eli Lilly and Company, the Indiana-based pharmaceutical manufacturer, acquired Cardiac Pacemakers Inc. A few years earlier, Villafana had departed CPI and started a new company, St. Jude Medical, to develop a new mechanical heart valve. With his departure, CPI had become technologically backward and insensitive to the market forces driving the pacemaker industry. Shortly after Eli Lilly's acquisition, CPI began losing market share to pacemaker companies that offered more sophisticated products. By 1985, CPI was losing a million dollars a month, and Eli Lilly was scrambling to staunch the flow of red ink. To become profitable, CPI would have to re-engineer itself and invest in a new device for preventing sudden cardiac death, the implantable defibrillator.

CHAPTER 7

Janet Parker was an active 55-year-old Vietnam War widow and grandmother who loved running. Weather permitting, she jogged every day and occasionally did half marathons. Regrettably, she could not afford a treadmill and there were no health clubs within easy driving distance of her home. After a seemingly endless winter in rural western Illinois, Janet looked forward to resuming her daily jogs in the county park nearby.

On the first warm day in the spring of 1978, Janet put on the red running shirt and pants that her daughter had given her for Christmas and started jogging toward the park. She became breathless after two blocks. She stopped. "Good heavens, I'm really out of shape," she whispered to herself. Janet walked for five minutes, recovered, and started jogging once more. After 100 yards, she dropped to her knees, gasping. Her heart was racing. She felt faint, and nearly blacked out. After a few minutes her breathing eased and the pounding in her chest stopped.

Janet returned home and called her daughter. Soon she was in the emergency room of the local hospital, but the doctor found nothing to explain her shortness of breath or rapid heart beating. Her EKG and blood tests were normal, as was her chest X-ray. The doctor told Janet she was deconditioned, instructed her to rest the remainder of the day, and to walk rather than jog the next morning.

Janet's daughter was not satisfied. She called her internist in Wheaton. He saw her the following afternoon. When the doctor placed his stethoscope lightly on Janet's chest just below her breast, he heard an extra heart sound. It was a low frequency vibration called a gallop, and it was indicative of heart disease. He explained his finding and suggested that Janet consult a cardiologist.

Several days later, I examined Janet in my office at Rush Presbyterian-St. Luke's Medical Center in Chicago. Janet looked several years younger than her age. Her brown hair was in a ponytail and she wore no make-up. She was five feet seven inches in height and weighed 123 pounds.

I probed for symptoms. "Mrs. Parker," I asked, "do you have stairs in your house?"

"Yes, from my basement to the first floor. I live in a ranch style house."

"Do you carry your laundry up those stairs?"

"Yes."

"Compared to a year ago, have you noticed anything different?"

"I'm a little short of breath."

"Do you have to stop on the stairs?"

"Sometimes, but I hardly get any exercise in the winter. I think I'm out of shape."

Janet's daughter interrupted, "Mom you've been getting short of breath just talking to me on the telephone. Tell the doctor about the fluttering in your chest."

Gradually Janet's symptoms formed the classic collage of congestive heart failure: unexpected fatigue, shortness of breath, occasional bursts of rapid heart beating, and weight gain without any changes in diet.

But what was the cause? All of the usual tests were normal. I needed more information about the structure and function of Janet's heart. Of particular interest was the condition of her left ventricle, the main pumping chamber, and the essential engine controlling blood flow. In the past, we would have obtained the information invasively, with a heart catheterization, but thanks to Dr. Harvey Feigenbaum we had a new diagnostic technique called *echocardiography.*

Harvey Feigenbaum was born of immigrant parents from Poland and England. He had planned to learn the violin and become a musician but changed his mind after winning a scholarship to study science. In 1955, he earned a bachelor's degree from the University of Indiana in Bloomington, and graduated from its medical school in 1958.

By 1963, Feigenbaum was a young staff cardiologist at the University of Indiana. One afternoon, he munched on a sandwich near the catheterization laboratory and browsed through his "junk" mail. One piece had an advertisement for an ultrasound instrument that claimed to measure the volume of blood in the left ventricle. This got his attention. He had become frustrated with the catheterization techniques he used to conduct his research because they were invasive, tedious and fraught with inaccuracies. Feigenbaum called the manufacturer, Biosonar, and learned that he could see and evaluate the instrument at the upcoming American Heart Association meeting in Los Angeles.

Sonar, a form of ultrasound, helped the Allied navies detect and intercept enemy submarines during World War II. When warships pulsed sound waves through the surrounding ocean and the sound waves encountered a solid object like a German submarine, they were reflected back to the sonar's oscilloscope. This ultrasound technology helped the Allies destroy the U-boats that were sinking ships loaded with food, supplies, and troops headed for Great Britain, Europe, and North Africa.

Feigenbaum was curious about the new ultrasound device he saw in the advertisement. He visited Biosonar's booth in the large exhibit hall in Los Angeles. The instrument was on display, and almost immediately he realized the company's claims were false: the device could not possibly measure the volume of blood in the left ventricle.

But instead of walking away in disgust, Feigenbaum asked the salesman if he could try the machine on himself. Placing the handheld ultrasound transducer against his chest, Feigenbaum sent invisible sound waves through his heart and watched the reflected signals appear on the small oscilloscope screen located on the front panel of the instrument. He was fascinated. The signal moved in concert with his pulse, and it appeared that it was reflecting off the back wall of his heart.

After returning to Indiana, Feigenbaum found an idle ultrasound machine in the hospital's neurology department where it was used to diagnose brain tumors. The machine was gathering dust because the brain images were poor. Feigenbaum "borrowed" the machine, placed the transducer on his chest and observed the same ultrasound echos that he saw with the Biosonar instrument.

At that moment, this junior cardiologist knew he should explore the possibility of using ultrasound to study the heart. It was like looking through a keyhole into a large room: no telling what was out of view on the other side. He resolved to find out.

However, Feigenbaum received little encouragement or financial support from the chief of his department. "He is young," the department chief told Feigenbaum's wife. "He will get over this thing." His close colleagues said he was jeopardizing a promising career. Feigenbaum dismissed skeptics and listened to the voice within himself.

His first breakthrough was the diagnosis of pericardial effusion, a condition in which fluid accumulates in the thin sac surrounding the heart. The fluid may be blood, infection, cancer, or simply serum. It may be innocuous or life threatening. In 1963, there was no reliable noninvasive test for pericardial effusion. Only the shape of the heart's shadow on a chest X-ray offered a cursory clue. The only definitive test for a pericardial effusion required inserting a long needle into the space around the heart and withdrawing the fluid. This "diagnostic tap" was risky—it could lacerate a coronary artery or lung—and the needle could miss the fluid altogether.

Feigenbaum found a patient in his hospital who had had a well-documented pericardial effusion for some time. He placed the ultrasound transducer on the patient's chest. Instead of one moving echo—the heart in motion—he saw a space behind the heart that did not reflect the ultrasound. This "echo free space" had to be fluid. Like sonar waves traveling through the ocean, the ultrasound beam did not reflect off fluid.

Moments like these occur rarely—if ever—in one's lifetime. Most important is the observer's recognition that what he or she is seeing is new and profound. Something clicked in Harvey Feigenbaum's brain that day. As with Mason Sones and coronary angiography, Feigenbaum knew that what he saw could be revolutionary. Here was a non-invasive method that could potentially visualize the heart in real-time and diagnose disease without exposing patients to needles, catheters, or radiation. It was risk-free and it could be repeated as often as necessary.

Feigenbaum confirmed his observations in the animal research laboratory. In a landmark 1965 publication, he reported that ultrasound was capable of diagnosing pericardial effusions. He named it "echocardiography."

To address the skepticism in the cardiology community, Feigenbaum made a key strategic decision: he decided to teach other cardiologists how to use and interpret echocardiograms. He started with the young cardiology fellows at the University of Indiana and then opened his program to any cardiologist who wanted to visit and learn. In 1968, he launched regular courses in echocardiography that hundreds of physicians attended from around the world. Feigenbaum published the first echocardiography textbook in 1972.

A growing cadre of echocardiographers and a tidal wave of new knowledge eventually silenced Feigenbaum's skeptics. By 1978, echocardiography was an accepted and widely used diagnostic tool. Moreover, the technology had advanced in giant leaps as manufacturers raced to introduce new echocardiogram machines with the latest features.

By 1979 It was possible to visualize a patient's beating heart in two dimensions and measure the velocity of blood flowing through the valves. No longer did we need to perform a heart catheterization to diagnose aortic or mitral valve disease, or measure the ejection fraction. It was all there to be seen on the echocardiogram in real time, and without invading the body. For the first time we were able to perform serial studies to follow the progress of hearts that were recovering from insults like heart attacks and infection.

An hour after I saw Janet in the clinic, she was laying on an exam table in the cardiology laboratory. A technician had Janet roll onto her left side and placed the ultrasound probe below her left breast. Janet and the technician chatted while the ultrasound probe gathered images and displayed them on a black and white video screen. After 45 minutes we had multiple views of Janet's heart recorded on videotape.

Janet's echocardiogram revealed an enlarged left ventricle with a low ejection fraction. The ejection fraction is the proportion of blood that the left ventricle pumps with each heartbeat. Her ejection fraction was 30 percent or about half the normal 55-65 percent. She had a condition called dilated cardiomyopathy, a disease of the muscle that crippled her heart's ability to pump enough blood.

The cause of Janet's cardiomyopathy was uncertain. A coronary angiogram revealed no evidence of coronary artery disease, but a biopsy of her heart muscle showed widespread scarring that could have been the result of a viral infection.

We could offer her no curative therapy. Hopefully the scarring would be self-limited and Janet's pumping function would improve with time. I treated her heart failure with the drugs that were available at the time—digoxin, furosemide, and spironolactone.

Every three months Janet's daughter drove her the 110 miles from her home to my clinic. By the third visit, she had made no progress. On the contrary, Janet's shortness of breath was worse at any level of sustained activity; she had given up doing laundry and rarely left home. At night she propped herself up on three pillows in order to breathe and slept fitfully. Her legs were swollen to the thighs with soft, mushy fluid and her weight at home was up 13 pounds since the previous spring. Her appetite had declined even more and she felt full after a few bites of food.

I repeated her echocardiogram. It showed that the four chambers of Janet's heart were enlarged and that her left ventricle's ejection fraction had fallen to 20 percent. Her heart disease was progressing rapidly. I admitted her to the hospital.

After three days of intravenous diuretics, Janet lost 12 pounds. Her shortness of breath improved and she could sleep comfortably on one pillow. The edema in her legs was nearly gone. Her daughter asked that I meet with them in Janet's room and discuss the options for her mother's future care.

I was frank. Janet's condition was deteriorating and the drugs had not slowed the inexorable decline in heart function. This downward trajectory was accompanied by worsening congestion, and now her other organs—especially the kidneys and liver—were exhibiting signs of low blood flow and fluid retention.

Janet needed a new heart, a transplant, and I recommended that we contact Dr. Norman Shumway at Stanford University in Palo Alto, California. In 1979, Shumway's heart transplant program was the only one in the country that was accepting new patients.

Dr. Norman E. Shumway was born in 1923 and grew up as an only child in Kalamazoo, Michigan. He entered the University of Michigan as a pre-law student but after a year was drafted into the Army during World War II. The Army sent him to engineering school in Texas.

One morning, Shumway and his training class marched into an auditorium where an officer announced, "All of you will take a medical aptitude test." This was the final test question: "If you pass this test would you prefer a career in medicine or dentistry?" Shumway figured that medical doctors would be needed more than dentists, so he checked "medicine". Years later, he wrote, "Sure enough, a little later the dental part of the program folded, and those poor guys who checked the wrong box were back in the infantry, while the rest of us continued in premed."

The Army enrolled Shumway in a nine-month pre-medical program at Baylor University in Waco, Texas. He went on to obtain his medical degree from Vanderbilt University in 1949. After two years in the Air Force, Shumway completed his surgical training with Dr. Owen Wangensteen at the University of Minnesota. He worked with Dr. F. John Lewis on hypothermia, earning a PhD in 1956. After practicing briefly in Santa Barbara, California, Shumway was recruited to start the new cardiac surgery program at Stanford Hospital in Palo Alto.

Early on, he met Dr. Richard Lower, a surgical resident assigned to Shumway's research laboratory. They began experiments to find better techniques for operating on the heart. While investigating hypothermia in animals, they removed the heart of one dog, cooled it, and implanted it into a second dog. Quite by accident, Shumway and Lower discovered that transplanted hearts functioned very well. They shifted the focus of their research from hypothermia to cardiac transplantation.

Lower became chief of cardiac surgery at the Medical College of Virginia where he continued heart transplantation in animals. One day in 1967 he greeted Dr. Christian Barnard, a young visiting surgeon from South Africa. Barnard was another Owen Wangensteen trainee who, for six months, served as chief resident at the University of Minnesota under Walt Lillehei. When Barnard left Minnesota for South Africa, Wangensteen was so impressed with the young doctor that he gave him a heart-lung machine to take back to Cape Town.

During his visit with Lower, Barnard watched a heart transplant on a dog. Four months later, on December 3, 1967, Barnard performed the world's first human-to-human heart transplant at Groote Schuur Hospital in Cape Town. The donor was an automobile accident victim declared brain dead. The recipient was Louis Washkansky, a 55-year-old grocer who was dying due to terminal heart failure.

Mr. Washkansky lived for 18 days and died of pneumonia. He had received high doses of steroids to dampen his immune system and prevent his body from rejecting the transplanted heart. The steroids also impaired his ability to battle pneumonia and other infections. This side effect of anti-rejection drugs would become a serious issue for many transplant patients.

Halfway across the world in Palo Alto, Shumway prepared to do his first transplant at Stanford. The problem was determining when potential donors were legally dead and their organs could be harvested. In the 1960s physicians in the United States could not declare a brain-injured patient dead until the heart stopped and breathing ceased. This could take hours or days during which the body's organs, including the heart, deteriorated and were not suitable for transplantation.

Thus there was a paradox: the need for both a living body and a dead donor. Eventually an ethical and legal definition of brain death was evolved and codified into law in every state; this milestone vastly increased the availability of healthy organs for transplantation. Today, brain death is defined as the irreversible loss of all functions of the brain. The three essential findings in brain death are coma, absence of certain reflexes, and failure to breath spontaneously.

However, a legal definition of brain death did not exist in 1968. Although Shumway was ready to perform a human heart transplant, he was stymied by the lack of a qualifying donor. Finally, in January of that year, a young woman in a nearby hospital was declared dead after suffering a ruptured brain aneurysm. She was kept alive until Shumway could remove her heart and transplant it into a 54-year-old steel worker, Mike Kasperak; he lived for 14 days and died of multiple post-operative complications.

The media coverage evoked by heart transplantation was astonishing. Soon many centers around the world were performing heart transplants. Every center with a heart surgery program seemed to feel that it had to do heart transplants in order to maintain its status in the community or on the national stage. Hospitals held live televised press conferences to announce their first transplant. Photographs of surgeons and their transplant patients appeared in local newspapers. Reporters scrambled to interview anyone remotely involved with the procedure. It was not one of medicine's finest hours.

Transplant surgeons were accorded celebrity status, and the charismatic Christian Barnard became the poster boy. A media frenzy surrounded Barnard, a debonair South African surgeon and the son of a poor Dutch Reformed Church minister. "It was, in many ways, a blessing that the focus was on Barnard," Shumway said, "because it allowed us to continue our work without so much folderol. That was truly an important thing for us, because there were still many more things that had to be done."

The challenge was not the surgery itself: the operation was relatively straightforward for an experienced heart surgeon. The problem was managing the patient after the transplant. The main issue was rejection, when the recipient's immune system attacked the new heart as it would any foreign protein.

The available antirejection drugs were azathioprine and corticosteroids. These were powerful drugs that not only fought rejection but also weakened the patient's ability to fight off infection. When patients took a turn for the worse, their doctors often did not know if the problem was rejection or infection. If the culprit was infection, giving azathioprine or steroids could be harmful. On the other hand, giving these same drugs was crucial if the patient's immune system was attacking the transplanted heart. Knowing what was wrong was absolutely critical to choosing the right therapy.

Even in Shumway's hands, heart transplant patients had only a 20 percent chance of living five years. Indeed, by 1971 the survival rates were so low that nearly every center in the United States had abandoned heart transplantation. The exceptions were Shumway at Stanford and Lower in Virginia.

Like so many great pioneers in medicine, Shumway persisted when others retreated. He decided to figure out rejection and overcome it. He attacked rejection on multiple fronts. Although monitoring the EKG was useful for identifying rejection, the technique was not specific and it was not very sensitive. Rejection of the transplanted heart could be far advanced before the EKG recorded any changes, and often it was too late for anti-rejection drugs. The immediate task was finding a better way for identifying rejection early enough so that prompt treatment could be initiated. Like fire prevention, it is always better to detect smoke before the flames take hold and begin to spread.

Dr. Matt Paneth, a London surgeon and old friend from the University of Minnesota, wrote Shumway that he had a bright young man who wanted to spend some time at Stanford. Shumway agreed and Dr. Philip Caves arrived on a British-American Heart Association fellowship. "Caves came out and was absolutely brilliant," Shumway recalled, "a hardworking, dedicated, highly motivated guy, and just a wonderful doctor."

Caves searched the medical literature and found a 1962 Japanese method for removing biopsy tissue from inside the heart. Together with an elderly German instrument maker, Caves fashioned a tool for accessing the interior of the right ventricle from the jugular vein in the neck. The tool was a long stainless steel forceps with a razor sharp scoop on the end.

Now they could remove tiny bits of heart muscle from transplant recipients and determine if there was evidence of rejection by examining the tissue under a microscope. This approach—heart muscle biopsy—led to more effective anti-rejection treatments and a doubling of the five-year heart transplant survival rate, raising it from 20 to 40 percent. The heart muscle biopsy methods developed at Stanford remained the gold standard for managing heart transplant patients.

Shumway's team also established methods for preserving hearts after they were removed from the donor and transported to Stanford. On one occasion, an Air Force F-4 Phantom fighter jet transported a heart from Fargo, North Dakota to Palo Alto when the medical team's Lear jet encountered equipment problems. The heart, preserved for eight hours in a special container of cold (4°C) saline, functioned perfectly in the desperately ill infant who received it.

Word reached Shumway in 1980 that a new drug, cyclosporine, successfully prevented rejection after kidney transplantation. Cyclosporine comes from a fungus found in Norway and Sandoz investigated it as a chemotherapy agent. Shumway sent one of his staff, Dr. Phil Oyer, to a medical meeting in Davos, Switzerland, to meet one of the investigators, Dr. Jean Borel. Oyer spoke with Borel while the two went skiing, and Borel arranged for Stanford to get cyclosporine from Sandoz. With the FDA's permission, Shumway began using the drug. Almost immediately, the one-year post-heart transplant survival rose to 80 to 90 percent, and the five-year survival rate increased to 70 percent. The dark days of cardiac transplantation were over.

Janet Parker flew to San Francisco with her daughter in February, 1979 and checked into the Holiday Inn in Palo Alto. She was evaluated in Shumway's clinic and placed on the transplant list. Several weeks later, she was admitted briefly to the hospital for worsening heart failure. For six weeks, she carried a pager in case a

116

donor heart became available.

But the call never came. On a Saturday in early April, almost a year to the day from the time I first met Janet, she collapsed while walking with her daughter near their rented apartment in Mountain View, California. Paramedics came, but her heart failed her. Like so many patients awaiting a heart transplant, Janet died suddenly, most likely due to ventricular fibrillation.

Shumway's meticulous attention to detail and his devotion to research made possible the emergence of heart transplantation as a safe and effective therapy for patients who otherwise had no future. Thousands of them have lived happy and productive lives because Shumway gave so much to mankind. He received multiple honors and awards during his lifetime. In the Wangensteen tradition, he trained a generation of cardiac surgeons, and many achieved international recognition and fame. A list of distinguished Shumway trainees, published when he died in 2007, included 18 University professors and heads of academic departments.

Many patients awaiting transplantation died suddenly due to ventricular fibrillation. Janet Parker was one of them. In 1985 a new device for preventing sudden cardiac death—the implantable defibrillator—would become available and prove to be a valuable bridge to heart transplantation.

CHAPTER 8

"She died in her sleep."

"He died on the golf course."

"She died waiting for a heart transplant."

"He died milking the cows."

"The youngster died playing hockey."

These people did not die because they suffered heart attacks. They died because the electrical systems in their hearts went haywire and abruptly caused ventricular fibrillation or rapid ventricular tachycardia. These lethal rhythms occur in hearts that are scarred, in hearts that are enlarged and weak, and in hearts that harbor genetic abnormalities that make them vulnerable to life-threatening rhythms.

This is *sudden cardiac death*: it is not a disease but a catastrophe that kills thousands of people who have known or unrecognized heart conditions. It strikes every day -- unpredictably, without warning. One minute the victim is alive and feeling well and the next he or she is dead. These are devastating events: people struck down in the prime of life, and families left without a mother or father. Sudden cardiac death even kills adolescents and young adults who inherit rhythm disorders from their parents and ancestors.

When I became a cardiologist in 1973, sudden cardiac death and out-of-hospital cardiac arrest were well recognized, but there was no effective therapy or means to identify patients at risk. Direct current defibrillation was available only to hospitalized patients or the few lucky individuals resuscitated by mobile emergency medical teams. It was clear, however, that prompt defibrillation within four to five minutes was necessary if victims were to survive with their brains and bodies reasonably intact.

Sudden cardiac death was a huge problem with no apparent solution until one extraordinary man accepted the challenge and made it his life's work.

Dr. Michel Mirowski was born Mieczyslaw Mirowski in 1924 in Warsaw, Poland. His parents owned a delicatessen and kosher factory. "My parents worked long hours," Mirowski later recalled. "I don't think my father ever took a vacation." Michel attended a Jewish private school because Jews in Poland, even before the Nazis, had limited access to public schools. At 11, he was learning French, Latin and Hebrew in preparation for the University. Mirowski preferred reading Paul de Kruif's *Microbe Hunters* and Jack London's *Martin Eden* rather than Yiddish stories about the small Jewish villages of Central and Eastern Europe. He was inspired by London's fictional character, Martin Eden, an outsider who overcame many obstacles before succeeding as a writer. However, unlike the imaginary Eden who committed suicide, Mirowski would utilize self-discipline and his native abilities to surmount personal and professional obstacles that would thwart most men.

Mirowski's odyssey began at the age of fifteen, three months after the Nazis invaded Poland in September 1939. Following his mother's death from heart failure, he resolved to leave Poland, refusing to wear the yellow Star of David. Mirowski was convinced that he had something to contribute in life. Together with a friend, he walked and rode 200 miles southeast to Lvov, which had been turned over to the Soviet Union under terms of the German-Soviet pact. By early 1940, thousands of Polish Jews had fled to Lvov. Mirowski left behind his father and 400,000 Warsaw Jews who would not survive the Holocaust.

When Germany invaded the Soviet Union in 1941, Mirowski fled east again, stopping in city after city, always keeping ahead of the Nazi invaders and the death squads. He was often hungry but always managed to find something to eat. Finally, he arrived in Andizhan with many other Jewish refugees. The ancient city was in Uzbekistan, 3,100 miles from Warsaw. He worked at several jobs and eventually became a non-combat junior officer in the Russian army. At the end of the war in 1945, he returned to Poland to find his family, discovering that they had vanished and their Warsaw ghetto had been destroyed.

Mirowski enrolled as a medical student at the University of Gdansk, but after a year he decided to leave Poland forever: "Many Poles still felt that Hitler hadn't finished the job [with the Jews]. Now I became a Zionist. After all that had happened and all that I had seen, the Jews had to have a country of their own to survive. Poland had become a cemetery for me."

After a brief stay in Tel Aviv where he worked as a shoe salesman, Mirowski decided to honor his father's last words: "Be a physician, Mieczyslaw; be a Jew." At the time, there were no medical schools in Israel, so in 1947 he returned to France where he entered medical school in Lyon. His class numbered 500 students and there was seven years of course work before graduation. Early on, Mirowski decided to specialize in the emerging field of cardiology. He graduated in 1954 and returned to Israel where he became a physician in training under Harry Heller, a brilliant internist at Tel Hashomer Hospital.

In 1950, Mirowski married Anna Rutkowski, whom he met through friends in Lyon. The first of their three daughters was born in 1959. After fellowships at the Cardiological Institute in Mexico City and Johns Hopkins Hospital in Baltimore, Mirowski and his growing family returned to Israel in 1963 for what he believed would be his last relocation. Mirowski had escaped the Holocaust in Poland, survived hunger in Russia during World War II, and found a way to secure his medical degree. His moral and intellectual fibers were woven into a steely fabric of grit, curiosity, and relentless drive. Mirowski would seek his life's work in the Jewish homeland.

Mirowski became a staff cardiologist in a community hospital outside Tel Aviv. He cared for patients and wrote scientific manuscripts that were published in the United States, Europe, and Israel.

In 1966, his mentor, Dr. Heller, died suddenly at home. Heller had been treated with quinidine and procainamide for ventricular tachycardia. The toxic effects of these two drugs were unknown at the time.

Heller's death forever transformed Mirowski's life. He felt a deep, personal loss and he dedicated himself to finding a way to prevent sudden cardiac death. Almost immediately, he concluded that the only practical solution was to build an implantable defibrillator, much like a pacemaker, that would automatically detect ventricular fibrillation and shock the heart back into normal rhythm.

Mirowski asked, "How could we have prevented Heller's death at that time: keep him in the coronary care unit, or follow him around with a defibrillator? Both solutions were obviously impossible. Implantable pacemakers were then becoming available. So I reasoned, let us create a similar kind of implantable device to monitor for ventricular fibrillation and automatically shock the patient back to sinus rhythm. It should be simple enough."

At that time, even "portable" defibrillators weighed 30 to 40 pounds. A defibrillator could not be as small as a pacemaker, the experts declared. "But I had been challenged by the problem, initially because of the death of a man I admired very much, but also because people told me it couldn't be done," Years later Mirowski said, "Thank goodness I wasn't an engineer because I would certainly have realized that the idea was crazy."

Mirowski had the concept, but the technology and funding were not available in Israel. He was 44 years old with a flourishing private practice, young family, and comfortable home in Savyon, the Beverly Hills of Israel. Was he prepared to risk all this for the chance to develop an implantable defibrillator? It was, after all, the medical equivalent of a Saturn moon shot. No one before him—not Lillehei or Starr or Greatbatch—had ever thought this far out of the box *and* succeeded.

The first essential step was to move to the United States. In 1968, Mirowski attended the American College of Cardiology meeting in San Francisco where he met Dr. Bernard Tabatznik, the chief of cardiology at Mount Sinai Hospital in Baltimore. Mirowski told Tabatznik about his implantable defibrillator idea.

Tabatznik and his boss, Dr. Albert Mendelhoff, the director of medicine at Mount Sinai, must have seen something very special in Mirowski and his concept for preventing sudden cardiac death. They offered Mirowski the position of Director of the Coronary Care Unit and promised him time and support to develop the defibrillator. Some years later Mirowski remarked, "In retrospect, moving back to America was one of the most reckless acts of my life...We sold what we owned and, after taxes, cleared $6,000 to start our new life."

The 44-year-old Michel Mirowski and his family arrived in Baltimore on September 3, 1968. He and a young Mount Sinai staff cardiologist, Dr. Morton Mower, began a life-long collaboration as they formulated various designs for the automatic implantable defibrillator, or simply "AID™." Mirowski believed that the AID™ would deliver its shock via a catheter—a lead—inserted through a vein into the heart much like a pacemaker. Mower thought otherwise: a steel plate on or near the heart would be required. They compromised and one of the first experiments used a steel plate under the skin of a dog and a catheter in the superior vena cava, a large vein in the chest just above the heart.

Mirowski and Mower prepared manuscripts that described the promising results of their defibrillator studies in dogs. They encountered skeptical editors and reviewers, and endured multiple rejections, but ultimately their articles appeared in print. Mirowski also protected his inventions with key patents filed with the U.S. Patent Office. His intellectual property portfolio grew rapidly.

In the early 1970s, Mirowski encountered many obstacles. "Everybody thought the project was unfeasible", Mirowski recalled. That was the technical side, but he was unprepared for the denouncement by Dr. Bernard Lown, a world famous cardiologist, who in 1972 wrote a critical editorial published in *Circulation*, the journal of the American Heart Association. Lown was, according to many including Mirowski, the "guru of sudden cardiac death." He was also an early proponent of the coronary care unit, co-developer of direct current defibrillation, and a distinguished Harvard professor.

"There is serious question whether an indication can be spelled out for the use of an implantable standby defibrillator," Lown wrote. "...In fact, the implantable defibrillator system represents an imperfect solution in search of a plausible and practical application." As if this statement was not sufficiently degrading, Lown concluded: "The rationale for some current biometric development is best exemplified by Edmund Hilary's reason for climbing Mt. Everest, 'Because it was there.' The same holds true for some electronic gadget manufacture: 'It was developed because it was possible.'" Lown and his co-author, Dr. Paul Axelrod, further criticized Mirowski's efforts as socially irresponsible and wasteful of "scarce health resources."

Mirowski published a reply to Lown's editorial; it was firm and reasoned but the damage was done. Medtronic, which had funded some of Mirowski's experiments, withdrew its financial support and, in an act the company would long regret, relinquished its rights to Mirowski's defibrillator patents.

Lown's editorial all but guaranteed that the usual federal and foundation funding sources would not be available. Mirowski was on his own, just as he was in 1939, a 15-year-old Jew who scrambled daily for food and shelter, a refugee who traveled thousands of miles to escape the Nazis. He may have been on his own but Mirowski was not alone: he had Anna and his three daughters, and a close-knit group of friends and supporters. Mower and Mendelhof never wavered, and they were joined by Dr. Arthur Moss, a New York cardiologist, who in the decades ahead would conduct many of the implantable defibrillator's pivotal clinical trials. They would survive Lown's shameful editorial and move on.

In 1979, I met Michel Mirowski at an international symposium in Montreal, Canada. He was medium height with a receding line of wavy hair and he wore glasses in thick frames. A dark silk purple tie highlighted his well-tailored gray suit. The Mirowski I met in this scientific meeting was all business, completely focused on his topic, which inevitably was the implantable defibrillator.

Mirowski had an AID™ ready for clinical trial. He had met Dr. Stephen Heilman in 1972 at a medical meeting in Singapore. Heilman, a physician and engineer, had formed a company called Medrad, based in Pittsburgh. The company manufactured powered X-ray dye injectors for use during angiography. The Medrad injector was commercially successful and Heilman, intrigued by the AID™ concept and Mirowski's vision, agreed to provide technical assistance. Eventually, they formed a company in Pittsburgh named Intec.

In Montreal, Mirowski showed a movie of the AID™ defibrillating a dog in ventricular fibrillation. It was a compelling and convincing demonstration of the AID™'s ability to automatically detect ventricular fibrillation and shock the heart back to normal. I was impressed and visited the Intec booth in the exhibit hall. The company was soliciting investigators to participate in the AID™'s initial clinical trial, so I signed up. But it would be four years before I could implant my first defibrillator.

Because Mount Sinai had no heart surgery program, the first human AID™ implant was performed at Johns Hopkins Hospital on February 4, 1980. The patient was a 57-year-old woman who had coronary artery disease and suffered numerous cardiac arrests despite multiple antiarrhythmic drugs. Her cardiologist was Dr. Roger Winkle at Stanford in Palo Alto, California. Winkle flew with her to Baltimore. They sat in the rear of a commercial jet with a portable defibrillator stored in the overhead compartment in case she had another cardiac arrest. The implant went smoothly, and Stanford became the second clinical trial site for the AID™.

During the clinical trial, a patient qualified for an AID™ only if he or she had documented ventricular fibrillation or ventricular tachycardia that could not be controlled by drugs. Early on, the AID™ did not always detect ventricular tachycardia. Consequently, the method used to detect ventricular fibrillation was modified so that a very rapid heart rate alone was sufficient to trigger a life-saving shock. Because the shock was synchronized to the patient's electrical heartbeat (QRS), the AID™ became the AICD™—the Automatic Implantable Cardioverter-Defibrillator. Some years later a generic designation was used in the scientific literature, and it became known simply as the *implantable cardioverter-defibrillator,* or *ICD.*

By September 1982, 52 patients received Intec's ICDs at Johns Hopkins and Stanford. The majority had coronary artery disease and weak hearts, and a few had genetic heart disease. As experienced accumulated, it became clear that the ICD was capable of recognizing dangerous rhythms and terminating them. Bottom line: Mirowski's invention worked, and we looked forward to implanting one at Rush Presbyterian-St. Luke's Hospital in Chicago.

I called Intec and reminded the company that I had signed up to be an investigator. Clearly, they had forgotten or misplaced my name but said Mirowski would call me. When Mirowski called, he was blunt: "I don't know you and I've never heard of you." At the time, I was the incoming president of the North American Society of Pacing and Electrophysiology but I could understand why Mirowski might not know my name. "Is there anyone at your institution who I may know?" he asked. I mentioned Dr. Pablo Denes, who had published numerous scientific papers on cardiac arrhythmias. Mirowski replied, "Yes, I know Dr. Denes. Have him call me." He hung up.

Pablo Denes' office was next to mine and I told him what had just transpired. He was amused and said, "Bob, you need a public relations agent."

Denes called Mirowski and arranged for him to visit and lecture at our weekly cardiology grand rounds. The meeting was a success and soon we were submitting the ICD study protocol to our Institutional Review Board. We would be the fourth center in the world to implant an ICD. All we needed now was a suitable patient.

I saw Jack Pearson in my clinic two months after Mirowski's visit. His fiancé, Barbara Shell who appeared half Jack's age, accompanied him. Jack was 53 and sold commercial real estate. He had been experiencing progressive fatigue and occasional episodes of lightheadedness. His wife-to-be thought it was his heart and made the appointment.

"Doctor Hauser, I am here because she made me come," Jack said, looking at Barbara. "I feel okay. I just get tired at the end of the day. Nothing, really, to get excited about."

"I disagree, honey," Barbara interjected. She then described his symptoms in great detail, including his struggles in the bedroom. "Doctor, I'm just afraid something is wrong and want him to have a thorough check-up before our wedding—before we have children."

I went through Jack's history, which was unremarkable. He never smoked, did not have high blood pressure or high cholesterol and he was not diabetic. His father had died of prostate cancer and his mother was still living in her 80s. Three siblings were healthy. There were no red flags.

I asked him to remove his shirt and sit on the exam table. I examined his eyes with an ophthalmoscope: normal vessels, no hemorrhages. I placed my stethoscope over his carotid arteries: no bruits (abnormal sounds suggesting plaque). His breath sounds were healthy: no wheezes, no rattles, no crackling. Then I had him lie down and placed the bell of my stethoscope over his heart. I expected to hear a regular rhythm and the crisp tones of the mitral and aortic valves. Instead, there were sounds that I had never heard before: thuds, random vibrations, silence, and more vibrations, like an erratic engine about to fail. I listened for a long time, trying to visualize what the heart must be doing to make these sounds.

"What's wrong?" Barbara asked anxiously.

I stepped back and removed the stethoscope from my ears. "I'm going to get an EKG," I replied.

She ignored what I said and pressed on. "You heard something, didn't you?"

By now, even Jack was interested. I looked at him and said, "Your rhythm is irregular. The electrocardiogram will tell us what it is." I left the exam room and asked our nurse to get an EKG.

Fifteen minutes later, I was sitting at my desk when the nurse placed the EKG in front of me. "What is it?" she asked softly. "I still have him connected if you want a longer recording."

I looked at the EKG and immediately understood what I had heard. His rhythm was paroxysms of rapid ventricular tachycardia interspersed with pauses and normal beats. It was the ugliest EKG I had ever seen outside the hospital.

I returned to the exam room. Jack was dressed and sat next to Barbara. I sat on a chair and regarded Jack. This was no time to deliver a soft message to a patient already in full denial. "You have a serious situation, Mr. Pearson," I said. "Your heart is going into and out of a rhythm called ventricular tachycardia. It comes from the bottom chambers of your heart. Frankly, I am surprised you're not having more symptoms. We should admit you to the hospital now and run tests."

"Like what? How long will I be in? I'm very busy right now."

"We'll start with an echocardiogram—an ultrasound of your heart. Tomorrow or the next day you will have a coronary angiogram. You will also see my partner, Dr. Denes, who specializes in these rhythms."

"Can't I do this next week?" he asked.

Barbara had heard enough. "Jack, this sounds serious! Do what the doctor says! I just knew there was something wrong. You need to listen!"

I called the emergency room for a cart and monitor and admitted Jack to the coronary care unit. Jack Pearson's echocardiogram revealed an enlarged and severely dysfunctional left ventricle; his ejection fraction was 20 percent (normal 55-60 percent). His coronary angiogram showed extensive plaque in all three of his major coronary arteries. The beginning of the right and left anterior descending had 90 percent blockages; the arteries beyond the blockages contained plaque but appeared suitable for surgical bypass.

Pablo Denes treated Jack's ventricular tachycardia with intravenous lidocaine and started a powerful oral drug—amiodarone—that would take a week or more to be effective. The FDA had not yet approved amiodarone and we, like many other U.S. medical centers, were covertly bringing it in from Europe and Canada.

Jack Pearson was in the operating room the following day. Dr. Marshall Goldin bypassed his left anterior descending and right coronary arteries. After placing the bypass grafts, Goldin defibrillated Jack's heart with a single shock. His heart began pumping but it was sluggish. His blood pressure was 60 to 70 mmHg. Goldin asked the anesthesiologist to start epinephrine. His blood pressure remained low because Jack Pearson's weak heart was not pumping enough blood.

"Get the balloon ready," Goldin said to the circulating nurse. Ten minutes later a technician wheeled the lime green intra-aortic balloon (IAB) console into the operating room. It had an oscilloscope and a dozen dials and switches on its sloping front panel.

Goldin made an incision in the femoral artery and inserted a long balloon that was mounted on a large catheter. He positioned the tip of the balloon in the descending aorta just below the left subclavian artery and connected it to the console.

"We're ready. Turn it on," Goldin ordered.

The technician flipped a switch and helium filled the catheter and inflated the balloon. A second later, the helium was forcibly withdrawn from the balloon, causing it to abruptly deflate. Inflate, deflate, inflate, deflate. It was all synchronized with Jack's heartbeat.

When it was inflated, the balloon obstructed blood flow to the lower body and thus augmented pressure and blood flow to the coronary arteries, bypass grafts, and arteries leading to Jack's brain. When the balloon abruptly collapsed, the sudden drop in resistance to blood flow allowed his heart to contract against a lower resistance, allowing his heart to eject a larger volume of blood. The output from Jack's heart increased by a third, and that was enough to bring his blood pressure up.

With the intra-aortic balloon supporting his circulation, Jack was gradually weaned off the heart-lung machine. Goldin closed the sternotomy incision with wire sutures. Later, in the intensive care unit, the balloon continued to augment Jack's blood pressure and blood flow. The next day Jack was taken off epinephrine and maintained a good blood pressure and urine output. Goldin adjusted the balloon so it pumped every other beat instead of every beat. This "weaning" process continued for another day when Goldin took Jack back to the operating room and removed the balloon.

While he was recovering in the hospital, Denes continued to give Jack oral amiodarone. The bursts of ventricular tachycardia decreased in frequency and finally disappeared altogether. However, Denes was not convinced that the tachycardia was controlled, so he scheduled Jack for an electrophysiology study that required a heart catheterization. Jack had recovered from his bypass surgery and wanted to go home. Once again, Barbara Shell intervened and convinced him to consent to the study.

The following day, Denes took Jack to the catheterization laboratory and inserted a temporary pacing catheter into the femoral vein in his groin. He advanced it to Jack's right ventricle. He connected the catheter to an electrical stimulator capable of rapidly pacing the heart with a programmed sequence of electrical pulses. Research had shown that failure to trigger ventricular tachycardia by rapid, programmed pacing was evidence that the antiarrhythmic drug was working. In Jack's case, the drug was amiodarone.

The study took only 30 minutes. Denes readily induced Jack's ventricular tachycardia with a sequence of three rapid pacing pulses. Jack blacked out and required two shocks to restore a normal rhythm. Denes called me from the laboratory. "Bob," he said, "Mr. Pearson is easily inducible into VT (ventricular tachycardia). He needs one of Mirowski's defibrillators. Otherwise, he is going to die."

Jack Pearson's left ventricle contained patches of scar tissue from multiple small myocardial infarctions—mini heart attacks. These scars were surrounded by live muscle that conducted electrical signals. The signals could not penetrate the scar tissue; instead they spread around it. Under certain conditions, the signals looped back on themselves, occasionally spinning out of control, generating the turbulent beats of rapid ventricular tachycardia. The tachycardia was like a tiger chasing its tail: it only stopped when the "tiger" was exhausted—or dead.

Drugs like amiodarone suppressed and slowed the signals that provoked and sustained the tachycardia. But the heart's biologic milieu is dynamic, subject to miniscule changes in acidity, potassium and sodium concentrations, and oxygenation. Consequently, a drug that works one day may not be effective the next day. Ventricular tachycardia can be fickle, vacillating, unpredictable, and resistant to targeted treatments like amiodarone. Jack needed a safety net, a therapy that would save his life when drugs failed. This therapy was the ICD.

A month earlier, Denes, Goldin and I had visited Intec in Pittsburgh to learn about the technical details of the device's operation. The ICD was much larger than I expected; it would be implanted in the wall of the abdomen. Two flexible metal patch electrodes would be sewn onto the surface of the heart through an incision in the chest; these electrodes would deliver the shock to the ventricles. Two pacemaker electrodes would be screwed into one of the ventricles; they would be used to detect the patient's heart beats.

When the ICD detected very rapid heart beats, which were most likely ventricular tachycardia or fibrillation, it would automatically charge its capacitors, like a flash camera, and deliver a high voltage shock (30 joules). If the tachycardia or fibrillation persisted, the ICD would shock the patient again and again, until it had delivered six shocks. At that point, it was assumed, the rhythm was no longer ventricular tachycardia or fibrillation, or the patient had died.

Denes and I went to Jack's room to describe what we proposed to do and why. Jack and Barbara were waiting for us. Denes began: "Mr. Pearson, we tried amiodarone and it seemed to be working, but today in the laboratory it was very easy to start up your tachycardia. You lost consciousness almost immediately and we had to shock you—twice. This suggests that your heart is very vulnerable. We cannot be sure the amiodarone is going to be enough to keep you alive. Doctor Hauser is going to tell you about a new device called an ICD—it stands for implantable cardioverter-defibrillator."

I sat on the bed next to Jack and removed a model of the Intec ICD from my lab coat pocket.

"My god," Jack said, "It's huge—and heavy. Where does it go?"

"Dr. Goldin will put it here," I said, pointing to the left side of his abdomen. "He will need to open your chest and sew two metal patches and two pacing leads on your heart. Then we will test the system and we're done. It'll take about an hour."

Jack took the ICD in his hand. "It's heavy too." I nodded. He paused, looked at Barbara and said, "I guess it's the right thing to do." Turning to me he asked, "You said it was experimental?"

"That's right. You'll have to read and sign this consent." I handed him a sheath of papers, which he immediately gave to Barbara.

"How long will it last?" Barbara asked.

"The company said the batteries should last two years, but that assumes only a few shocks. If you get a lot of shocks, the battery will run down faster and it will need to be replaced sooner."

"What happens when the battery runs down?" Jack asked.

"We bring you in the hospital and replace it."

"What happens if I get a shock?

"Most patients are unconscious when they get shocked, so you won't feel anything. If you're awake, it will feel like a horse kicked you in the chest."

Denes interjected. "We'll keep you on amiodarone. It will help keep the tachycardia under control. The likelihood that you'll be shocked is low."

"Then why do I need this thing?" Jack asked.

"Because you are at high risk for dying suddenly," Denes replied firmly. "It could be ventricular tachycardia, or your ventricles may fibrillate. Either rhythm could happen at any time—in your sleep, during the day, on an airplane, wherever. The ICD is a safety net—it will monitor your rhythm 24 hours a day and rescue you when you need it."

I asked, "Do you want to think about it? We can come back."

Jack raised his arms and gestured with both hands to stop. "No, no, the sooner we do this the sooner I'll get out of here. Give me the papers, Barbara. I'll sign now." I gave Jack a pen and showed him where to sign the consent.

The ICD we were about to implant in Jack Pearson had to do two things without fail: 1) detect ventricular tachycardia or fibrillation, and 2) promptly deliver a shock to his heart that would restore a normal or life-sustaining rhythm.

There was no margin for error. Like a parachute, the defibrillator had to work every time; unlike the parachute, the defibrillator had no reserve parachute.

The operating room was crowded with staff and technical representatives from Intec. Goldin and I sutured two pacing wires and two patch electrodes to the surface of Jack's heart and connected them to the bulky ICD pulse generator. When all was ready I put Jack's heart into ventricular fibrillation using a high-frequency electrical current from a common battery charger. Everyone in the room watched the EKG monitor. Jack's heart was fibrillating but we had to wait for the ICD to recognize the fibrillation and hopefully shock Jack's heart into a normal rhythm.

Doctors and nurses are not used to passively watching ventricular fibrillation. The tension in the room was palpable as we waited for the ICD to respond. I felt a hollowness in my chest: my heart was pounding and rivulets of sweat rolled down my neck and back.

Finally, after 42 seconds --an eternity -- we heard the whine of the ICD charging its capacitors. Seconds later it delivered a shock through the two patch electrodes on Jacks' heart. All eyes were on the EKG monitor. Slowly, very slowly a marvelous normal rhythm appeared. A restrained cheer erupted in the operating room.

Jack Pearson left the hospital four days after receiving his ICD. Five weeks later, almost to the day, he blacked out and collapsed on the floor of his expansive office in the Sears Tower. Alone at the time, he awoke after a few minutes and telephoned Barbara who called me at the clinic. I suspected that Jack had experienced an episode of rapid ventricular tachycardia and that the ICD had saved his life, just as we said it would.

An hour later, Jack sat on an exam table in our cardiology clinic. He looked relaxed and dapper in his three- piece suit complete with matching tie and handkerchief. His EKG was normal, as was his blood pressure. All of his incisions were healing nicely. Using a donut-shaped magnet to activate the ICD's electronic memory, I interrogated the implanted device's shock counter with a handheld unit called an AID-Check™. It indicated that Jack had received just one shock from his ICD.

"Should he be admitted to the hospital?", Barbara asked.

I looked at her and back to Jack, and replied, "I don't think that is necessary. If there are more shocks, then yes we would want to run some tests and I would want Dr. Denes to see you. Right now I suggest you go home and take the day off."

It was the only shock Jack Pearson ever received. He and Barbara married and moved into a high-rise on Lake Shore Drive next to the Drake Hotel. They would have no children. Two years after his surgeries, Jack developed heart failure. He refused to consider heart transplantation, sold his real estate business, and moved to Fort Lauderdale, Florida, where he died in 1989 when his heart simply stopped. Bypass surgery and the ICD had added six years to Jack's life. Severe congestive heart failure due to the residual scars of coronary artery disease ultimately prevailed.

Yes, we could prevent sudden cardiac death with the ICD, but the condition of Jack's heart pump was the fundamental, life-limiting problem. New treatments for heart failure were on the horizon, including drugs, mechanical assist devices, and a novel pacing system. However, these advances would require years of development and testing before they would become available in the new millennium.

Even after FDA approval in 1985, the ICD remained a treatment of last resort, and it was implanted only in patients who had survived a cardiac arrest or its equivalent. Yet, the majority of victims did not survive their first cardiac arrest. The key was to identify people who were at high-risk for sudden cardiac death and implant an ICD *before* catastrophe struck. This was *primary prevention*, aimed at saving the most lives, and it had been Mirowski's original vision when he conceived the implantable defibrillator after Dr. Harry Heller's death in 1966. Before primary prevention trials could begin, ICD technology had to be safer and more acceptable to patients.

Eli Lilly and Company purchased Intec in 1984 for $68 million and a royalty agreement. The ICD technology was transferred to Lilly's Cardiac Pacemakers Inc. (CPI) division in St. Paul, Minnesota. CPI's immediate challenge was to manufacture an ICD that was reliable and profitable. Soon thereafter Medtronic began its defibrillator development program, initially without the benefit of Mirowski's intellectual property portfolio. Eventually Medtronic and other manufacturers would receive licenses to use his patents, and for years they would pay the Mirowski family millions of dollars for the privilege.

Ahead were years of costly technology development and clinical testing. The ICD would follow the same development path that had been taken by the pacemaker: a lead that could be inserted through a vein rather than opening the chest; sophisticated electronics that could pace as well as shock the heart; and long-lived batteries sealed in a small titanium metal can that could be implanted below the collarbone like a pacemaker.

Although the engineering challenges were daunting, a pacemaker-like ICD became available by the late-1990s. A series of primary prevention trials in the United States and Europe involving thousands of subjects showed that certain patients benefited from prophylactic ICD implantation because they were at high risk for sudden cardiac death. Hundreds of thousands of these high-risk patients are alive today because their ICDs have saved them, and often on more than one occasion. After four decades, Mirowski's goal was achieved.

However, Mirowski would not live to see his full vision realized or to enjoy the fortune he earned. He died at 65 in 1990 of multiple myeloma. As his health was failing, a group of physician friends held a dinner in his honor in Baltimore. In attendance were his family, several boyhood classmates from Warsaw, and close colleagues. The White House sent a telegram to Mirowski and his family, and it was read to Mirowski and the dinner guests. In it, President George H.W. Bush thanked Michel Mirowski on behalf of the American people for his contributions to medicine and mankind. He had climbed a tall and treacherous mountain, and at last he stood on the summit.

CHAPTER 9

On a summer morning in 1986, 56-year-old Harold Swanson showered and dressed for work. Having sold his family's restaurant to Doris Hart, he was now the founder, owner, and chief executive officer of Swanson's Subs, a national chain of sandwich shops. Harold and his wife, Jean, lived in Lake Forest, Illinois, with their three children.

While tying his shoes, Harold felt a squeezing discomfort in the middle of his chest. He broke out in a profuse sweat, drenching his lightly starched, white dress shirt. Harold looked in the bathroom mirror. He was pale and beads of perspiration glistened on his forehead. Next came a wave of nausea and lightheadedness. He leaned against the sink. Harold thought he had the flu. The chest discomfort spread to both his arms; they ached and felt heavy. The air was thick. He could not take a deep breath. "This isn't the flu," he whispered to himself.

An inflamed cholesterol-rich plaque had cracked inside Harold's left anterior descending coronary artery, releasing a cascade of chemicals that hastened formation of a blood clot. The clot—a thrombus—rapidly snowballed and obstructed blood flow to a vast and vital expanse of Harold's heart. The thrombus contained thin strands of fibrin, a protein, and clumps of tenacious platelets that circulate in the blood to form clots. A major section of Harold's left ventricle had begun to weaken and die. Harold was having an acute anterior myocardial infarction, the most lethal form of a heart attack.

Harold awoke Jean.

"I don't feel right," he said, sitting on the edge of the bed. "My chest is tight."

"Oh, you look awful," she said, placing her hand on his forehead. It was cool and moist. Reaching for her robe, she said, 'I'm calling an ambulance."

"No, no, don't do that. Maybe it's that chili spaghetti we had for dinner last night." Harold lay on the bed.

"I had the same food and I feel fine." Jean picked up the phone on the bedside table and called the operator. "Operator, we need an ambulance. I think my husband is having a heart attack."

Sixteen minutes later three paramedics arrived in an ambulance. They connected Harold to a Physio-Control™ portable defibrillator and placed an oxygen cannula in his nose. The EKG on the defibrillator's monitor showed ST segment elevation—an acute heart attack. "We're taking him to Lake Forest Hospital," the paramedic told Mrs. Swanson. "He's having a heart attack, for sure."

At that moment, Harold Swanson's ventricles fibrillated and he lost consciousness. A paramedic tore open Harold's shirt and started CPR, compressing the left side of Harold's chest with clenched hands. The downward thrusts were rapid and vigorous. Another paramedic slipped a plastic airway into Harold's mouth, and started ventilating him with a facemask. The third paramedic removed the metal paddles from the defibrillator and coated them with a conductive gel.

"Ready!" the paramedic called out. Everyone stepped back. The paramedic placed the metal paddles on Harold's bare chest and yelled "Clear!" A second later, he pressed a button on the paddles and a 360-joule shock embraced the fibrillating heart with millions of electrons. Harold's entire body seized. Jean covered her face.

The energy from the shock abolished the electrical wavelets of ventricular fibrillation. After three seconds, his heart relaxed, releasing a slow, regular rhythm. "I've got a pulse," said the paramedic at the head of the bed. His fingers were on Harold's carotid artery. Harold started to breath and opened his eyes, groaning, "Waa...whoa?" He tried to sit up.

"You're okay, Mr. Swanson, we had to give you a shock," a paramedic said. "You're fine now." Through an intravenous catheter, Harold was given 100 mg of a lidocaine solution to suppress premature (extra) beats coming from his left ventricle.

Three-year-old Danny Swanson came into his parents' bedroom and stared at his father lying helpless on the bed surrounded by uniformed men. He thought they were Star Wars droids and started to cry. Jean whisked him back to his room and told him daddy had to go to the hospital. She woke her other two children and explained what was happening to their father. They would stay home from school until their mother called them from the hospital.

The paramedics placed Harold on a gurney and carried him down the stairs and through the front door to the ambulance parked in the driveway. A heavy mist hovered over the lawn. The Swanson's neighbors stood motionless and silent on the sidewalk as the ambulance's flashing red lights reflected off their faces. Harriet Beller crossed the lawn from her home and said she would stay with the children.

Fifteen minutes later, Harold was in the emergency department of Lake Forest Hospital. He was still having the chest pain that had started 55 minutes earlier. Dr. Ralph Sims, the emergency room physician, checked his blood pressure, had him chew an aspirin tablet and gave him two milligrams of morphine. A technician placed electrodes on Harold's chest and recorded an electrocardiogram.

Sims examined the EKG and said, "Mr. Swanson, you're having a heart attack. I want to give you a drug that can dissolve the blood clot that is causing it. The drug is called streptokinase. We will give it to you through your vein. Do you have any bleeding tendencies, any recent surgery, or history of stroke?" Harold replied, "No."

Jean asked, "Are there any risks?"

Sims replied, "He could bleed anywhere—including in his brain. Some patients have a type of allergic response. But the greatest risk is to do nothing." He looked at Harold and said, "This is a significant heart attack. We should get going."

"Okay," Harold said. "You know I had bypass surgery in 1969?"

"No, but I do now." Sims nodded to the nurse holding the bag of streptokinase. She hung it on the iv pole and started the infusion. "It will take about an hour to give you a full dose, Mr. Swanson. We'll get a bed for you in the coronary care unit. I'll call cardiology and let them know you're here."

As the streptokinase entered Harold's bloodstream, it attacked the thrombus in his left anterior descending coronary artery by activating plasminogen, a naturally occurring substance that dissolves blood clots. Harold's entire body entered into a "lytic" state, a churning chemical factory focused on cleaving the fibrin mesh that formed the bulk of the thrombus blocking his coronary artery. Gradually the fibrin strands were cleaved into fragments and carried away in the blood stream.

Bit by bit the clot shrank until it gave way, like a dam breaking, and blood rushed forward to the mass of muscle that had been deprived of oxygen and nutrients for nearly four hours. Despite the numbing effects of morphine, Harold sensed easing of his chest discomfort: the gripping pressure was gone, his breath came easier, and the nagging sense that he was being assaulted left him.

The coronary care unit nurse noticed that Harold's EKG had changed. The bedside monitor showed that the ST segments were no longer shaped like tombstones. Some extra beats appeared. She asked Harold, "How's the pain?"

"It's gone," he replied.

"Good," she said. "Your EKG looks better too. I'll call Doctor Billingham."

"Who's he?"

"Your cardiologist. And I'll let your wife know. She's in the waiting room."

Streptokinase is an enzyme produced by the Group A beta-hemolytic streptococcus, the same bacteria that causes strep throat, ear infections, and rheumatic fever. William Smith Tillett, an internist and microbiologist, discovered streptokinase with brilliant deductive reasoning, and a little luck, while working in his laboratory at Johns Hopkins in 1933. He found that cultures of beta hemolytic streptococcus dissolved clots in test tubes and he guessed that the streptococcus bacteria produced an enzyme that broke down the fibrin in the clot. The enzyme was streptokinase and Tillett called clot dissolution *thrombolysis*.

From the beginning, Tillett believed that streptokinase could treat thrombosis. In the mid-1950s, Dr. Sol Sherry in St. Louis treated 22 acute myocardial infarction patients with intravenous streptokinase and reported success in the majority. Importantly, he observed that a patient was more likely to live the earlier streptokinase was given. This was a seminal discovery: elapsed time to treatment was crucial, and eventually it would prove to be true for strokes as well as heart attacks.

Sherry's study should have inspired larger clinical trials, but interest in streptokinase was modest. Not everyone agreed that clots played a central role in acute myocardial infarctions. Most cardiologists thought the clots seen at autopsies were the result, not the cause of heart attacks. We believed that progressive plaque build-up--gobs of cholesterol and calcium piling up like trash in a culvert until blood could no longer flow—caused heart attacks.

Instead of attacking the root cause of heart attacks—blood clots—we concentrated on treating the consequences. Elaborate efforts to repair the heart after irreversible muscle damage occurred were rarely successful. So too were therapies intended to preserve heart muscle on the periphery of a heart attack. The most we could do was make the surviving muscle more efficient and try to keep it from contorting and reshaping itself into a feeble, inefficient ball. Tens of millions of dollars, armies of scientists, and thousands of meetings and conferences were all for naught because we were focused on the wrong target.

Our awakening came in 1980 when a group of cardiologists and cardiac surgeons in Spokane and Seattle, boldly performed coronary angiograms on 322 patients with acute myocardial infarction. They found that a blood clot—a thrombus—was blocking blood flow in 90 percent of the patients. They had also performed emergency coronary bypasses on patients with acute heart attacks. During surgery, they found fresh clots in the affected arteries in the vast majority of patients. This was a momentous discovery, and the results were published in the *New England Journal of Medicine.* This study would forever change how we treated heart attacks. The chief culprit in heart attacks was the clot, and at long last it was in the crosshairs of clinical research.

Physicians in Europe and the United States reported success with the direct injection of streptokinase into coronary arteries that were obstructed by blood clots. However, such an approach in 1980 was impractical because it would require an emergency heart catheterization for thousands of heart attack victims and there were too few catheterization laboratories and too few qualified cardiologists. We tried to do it at Rush, but the effort fizzled when our catheterization teams became exhausted with the round-the-clock effort.

Then in 1983, a group of Italian physicians decided it was time to conduct a trial with intravenous streptokinase, which could be given in any hospital 24 hours a day. The trial was designed to answer three questions: 1) Does intravenous streptokinase save lives, i.e. decrease near and long-term heart attack mortality? 2) How important is the time from the onset of chest pain to the injection of streptokinase? 3) Are the risks associated with intravenous streptokinase acceptable?

The Italian study was called GISSI-1 (first study of Gruppo Italiano per lo studio della strepochinasi ell'infarto Miocardio). It included 11,806 heart attack victims in 176 Italian hospitals. Each patient was randomized to one of two treatment groups. The first group received 1.5 million units of streptokinase through a vein in the arm over one hour, and the second group did not receive streptokinase. All patients were treated within 12 hours after the onset of their symptoms. Other than streptokinase, patients in each group were treated the same.

The study showed that patients who received streptokinase had a highly significant 18 percent better chance of surviving their heart attacks than those who did not get streptokinase. The study also found that the sooner streptokinase was given after the onset of symptoms, the more likely the patient would live—precisely what Sol Sherry found in the 1950s. Only four percent of patients had side effects attributed to streptokinase, including fever and bleeding. These risks were acceptable given the drug's ability to improve early heart attack survival.

Harold Swanson received streptokinase in a small community hospital in Illinois because a group of Italian doctors had the foresight to conduct a decisive and pivotal clinical trial. His left anterior descending coronary artery was open, delivering oxygenated blood to the mass of heart muscle that had been starved for oxygen and nutrients for nearly four hours. A small fraction of his heart muscle would die, but most of it would be salvaged and its pumping function preserved.

Jean would not be a widow this day, and Danny and his two sisters would have a father to nurture them to adulthood. Harold benefited from the serial advances in cardiac care that began with cardiopulmonary resuscitation and defibrillation and now included revascularization with coronary bypass, angioplasty, and thrombolysis.

CHAPTER 10

Dolph Bachmann was a 37-year-old Swiss chain-smoking insurance salesman in good physical condition. For some time, he had been experiencing angina pectoris (heart pain) with exertion. It was getting worse, occurring with less and less effort and lasting longer. He took nitroglycerin frequently. On September 15, 1977, he came to the University Hospital in Zurich complaining of increasing bouts of angina.

Cardiologist Dr. Bernhard Meier performed an angiogram and found a discrete, short, severe blockage at the beginning of Bachmann's left anterior descending coronary artery, often called the "widow maker." This artery supplied much of the blood to his left ventricle, the main pumping chamber. Bachmann's other arteries were free of disease and his left ventricle was not damaged. The next day, he would undergo urgent coronary artery bypass surgery.

That afternoon the young, vigorous Bachmann became increasingly unhappy at the prospect of having his breastbone split open and being connected to a heart-lung machine while his heart was stopped. Worse, he would be laid-up for weeks after the surgery. He had a successful business and did not want to be absent from his office or customers.

Meier offered another option—a new untested technique called coronary angioplasty—and he asked Bachman if Dr. Andreas Gruentzig could explain the procedure. Bachmann readily agreed.

A Hollywood director could have cast Dr. Andreas Gruentzig as Doctor Zhivago or James Bond. The wife of a colleague once remarked, "Some women just threw their clothes off at the sight of him." Indeed, Gruentzig was a dashing dreamer, larger than life, and he was destined to change the treatment of coronary artery disease forever. His innovations proved to be critical for millions of patients, including Harold Swanson. No one would have a more profound impact on cardiovascular care in the 20th century than this gentle, flamboyant, dark-eyed cardiologist. One of his close associates wrote, "...he came into our lives like a comet...and ignited the imagination of others throughout the world."

Andreas Gruentzig was born in Dresden in 1939, a few months before the start of World War II in Europe. His father, a chemist in civilian life, never returned home after the war. His mother, Charlotte, a teacher, struggled to raise Gruentzig and his older brother, Johannes, in what was then communist East Germany. In 1950, Charlotte took her two sons to Argentina for a year to live with relatives, but returned to Leipzig a year later so the boys could attend German schools.

Children of working parents in East Germany were not allowed to attend University, so Andreas followed his brother to West Germany where he graduated from Heidelberg University medical school in 1964. He completed his internship and a fellowship in epidemiology and statistics, and studied vascular disease at the Ratchow Clinic in Darmstadt, Germany where he learned and first performed peripheral angiography. Eventually he secured a position in the vascular department at the University Hospital in Zurich, Switzerland.

In 1971, Gruentzig visited the Aggertal Clinic in Engelskirchen, Germany to watch Dr. Eberhart Zeitler open clogged arteries in patients' legs. Zeitler used catheters developed by Dr. Charles Dotter, a well-known radiologist at the University of Oregon. Dotter had performed the first vascular angioplasty in 1964 by inserting progressively larger catheters into diseased arteries in order to compress the fat-laden sclerotic plaque that was obstructing blood flow.

Dotter's first patient was an 83-year-old woman, Laura Shaw, whose foot was gangrenous from lack of blood flow. She resisted amputation in spite of the intense pain. Dotter did an angiogram that showed a severe blockage in a major artery above Laura's knee. He inserted a series of tapered Teflon catheters through the blockage and managed to open the artery and restore blood flow to her gangrenous foot. The artery remained open and her foot healed. The pain was relieved and she kept her leg.

Dotter treated other patients and published his work, but physicians in the United States did not adopt his techniques. They were skeptical and surgeons did not like a radiologist invading their turf. However, specialists in Europe embraced and expanded Dotter's methods. One of them was Zeitler who employed a variety of other tools to open clogged arteries, including thrombolytic agents like streptokinase, and inflatable balloons.

Gruentzig told Zeitler he wanted to treat coronary artery disease using an inflatable balloon to perform angioplasty. He approached several companies to build a balloon on a catheter that was stronger than the relatively soft latex balloons Zeitler used. None of the companies were willing to help, so Gruentzig decided to build his own.

Nearly every night for two years, after finishing his hospital duties, Gruentzig worked on the catheters in the family kitchen, while his psychologist wife, Michaela, consulted with patients in the living room of their small apartment. At times, the challenges for Gruentzig appeared insurmountable with technical barriers, and dead ends. The major obstacle was finding a balloon material that was strong enough to compress the tough, often calcified plaque that was typical of severe atherosclerosis.

The solution came from an unexpected source: a retired high school organic chemistry teacher, Heinrich Hopff. He suggested that Gruentzig try polyvinyl chloride (PVC), a synthetic polymer used for insulation and waterproofing. Gruentzig built a catheter with a balloon made with PVC and in 1974 he used it for the first time to open a severe femoral (leg) artery blockage. The patient was Fritz Ott, a 67-year-old man who suffered incapacitating pain in his thigh and calf whenever he walked a few feet. Gruentzig inserted the angioplasty catheter into Ott's artery and positioned the balloon across the blockage using fluoroscopy. Then he inflated the balloon with high pressure, compressing the plaque and opening the artery so that blood flowed freely. Mr. Ott was able to walk without pain. The PVC balloon was an unqualified success.

Gruentzig went on to perform 270 angioplasties in peripheral arteries. He custom-made each PVC balloon angioplasty catheter in his kitchen, sizing every balloon to fit each artery based on measurements made from the patient's diagnostic angiogram. Two years after Gruentzig made his first balloon catheter, the local Schneider Company began manufacturing them.

The catheters Gruentzig used in the legs were too large for coronary arteries, so he went back to his family-kitchen-turned-laboratory. He worked with his wife, his assistant, Maria Schlumpf, and her husband Walter. The catheter had to be small but it also had to have two channels or lumens: one channel for measuring pressure and injecting dye and one for inflating the balloon.

Gruentzig was a man on a mission and a friend said he possessed a "sacred fire." Gruentzig was so focused that he drew people into his vortex. Maria Schlumpf was with him constantly in the kitchen, late at night, fabricating catheters and balloons, and experimenting with various materials. The kitchen table was a rat's nest of implements, adhesives, tubes and wires.

By 1976, Gruentzig believed he had a balloon tipped catheter that was suitable for coronary arteries. He tested them in cadavers and dogs and submitted a summary of his work to the American Heart Association for presentation at the annual scientific meeting in November. I remember that meeting. The weather in Miami was magnificent and the hotels were crammed with 30,000 cardiologists, cardiovascular surgeons, nurses, technicians and industry personnel. This was the first big scientific meeting of the academic year.

Gruentzig presented his research at a poster session entitled "EXPERIMENTAL DILATATION OF CORONARY ARTERY STENOSIS" in a congested exhibit hall where dozens of other posters on 30x60-inch corkboard were similarly displayed. Gruentzig stood in front of his poster and, at the appointed hour, described his research to the more than 50 cardiologists and surgeons who attended his presentation. He wore a jacket and ascot that immediately distinguished him from the plain ties, button-down shirts, sport coats and slacks worn by his mostly American audience.

Gruentzig explained to the group that his study showed it was feasible to dilate coronary blockages in dogs with his balloon tipped angioplasty catheters. Moreover, the dilation did not result in heart attacks or damage to the lining of the arteries. Gruentzig boldly stated that his study was the prelude to performing coronary angioplasty in humans.

Dr. Spencer King, a young cardiologist at Emory in Atlanta listened and thought, "This will never work." However, another cardiologist, Dr. Richard Myler from San Francisco, was dazzled by Gruentzig's presentation. The following March,

Myler attended a conference in Nuremberg where Gruentzig presented more data. Again, Gruentzig declared that coronary angioplasty would be done in humans—and soon.

Myler offered to bring Gruentzig to his hospital in San Francisco. There were distinct advantages, Myler said, including a large volume of patients and an environment that was far more receptive to novel ideas than the hospital in Zurich where Gruentzig struggled daily. Gruentzig, his wife and infant daughter, Sophia, flew to San Francisco in May 1977.

Myler arranged for Gruentzig to test his angioplasty catheters in patients who were undergoing coronary bypass at Saint Mary's Hospital. The catheters and balloons performed well and Gruentzig realized he was ready at last. All he needed was an appropriate patient. He decided to choose a patient who was otherwise healthy and ideally suited for balloon dilatation, rather than a very sick patient for whom angioplasty was the last resort. He returned to Zurich with his family.

What Andreas Gruentzig proposed could vastly disrupt the treatment of coronary artery disease. Angioplasty could supplant coronary artery bypass surgery and end the reign of cardiac surgery as the dominant clinical and economic force in many major medical centers. Vascular surgeons had thwarted Dr. Charles Dotter; cardiac surgeons could have done the same to Gruentzig, even before he performed his first coronary angioplasty.

The one man whose support Gruentzig desperately needed was Dr. Ake Senning, a world-famous heart surgeon and Director of the Department of Surgery at the University Hospital in Zurich. Senning was born in Rättvik, Sweden in 1915. He graduated from the University of Uppsala medical school in Stockholm, and in 1948 trained under the renowned cardiovascular surgeon, Dr. Clarence Crafoord, at the Karolinska Institute. During the next 15 years, Senning was a prolific innovator: he developed an oxygenator, devised operations for congenital heart disease (called "the Senning repair"), and implanted the first heart pacemaker (it failed shortly after the surgery). In 1961, he moved to Zurich to become Director of Surgery at the University Hospital. There he helped to promote coronary artery bypass surgery throughout Europe.

To perform angioplasty, Gruentzig needed a cardiac surgeon to standby in case of a complication that would require an emergency operation. Would Senning allow his department to do this? Would he permit an operating room to be open in case the angioplasty failed? Did this heart surgeon want to help someone develop a technique that could make coronary bypass surgery obsolete or a second-line therapy?

Gruentzig did not hesitate when Dr. Bernhard Meier told him about Dolph Bachmann. He went to Bachmann's hospital room and described what he proposed to do. As Meier later recalled, Gruentzig held nothing back. He told Bachmann that he would be the first patient in the world to undergo this experimental procedure called angioplasty, and that he could suffer a heart attack and die. Emergency bypass surgery might be required if the angioplasty went wrong. Bachmann listened and consented, eagerly.

Immediately, a firestorm erupted when Gruentzig scheduled Bachmann's angioplasty for the following day. University Hospital doctors called an emergency meeting to debate whether Gruentzig should be allowed to go forward with the procedure. Nearly everyone in the room, including the heads of medicine and cardiology, opposed Gruentzig. For months, these same physicians had been very vocal, declaring that coronary angioplasty was crazy, unethical, and fraught with risks. It appeared that Dolph Bachmann would have to settle for coronary artery bypass.

Then chief surgeon Ake Senning rose from his chair. He was an imposing presence, tall and distinguished. "Let him do it," Senning said. "What's to worry about? If something goes wrong, I will operate." The room fell silent. Gruentzig had been given the green light.

The following afternoon, Dolph Bachmann was wheeled into the catheterization laboratory at the University Hospital. He was awake and lightly sedated. The room was crowded with observers. Several cardiac surgeons were present in the event emergency bypass surgery was needed. It was September 16, 1977.

Gruentzig punctured Bachman's right femoral artery and advanced a large diameter catheter up the aorta into his chest. He guided the catheter around the aortic arch and maneuvered its tip into the opening of the left coronary artery. This catheter served as the conduit through which he inserted his homemade angioplasty catheter. Using the X-ray fluoroscopy, Gruentzig carefully positioned the deflated balloon on the tip of the angioplasty catheter across the severe blockage in Bachmann's left anterior descending coronary artery. He measured the pressures on either side of the blockage and calculated the difference between the two pressures. As expected, the pressure beyond the blockage was much lower than the pressure before it. If the angioplasty was successful, the pressure difference should fall to near zero.

Not knowing what was going to happen—*he could very well kill this young man*—Gruentzig inflated the balloon. The walls of the high-pressure PVC balloon engaged the plaque and split it, forcing the cholesterol rich tissue outward, stretching the artery's elastic tissue, winding it like a spring that could recoil when the balloon was deflated.

While the balloon was inflated, all blood flow to the front of Dolph Bachman's left ventricle ceased. Gruentzig feared that the EKG might show signs of a heart attack, but the EKG did not change. He worried that Bachmann's heart might fibrillate, but his rhythm remained stable.

When he deflated the balloon, the plaque did not snap back; rather, the plaque remained compressed, allowing blood to flow freely. Gruentzig measured the pressure gradient across the blockage and found it near zero. The balloon inflation had worked!

One observer, however, thought there was a narrowing in the diagonal branch that arose at a point just beyond the blockage, which Gruentzig had just dilated. Gruentzig agreed and advanced the balloon catheter into the diagonal branch. Once again, he inflated the balloon and the blockage seemed to go away. (Afterward, when Gruentzig reviewed the actual X-ray films, there was no blockage in the diagonal branch and the second balloon inflation had been unnecessary).

Next, Gruentzig injected dye onto the left anterior descending coronary artery. Both the artery and the diagonal branch were wide open and blood flowed unimpeded. Andreas Gruentzig's first coronary angioplasty was a stunning success.

After returning to his room, Dolph Bachmann was so elated that he telephoned the local newspaper from his hospital bed. When the reporter called the hospital,

Gruentzig pleaded with him not to publish the story. It was a heated discussion. One successful angioplasty, he argued, did not constitute proof of safety or efficacy. Premature publicity, especially in Zurich, could destroy Gruentzig's reputation and his ability to treat more patients. The reporter reluctantly dropped the story.

Bachman's angina was gone. He no longer needed the nitroglycerin tablets. A month later Bachman had a follow-up angiogram. The site where the angioplasty had been performed looked good: the blockage had not returned.

During the next few weeks, Gruentzig performed three additional angioplasties and all of them were successful, including two patients who had severe disease in the left main coronary artery. In retrospect, Gruentzig and his patients were fortunate, because subsequent experience with left main coronary artery angioplasty proved that lesions in this location were prone to catastrophic complications, including abrupt closure and immediate death.

In November 1977, Gruentzig presented his four angioplasty cases to a rapt audience at the 50th Scientific Sessions of the American Heart Association in Miami. As he described the fourth case -- a severe lesion in the left main coronary artery -- the audience applauded – an almost unprecedented response during a scientific presentation. Afterward I heard about Gruentzig's presentation from a Rush colleague: "Hey Bob," he told me. "Some crazy Swiss guy is blowing up balloons in the coronary arteries!"

Mason Sones, the father or coronary angiography and Rene Favaloro's close friend, approached Gruentzig after his presentation. Sones was thrilled and asked Gruentzig to show him his results. Gruentzig had the angiogram films of his four patients in his briefcase. Sones, who had dabbled with dilating coronary arteries a decade earlier, had tears in his eyes. "It's a dream come true," he said.

Five months later, in March 1978, Richard Myler in San Francisco and Simon Stertzer in New York City performed the first coronary angioplasties in the United States. Shortly thereafter Dr. Robert Van Tassel did the first angioplasty in Minnesota. Cardiology would never be the same.

Andreas Gruentzig became a willing and skilled teacher. He trained and mentored hundreds cardiologists who learned to perform coronary angioplasty correctly and safely. Nevertheless, he continued to encounter obstacles in the Swiss and European medical communities. The list of patients awaiting angioplasty at his hospital grew longer and longer, but the hospital restricted him to two angioplasty cases a week.

He left Zurich and moved his family to Atlanta, where he joined the faculty of Emory University. There he could perform two angioplasties a day.

I was in the midst of teaching rounds in the spring of 1985 when Dr. Joe Messer, the Chief of Cardiology, paged me. I called his office.

"Bob," he said, "I'm here in the clinic with Harold Swanson who I am going to admit to your service. He's 55 and had coronary bypass in 1968 or '69. I think Hassan Najafi did the surgery. A year ago, he had an anterior MI (myocardial infarction, heart attack) and received streptokinase at Lake Forest Hospital. Now he's having angina, primarily with effort, but this morning he awoke with it. He needs an angiogram. I'll send his records along."

When I entered his hospital room, Harold Swanson looked vaguely familiar, but I did not connect him to the balding young man I saw as an intern 16 years before. I introduced myself, and he said, "I think you took care of me back in 1969 when I had my bypass." I looked at his face carefully and shrugged, "That could be. I was an intern then." He smiled, "I know it was you."

Harold Swanson's red hair was now gray and he was mostly bald. He appeared in good shape, not heavy, with good muscle tone. I reviewed the hand-written notes Joe Messer had sent along together with his medical records from Lake Forest. "How long have you been having the chest discomfort?" I asked.

"It started this winter," he said. "I first felt it when I was late for a flight at O'Hare in February. I boarded the plane and noticed the pressure. It let up after a minute and I decided to continue with the trip. Probably not smart, but I was meeting with some bankers in New York and—--well, I did okay. When I got back, I saw my internist. He put me back on propranolol—I hate that drug—and gave me a new prescription for nitroglycerin tablets."

"Then what happened?"

"I got it again a few weeks later while doing some cross country skiing near our home. I stopped, but it took a while to go away. I went back home and told my wife. She called the internist. He set me up with Doctor Messer, and here I am."

The door to the room opened and Jean Swanson entered with a small suitcase. "I'm Jean Swanson," she said, extending her hand.

"I'm Doctor Hauser, Mrs. Swanson—one of Doctor Messer's associates."

"Will you be doing the angiogram?" she asked.

"No. I believe it will be Doctor Ruggie. I'm sure Doctor Messer will be there too."

She looked at her husband and back to me. "Did he tell you about the pain last night and this morning?"

"Not yet," I replied. "We were getting there when you came in. Doctor Messer filled me in on the phone. There is no question that your husband should be in the hospital and have an angiogram. We'll get it done tomorrow."

Jean sat next to Harold on the bed. "You know, there's been a lot of heart trouble in his family," she said. "All the men going back to his grandfather, uncles, and father. I'm worried about our children."

I nodded, and turned to Harold. "Have you had your cholesterol checked?"

"It's high—over 350—but I just can't take that drug—Name starts with a 'Q'—tears up my gut."

Harold was referring to cholestyramine, also known by the trade name Questran®. Cholestyramine causes constipation and abdominal discomfort, and it has to be taken frequently during the day. Harold's side effects were common, and very few patients took the recommended daily dosage.

"Cholesterol was controversial," I said. "But 350 is much too high. We need to find ways to get it down."

The following morning, Dr. Neal Ruggie performed Harold's coronary angiogram. The plaque build-up at the beginning of his left anterior descending coronary artery had narrowed the lumen (channel) by more than 90 percent. This very severe blockage was responsible for Harold's symptoms. Luckily, the blockage was discrete rather than long—in fact, similar to the plaque in Dolph Bachmann's artery. The artery beyond Harold's blockage had mild plaque, but none of it was compromising blood flow. The vein bypass that Hassan Najafi had performed in 1969 was open and supplying blood to Harold's moderately-sized right coronary artery. The third major artery—the circumflex—had mild plaque but no obstructions.

Ruggie called Messer into the laboratory and asked him to review the angiogram. Messer said he was satisfied with the images and asked Ruggie to obtain a left ventriculogram. The ventriculogram revealed that Harold's left ventricle was normal in size and shape and his ejection fraction was good at 60 percent. However, his heart attack a year earlier had compromised the front or anterior wall; it was not squeezing as vigorously as the rest of his heart. This could be due to scarring from the heart attack, or lack of adequate blood flow through the left anterior descending artery.

Ruggie removed the catheters and applied pressure with his fingers to the femoral artery. He told Harold, "We'll develop the films and review them with Doctors Messer and Hauser. Then we will come talk to you about the options. Your bypass looks good, but you have significant blockage on the left side. We'll know more after looking at the films." A nurse stepped in to hold pressure on the artery.

Ruggie stripped off his gown and gloves, and asked, "Any questions, Mr. Swanson?"

"When do you think you'll be up to my room? I want my wife to be there."

"We'll get you something to eat and we should be up around two o'clock."

When we began the angioplasty program at Rush, Messer wisely established a protocol to ensure that the procedure would be limited to patients who clearly needed it and would benefit at the lowest possible risk. Any cardiologist who wished to perform coronary angioplasty in his department had to be a member of a collaborative team of private practice and full-time cardiologists. It was an enlightened approach, and patients benefited from the team's collective expertise.

Coronary plaque is not uniform in shape or hardness. It may be inflamed like a wound or sore. It may contain liquid fat, calcium, and red blood cells and platelets that form tiny clots. When the angioplasty balloon inflates inside the artery, it compresses and mechanically disrupts and fractures the diseased tissue. The balloon also stretches the artery and imparts energy that is stored in the vessel's elastic components. When the angioplasty balloon deflates, the compressed tissue usually remains stable. Occasionally it collapses or recoils, like a tunnel caving in or a roof falling. Blood flow ceases, obstructed by biologic trash and fresh clot. Sudden or *abrupt closure* is a violent event, and it can cause a heart attack, ventricular fibrillation, shock, and death.

The threat of abrupt closure pervaded every angioplasty procedure. Of Gruentzig's first 76 patients, seven (nine percent) required urgent coronary artery bypass surgery. Statistically, abrupt closure occurred in one of every 15-20 angioplasties; sometimes it could be treated successfully with another balloon inflation. We avoided angioplasty in patients who had plaque that looked unstable or were causing an acute heart attack. Also dangerous were highly calcified plaques and those that were long or located in a small or tortuous artery. With every angioplasty, an operating room was reserved and a cardiac surgeon was always on emergency standby in case immediate bypass surgery was necessary.

Messer, Ruggie, Hassan Najafi, and I stood in front of the angiogram film viewer outside the catheterization laboratory. Ruggie loaded Harold Swanson's angiogram film and played it back and forth so all of us could watch the dye flow down each artery. The 90 percent blockage in Harold's left anterior descending coronary artery was responsible for his angina. It was relatively short with sharp borders and the artery beyond it was a reasonable size with no significant plaque build-up. Najafi was happy with the right coronary artery vein bypass he had done in 1969: it was one of his first.

Joe Messer took over the film viewer's controls from Ruggie. He viewed the blockage frame by frame. "What do you think, Neal?" he asked.

"I think it's doable with a reasonable chance of success," Ruggie responded.

"It's a bit eccentric [not uniform], don't you think?" Messer said, pointing to the blockage on the screen.

"Yes, it is, but it's fairly short and there's no calcium, at least that we can see," Ruggie replied.

Messer looked at Najafi, "Hassan, any thoughts?"

"Well, we can certainly bypass the artery," Najafi said. "I would use the internal mammary. I can schedule an operating room to be open tomorrow and I'm available all day."

Messer asked me, "What do you think?"

"There's a lot of myocardium (heart muscle) at risk and there is already a bit of scar there from his previous heart attack," I said. "But he's had one surgery already. If Neal feels confident, then I favor angioplasty."

Messer lighted his pipe and turned to Ruggie, "I think we should go ahead with angioplasty. Tomorrow?"

"Tomorrow morning—if that's okay with you, Doctor Najafi." Najafi agreed. Messer, Ruggie, and I went to Harold Swanson's room.

Neal Ruggie explained the procedure and the risks to the Swansons. Harold was enthusiastic, but Jean had many questions. Wives usually do.

"Has anyone died?" she asked.

"Yes, we have had one death and we have done about 75 procedures," Ruggie replied. "That patient died in the operating room."

"Will the angioplasty last? How long?"

"Great question. The angioplasty could last days, months, or years. About one in three patients will need another angioplasty during the first 12 to 24 months. We have not been able to predict with any accuracy who will have the best results, but your husband's blockage is not complex. I'm optimistic that we'll get a good result."

Jean was persistent. "Is there anything we can do to keep the plaque from coming back?"

Messer answered, "He'll take an aspirin a day, and we need to get his cholesterol down, however difficult that might be with Questran®. There are some new drugs in clinical trial, but they are not FDA-approved yet."

The next morning, Neal Ruggie successfully dilated the 90 percent blockage in Harold Swanson's left anterior descending coronary artery. The angioplasty required three balloon inflations and the remaining stenosis was less than 10 percent. It was an excellent result. Harold left the hospital the following day.

Six months after Harold Swanson's angioplasty, in October 1985, Andreas Gruentzig and his wife were killed when the private plane he was flying crashed during a storm in Monroe County, Georgia. He was 46. His colleague, Spencer King, wrote, "He was a dreamer but, unlike most, he dared to act on his dreams. He acted when others would not dare." Like Michel Mirowski, Andreas Gruentzig succeeded because he was a visionary who persisted despite seemingly insurmountable obstacles that would have deterred most people. He was also a scientist who paid exquisite attention to detail and who was willing to teach and mentor his colleagues.

Gruentzig's legacy has endured: coronary angioplasty is an established therapy that doctors perform safely in thousands of patients daily in every major medical center in the world. Angioplasty was successful because Gruentzig's disciples including Richard Myler, Simon Stertzer, Spencer King and many others refined the techniques and subjected them to rigorous examination and scientific study.

The revolution Gruentzig started continued to evolve and it achieved heights no one could have foreseen. The two persistent challenges were the management of abrupt closure and the reappearance of a blockage at the angioplasty site, known as *restenosis*. Both are responses to the injury created by inflating the angioplasty balloon in diseased coronary arteries.

Abrupt closure was a grave event that usually happened in the catheterization laboratory; emergency bypass surgery was often required to save a patient's life. Restenosis was a delayed phenomenon, and could manifest itself after weeks or years in the form of angina, shortness of breath, profound fatigue or a heart attack. Some patients, like Dolph Bachmann, had no evidence of restenosis, even decades after their angioplasty. Others, however, suffered recurrent restenosis and were "frequent flyers" in the catheterization laboratory. These two challenges stimulated intense basic and clinical research and technology development that has continued well into 21st Century.

Harold Swanson returned to work within a week after his angioplasty. Despite every effort, including diet, exercise, and as much cholestyramine (Questran®) as he could tolerate, Harold's cholesterol remained above 300. While bypass surgery and angioplasty had restored blood flow and relieved his angina, the cholesterol in Harold's blood continued to feed the inflammatory process associated with progressive coronary artery disease. No longer did we view plaque build-up as a physical or anatomic phenomenon. It was a sequence of biochemical reactions that corrupted the artery's layers and destroyed friendly molecules. The thin sullied tissue that comprised the artery's inner lining was stripped of its normal defenses, creating a fertile breeding ground for inflammation, clot formation, and thrombosis.

Providentially, 1985 was the year when the controversy surrounding cholesterol's role in atherosclerosis was approaching resolution. A large clinical trial, sponsored by the National Institutes of Health, finally demonstrated that lowering cholesterol helped patients who had coronary heart disease.

CHAPTER 11

We learned during a century of population studies that cholesterol promotes the development of coronary artery disease, and lowering cholesterol benefits patients. Diets low in cholesterol and saturated fats are helpful but diet alone often does not adequately lower blood cholesterol for many patients. Harold Swanson was particularly vulnerable because he had very high cholesterol, and there were millions of patients like him.

The problem was the absence of a highly effective drug that lowers cholesterol and has few side effects. The pharmaceutical company Merck developed cholestyramine in the late 1950s; it is a powder that is taken by mouth several times a day and lowers cholesterol by acting in the intestine to bind bile acids and excrete them in the stool. The liver thus has to manufacture more bile acids and it does this by removing cholesterol from the blood. Consequently, blood cholesterol levels fall. The problem for Harold Swanson and many other patients was that it caused severe constipation. Few people can take all the necessary doses.

The quest for a more effective and tolerable drug began in earnest during the 1960s after two German-born biochemists, Konrad Bloch and Feodor Lynen, discovered how the body made cholesterol. In 1964, they received the Nobel Prize for their work. The challenge was to find a well-tolerated drug that could interrupt this natural pathway without doing harm. The discovery of such a drug occurred in an unlikely place, and it became the most important advance in the prevention and treatment of atherosclerosis in the 20th Century.

Akira Endo was born in 1933 on a farm in Akita, Japan. It is a mountainous region in northern Honshu famous for its rice and sake breweries. Growing up, Endo's grandfather spawned his interest in molds.

Endo was inspired by Alexander Fleming's discovery of penicillin. In 1928, Fleming returned from holiday to his laboratory at Saint Mary's hospital in

London. To his dismay, he found that a rare mold called *Penicillium notatum* had contaminated one of his *Staphylococcus* bacterial cultures. Fleming could have thrown the cultures away, but instead he noticed a zone around the blue-green mold that was free of the bacteria. It was one of those mystical moments in medicine: Fleming deduced that the mold was secreting a substance that inhibited bacterial growth. He was correct: the substance, penicillin, later transformed the treatment of bacterial infections and launched the antibiotic era.

Endo pursued a career in research and he earned a PhD in biochemistry from Tohoku University. After graduation, he went to work for Sankyo, a Tokyo-based pharmaceutical company. There he studied fungi in search of an enzyme to make fruit juice less pulpy. After searching more than 250 species of mold, he found an enzyme that worked. Sankyo rewarded Endo by sending him to the Albert Einstein College of Medicine in New York to study under the great biochemist, Bernard Horecker.

While living in New York, Endo was dismayed by the number of his neighbors who were dying of heart attacks. He was interested in cholesterol because population studies showed that the incidence of heart attacks rose with increasing levels of cholesterol. He also knew that Konrad Bloch and Feodor Lynen had worked out the biochemical pathway through which the body synthesized cholesterol.

The critical step in this pathway was *HMG coenzyme A reductase*. Remembering Fleming's discovery of penicillin, Endo asked himself: Is there a mold that produces a substance that will inhibit HMG coenzyme A reductase? Endo was looking for a penicillin equivalent that could treat high cholesterol. While other scientists experimented with vastly different ways to lower cholesterol levels, Endo turned to nature.

Working in Sankyo Research Laboratories, Endo cultured more than 6000 strains of fungi. His team worked long hours in a dreary laboratory next to a train depot in south Tokyo. He later recalled, "We were doing grunt work every day until we got sick of it." After a year, he found a substance called citrinin that inhibited HMG coenzyme A reductase and lowered cholesterol levels in rats. Regrettably, citrinin turned out to be toxic to the kidneys and Endo had to begin again. "The experience with citrinin gave us hope and courage that we might be able to discover much better active substances in the future," Endo later wrote.

In 1972, Endo obtained a sample of rice at a grain store in Kyoto, a beautiful and historical city south of Tokyo. From the sample, he isolated a blue-green mold, *Penicillium citrinum*, which contaminates fruit including melons and oranges. It took a year of experimentation for Endo's team to extract a compound from the mold that they named *compactin*. Further work showed that compactin was an extremely potent inhibitor of HMG coenzyme A reductase. Endo had discovered the very first statin.

"I had set my sights on finding a competitive inhibitor of HMG coenzyme A reductase, and compactin seemed to be a wonderful gift from nature," he said about the discovery in 1973. It was also the second gift from the genus *Penicillium* to the species *Homo sapiens*.

Endo was disappointed when studies suggested that compactin did not appear to lower cholesterol in rats. He could have given up, but he spent the next two years figuring out how compactin worked and why it was ineffective in rats. It turned out that rats have very low levels of LDL—low-density lipoprotein—and high levels of HDL—high-density lipoprotein. Compactin worked to lower the LDL, but not the HDL, so the total cholesterol in rats was not significantly affected. LDL is the "bad cholesterol," a lipoprotein responsible for causing plaque build-up in the coronary arteries. HDL is the "good cholesterol" because it removes LDL from the circulation. Compactin did exactly what it needed to do: reduce the bad cholesterol—LDL—while leaving HDL, the good cholesterol, alone. Never mind the rats.

Endo gave compactin to hens, dogs, and monkeys. In these animals, compactin proved to be a strong cholesterol-lowering agent, and in 1976, Sankyo decided to launch a project aimed at developing compactin for humans. This winding road had another detour for Endo. A toxicology study seemed to show that compactin caused strange deposits in the liver cells of rats. The deposits turned out to be bogus, but Endo had lost another nine months.

In 1978, Endo secretly arranged a human study on his own at the University of Osaka where Dr. Akira Yamamoto found that compactin lowered cholesterol by an average of 27 percent in patients who inherited genes that caused severe hypercholesterolemia and atherosclerosis. By this time, Endo was communicating with two American scientists, Drs. Michael Brown and Joseph Goldstein, at the University of Texas Southwestern Medical Center in Dallas. The three of them—Endo, Brown, and Goldstein—published a paper describing the effects of compactin on HMG coenzyme A reductase. It was the first paper on a statin published outside Japan, and Brown and Goldstein sent it to Dr. Roy Vagelos, head of research at Merck, Sharp, & Dohme, the giant pharmaceutical company.

Merck already knew of Endo's work. In fact, Merck had signed a one-page confidentiality agreement with Sankyo in 1976 and obtained samples of compactin. Studies by Merck's scientists confirmed Endo's discoveries and they used his methods to create its own statin drug from the fungus *Aspergillus terreus*. Merck named the drug lovastatin. Around the same time Endo also discovered lovastatin, which he derived from *Monascus ruber*, a fungus used to make rice wine and red rice.

As Roy Vagelos wrote in his book, *Medicine, Science, and Merck*, lovastatin created a lot of excitement. Vagelos was the son of Greek immigrants who ran a luncheonette and ice cream factory in Westfield, New Jersey. As a youngster, Vagelos worked in the luncheonette and listened to many of the Merck scientists who ate there during their noon break. Vagelos majored in chemistry at the University of Pennsylvania and graduated from the Columbia College of Physicians and Surgeons in 1954. While interning at Massachusetts General Hospital, the head nurse told Vagelos that he should look into a fellowship at the National Institutes of Health (NIH) where her fiancé worked.

Vagelos flew to the NIH and met Earl Stadtman, a PhD biochemist, who was doing leading edge basic science research on enzyme molecules. "I've never taken on an M.D. as a postdoctoral fellow," Stadtman told Vagelos. In his soft-spoken way Stadtman explained his research in fatty acid metabolism and Vagelos became increasingly excited. Stadtman saw something special in Vagelos. He took him on and Vagelos' career began its shift from medicine to biochemistry.

Stadtman allowed Vagelos to work independently and never tried to control him or take ownership of his work. "He was a wonderful developer of young people, very loyal and supportive," Vagelos said. Many of Stadtman's trainees became renowned academic biochemists and one became a Nobel Laureate.

Vagelos had clinical duties in the cardiology department at the NIH, but his basic science research became his passion under Stadtman. Eventually, Vagelos had his own NIH research laboratory. In 1959, he brought in Al Alberts, a top scientist from the University of Maryland and the two men, whose personalities were quite different, began a highly productive decades-long collaboration.

Vagelos moved from the NIH to St. Louis in 1965 where he became Chairman of Biochemistry at Washington University Medical School. His basic research increasingly focused on the metabolism of fats and cholesterol. In 1974, he received a call from a vice president in Merck Research Laboratories (MRL). Merck had decided to make fundamental changes in its research strategy and wanted Vagelos to head up the transformation. Vagelos took the job and initiated a process focused on developing drugs to inhibit critical enzymes, including HMG coenzyme A reductase. Two years later in 1976, Merck signed its confidentiality agreement with Sankyo and Merck received Sankyo's samples of compactin.

Based on Akira Endo's work and the results of Merck's own basic research, the statins appeared to be potent cholesterol lowering agents and they were not toxic to laboratory animals. They were ready for human trials. By 1980, Merck's early clinical trial results were very promising: lovastatin dramatically reduced cholesterol levels, especially LDL—the bad stuff. No other drug had even come close, and lovastatin's side effects were minimal and acceptable. Vagelos thought Merck had a blockbuster drug ready for a multibillion-dollar market. They even had a brand name ready—Mevacor®.

During Mevacor®'s early clinical trial, Vagelos took a phone call from one of Merck's executives in Japan. He said Sankyo had shut down its own clinical trial of compactin because it appeared to cause tumors in animals. "This news was devastating," Vagelos wrote, "We knew that the Sankyo drug and Mevacor® functioned through the same mechanism of action: both blocked the enzyme HMG coenzyme A reductase. If compactin caused tumors through its activity as a HMG coenzyme A reductase inhibitor, then all drugs inhibiting that enzyme were likely to be toxic as well. We had no way of knowing."

Vagelos did the right thing: he shut down Mevacor®'s clinical trial and informed the FDA. "We couldn't allow anyone to use our compound if there was the slightest possibility it might be carcinogenic," Vagelos wrote. He also called Sankyo, but the Japanese company refused to give him any information, claiming industrial secrets. Vagelos offered to share Mevacor® with Sankyo and to include them in the development of the next generation statin. However, Sankyo declined, repeatedly, even though the issue had enormous implications for millions of patients. The reason for Sankyo's obstinacy remains a mystery.

Vagelos launched extensive toxicology tests in animals and initiated a search for another statin. Meanwhile the physicians who had participated in Mevacor's clinical trial were concerned and impatient. High cholesterol was killing their patients and the NIH cholesterol study using cholestyramine had shown that for every percentage point reduction in cholesterol, there was a two-percentage-point drop in heart attack risk. The physicians felt Mevacor® was a far better cholesterol drug than cholestyramine: it had lowered total cholesterol 18 to 34 percent. They exhorted Vagelos to resume Mevacor®'s clinical trial.

By 1983 Merck's animal studies showed that Mevacor® did not cause cancerous tumors. Meanwhile, Joseph Goldstein, who together with Michael Brown had collaborated with Akira Endo, spoke with Endo during a trip to Tokyo. Endo was convinced that compactin, like Mevacor®, had not caused tumors at all; rather, he believed Sankyo's pathologists had misinterpreted the specimens because the dye they used had stained an innocent cell membrane and not a malignancy. In other words, Sankyo's scientists got it wrong. Merck's own research and Endo's insight debunked the tumor scare and Vagelos resumed Mevacor®'s clinical trial.

The FDA approved Mevacor® in 1987. Soon thereafter Harold Swanson started taking the maximum dose. After three months, Harold's total cholesterol had fallen to 218 and his LDL was 128—not ideal but a major improvement. Merck had another statin—simvastatin--in clinical trials. In fact, Merck's chemists developed simvastatin as a direct result of the Sankyo tumor scare.

Simvastatin was studied in a groundbreaking clinical trial at 94 centers in Scandinavia involving 4,444 patients who had a history of coronary heart disease manifested by angina or a previous heart attack. Half the patients received simvastatin and half received a placebo. When the results were published in 1992, not only did simvastatin reduce coronary deaths but it also decreased death from any cause. There were over 40 percent fewer coronary deaths in the simvastatin treated patients over five years. Also, the patients who took simvastatin had fewer heart attacks and required fewer coronary bypass surgeries and angioplasties.

The simvastatin study was a victory with enormous implications for preventing the deadly effects of hypercholesterolemia—high cholesterol—in millions of patients like Harold Swanson. It was also a milestone in cardiology because it underscored the value of large randomized clinical trials that provided the evidence needed to guide appropriate therapy in high-risk populations.

A key question lingered: would a statin reduce death and heart attacks in people who had high cholesterol but no history of a heart attack? Seven thousand such men in Scotland were given pravastatin * or a placebo at random and they were followed for five years. The pravastatin patients experienced over 30 percent fewer deaths and heart attacks. These results, reported in 1995, showed that lowering cholesterol with a statin saved lives even in patients who had high cholesterol but no evidence of a prior heart attack. At last, we had a class of drugs that could extend life and prevent heart attacks—and we had the data to prove it. That is, at least in men. Women were not included in these trials because, at that time, we were blind to gender differences.

The FDA approved simvastatin in 1992 and Merck marketed it under the name Zocor®. Harold Swanson was treated with Zocor® and his bad LDL declined to less than 100. Eventually stronger statins were produced, including atorvastatin (Lipitor®) and rosuvastatin (Crestor®). By 2012, 28 percent of Americans—about 11 million people—over age 40 were taking a cholesterol-lowering drug and 93 percent of them were taking a statin. Drugs like cholestyramine were reserved for the low percentage of patients who experienced serious side effects on statins.

In 1985, Michael Brown and Joseph Goldstein received the Nobel Prize for their discoveries focused on the regulation of cholesterol. In 2004, these Nobel Laureates wrote:

"None of this [statins] would have happened if Akira Endo had not conducted his relentless search for a fungal product that would

inhibit cholesterol synthesis, and if he had not shown convincingly that ML-236B [compactin] inhibits HMG coenzyme A reductase. Without Endo, the statins might never have been discovered, and without Alberts, Vagelos, and Scolnick at Merck, statins might never have become approved drugs…The millions of people whose lives will be extended through statin therapy owe it all to Akira Endo and his search through fungal extracts at the Sankyo Co."

In 2008 Akira Endo received the prestigious Lasker-DeBakey Medical Research Award for his discovery of statins.

Drugs that reduce cholesterol and blood pressure and control glucose (sugar) levels have improved outcomes in patients with cardiovascular disease. Still, drugs are not a substitute for healthy living that combines a nutritious diet with daily exercise and abstinence from tobacco. Yet we as a society have not embraced common sense healthy living as a national strategic health objective despite its obvious benefits. Not that government and many non-profit organizations have not tried: they have, spending millions of dollars on prevention, public education campaigns, and school programs.

In 2009, Dr. Kevin Graham at the Minneapolis Heart Institute™ boldly asked: Is it possible to reduce death and disability caused by heart disease in a community through a focused and sustained effort to improve the health habits of its citizens? Together with the Minneapolis Heart Institute Foundation (MHIF) and Allina Health, he approached community leaders and physicians in New Ulm, a Minnesota town 100 miles southwest of the Twin Cities. New Ulm was known for its beer and brats, and coronary artery disease was prevalent amongst its 8,000 citizens.

Graham asked New Ulm to join with him and MHIF/Allina Health to promote healthy living with the 10-year goal of reducing the number of heart attacks and deaths due to cardiovascular disease. The community agreed, enthusiastically, and New Ulm formed its heart healthy program called "Hearts Beat Back™."

In 2016, "Hearts Beat Back™" can boast of many accomplishments, including reductions in blood pressure and cholesterol, especially in its citizens who are at highest risk for heart attacks and strokes. New Ulm restaurants and grocery stores have added and improved their choices of healthy foods. Recreational exercise programs have been created where previously none had existed. More people are taking aspirin appropriately for preventive purposes. Neighbors are encouraging each other to forego the burgers and brats and see their health care providers for annual preventive check-ups.

It is too soon to know if heart attacks or coronary deaths have been reduced in New Ulm, but at a minimum "Hearts Beat Back™" can claim that its participants feel and look better. Preventing heart disease is cardiology's holy grail, and community efforts like the one in New Ulm could shorten the journey.

CHAPTER 12

I met Helen Robertson, age 50, at 2 a.m. on a Sunday morning in November 1992. Her husband brought her to the Abbott Northwestern's emergency room after she awoke from sleep with a vague fullness in her upper abdomen. She was nauseated and had a little diarrhea. Her EKG and blood tests were normal. Helen's husband thought a cardiologist should see her, and I was awakened in the hospital's on-call room. The emergency room doctor was apologetic. He said Helen probably had gastroenteritis, but her worried spouse asked for a cardiologist.

Mrs. Robertson rested on a gurney in the emergency room. Her husband, Jim, sat on a folding chair beside her. Both of them looked like most of us do in the middle of the night: hair mussed, eyelids at half-mast, and a little crabby. I introduced myself and delved into her symptoms. Helen had been tired for several weeks, but nothing remarkable had happened until the previous evening when she became short of breath as she took out the garbage. "How heavy was the garbage bag?" I asked.

"We have a trash compactor, so it was heavy," she said. "Jim usually does it but he was in the basement doing something else." She looked at her husband, a little irritated.

"Then what happened?"

"I went to bed—I was so tired that I didn't hear Jim when he came to bed."

"It was around midnight I guess," Jim offered. "I lay there about ten minutes when Helen woke up complaining of pressure in her stomach."

Helen continued: "That's when I got up, went to the bathroom, and had some diarrhea. Now I'm just tired, washed out, but no pain anywhere."

Helen had high blood pressure and diabetes for five or six years; both were supposedly under good control. She stopped smoking cigarettes with her first pregnancy. Her grandmother had died of a heart valve problem and both of her parents died of cancer. Helen did not know her cholesterol levels, but said her primary physician indicated they were "okay". Helen had completed menopause and was taking an estrogen pill.

Mrs. Robertson's vital signs (heart rate, blood pressure, respiratory rate, temperature, oxygen saturation) were normal. She was a little overweight and looked her age, and indeed appeared quite fatigued even for three o'clock in the morning. There was nothing else unusual—her lungs were clear, she had no abnormal heart sounds, her belly was soft and her legs and calves were not swollen or tender. I reviewed the EKG taken shortly after midnight when Helen arrived: it showed some minor abnormalities. Nothing suggested a heart attack.

I told Helen and her husband that I wanted another EKG and left the exam room. "What do you think of Mrs. Robertson?" the emergency room doctor asked me in the charting area. "She has two risk factors for coronary artery disease—hypertension and diabetes," I said, "and her physical exam, EKG, and blood tests are normal. The fatigue and recent shortness of breath are concerning. We should repeat her EKG."

I left the emergency room and checked on a patient in the surgical intensive care unit. When I returned, the emergency room doctor handed me Helen Robertson's second EKG. It was no longer normal: the "T-waves" had flipped and were pointing downward. I looked up and said, "Let's get another set of [heart] enzymes." He asked, "Do you want to admit her? She's been here for four hours."

"Let's put her on Station 44," I said and paged the cardiology technician to come in from her home and do an echocardiogram. I wanted to know how her heart was functioning.

After explaining my plan to the Robertsons, I went back to the on-call room, hoping to get some sleep. It was not to be. First, I received a page to call the emergency room in Hutchinson, Minnesota, a town 70 miles west of Minneapolis. A 69-year-old man was having a classic heart attack—an acute inferior wall myocardial infarction—and had received tPA, a new thrombolytic agent (clot buster). They wanted to transfer him for further management. I called Station 45, the cardiac intensive care unit, and told the charge nurse to expect a patient arriving by ambulance from Hutchinson in several hours.

I hung up the phone and closed my eyes. Five minutes later, the phone rang. It was Darla Schmidt, the senior echo technician who had finished Helen Robertson's echocardiogram. She sounded concerned. "The echo shows that this lady's anterior wall is not moving," she said. "The nurse said her blood pressure is low and you need to see her. She's doing another EKG."

Ten minutes later, I was on Station 44. Helen Robertson was pale. Her husband was standing at the bedside holding her hand. "She's not feeling too good, doctor," he whispered.

The nurse handed me the new EKG. Now it showed a typical heart attack affecting the front side of her main pumping chamber that was supplied by her left anterior descending coronary artery. Helen was quietly staring at the ceiling lights above her.

The nurse said, "Her blood pressure is 68."

She was in shock. I started levophed to increase her blood pressure, and asked the nurse to page Dr. Jim Madison, the on-call interventional cardiologist.

Madison was at home in White Bear Lake, a suburb 20 miles northeast of the hospital. I told him about Mrs. Robertson. Our choices were to give her intravenous tPA, the clot buster, or perform immediate angioplasty. Angioplasty would be the most certain way to get her blocked artery open quickly. Madison said he could be at the hospital in a half hour and asked me to call in the catheterization laboratory team. Meanwhile, I gave Helen aspirin and started intravenous heparin, a blood thinner.

Thirty minutes later, Helen was on the X-ray table in the catheterization laboratory. She was barely responsive and breathing oxygen from a two-pronged plastic cannula in her nose. The circulating nurse shaved her right groin and the scrub nurse was preparing the angiogram catheters. A technician entered with an intra-aortic balloon console in case we needed it to support her circulation. Madison scrubbed at the sink outside the room. I sat next to the radiology technician behind a leaded window that shielded us from radiation.

Jim Madison was director of the catheterization laboratory and an experienced interventional cardiologist, a new subspecialty devoted to coronary angioplasty. In 1992, the angioplasty balloon catheters were smaller and more steerable than the ones available to Gruentzig and his colleagues in the 1980s.

My pager beeped. The patient from Hutchinson had arrived. His chest discomfort was minimal and the EKG indicated that the thrombolytic agent—tPA—had dissolved the clot obstructing his coronary artery. We could expect ventricular arrhythmias when blood began flowing to his oxygen-deprived heart muscle. I asked the nurse to give him metoprolol, a beta-blocker, intravenously; it would help prevent ventricular fibrillation.

Madison anesthetized Helen Robertson's groin area and quickly inserted a plastic sheath into the femoral artery. Using the fluoroscope, he placed a thin wire through the sheath and guided it up to the arch of the aorta in her chest. Next, he placed an angiogram catheter over the wire and advanced it to the tip of the wire. He removed the wire, allowing it to take its preformed shape, and aspirated any residual air into a syringe. He then flushed the catheter with heparinized saline to prevent clots from forming in the catheter.

Dr. Melvin Judkins developed the catheter that Madison was using to perform Mrs. Robertson's angiogram. Judkins was a farm boy from southern California, who became a radiologist at the University of Oregon in Portland. In 1965, he studied radiology at the University of Lund in Sweden, where he developed a method to pre-shape angiography catheters. Upon returning to Portland, Dr. Albert Starr wanted coronary angiograms in all of his patients over age 50 who were having heart valve surgery.

Judkins accepted the challenge and he soon developed pre-formed catheters for coronary angiography that could be inserted rapidly from the femoral artery. They were effective and easy to use. The user-friendly Judkins technique largely displaced the catheters created by Dr. Mason Sones, and they remain in use today.

Helen was mildly sedated and unaware of what was happening. Madison slid the catheter into her left coronary artery and injected X-ray dye. I watched the X-ray monitor as the dark dye filled the left main coronary artery. What I saw astounded me. Her left main coronary was almost completely blocked.

Madison looked at me through the glass and said what I already knew: "Get a surgeon—fast."

Helen Robertson needed emergency coronary bypass surgery. I picked up the phone and called the cardiac surgery answering service. Dr. Frazier Eales would come directly to the catheterization laboratory. Meanwhile Madison exchanged catheters and injected dye into her right coronary artery; it was normal and we could see dye from the right coronary artery filling the left anterior descending coronary via small channels called collaterals—it appeared to be free of plaque, a good sign.

Madison asked for an intra-aortic balloon (IAB) and a Swan-Ganz™ catheter. The IAB would support Helen's blood pressure and make it easier for her damaged left ventricle to pump blood. The Swan-Ganz™ catheter, inserted via the right internal jugular vein, would monitor the pressures inside her heart and measure the amount of blood her heart was pumping. It was invented by Drs. Jeremy Swan and William Ganz. Swan, a charismatic cardiologist from Ireland, trained at the Mayo Clinic before becoming Chief of Cardiology at Cedars-Sinai in Los Angeles where Ganz also practiced. In 1970, they fashioned an inflatable balloon on the tip of a flexible catheter so it would float easily through the right side of the heart into the pulmonary artery without X-ray guidance.

Frazier Eales arrived at the catheterization laboratory. He was a highly skilled surgeon who communicated well with patients. Born in Minnesota, he was tall, an amateur pilot, and president-elect of the hospital medical staff. We were glad to see him. "What's going on?" he asked. I showed him the angiogram while relating Helen's history. "The echo shows what you might expect: the anterior wall is not contracting and the ejection fraction is about 20 percent," I said.

"Okay," Eales said. "I'll get the operating room ready. Is there family?"

I replied, "Her husband, Jim. He's in the waiting room. I'll speak to him and tell him to stay there until you can see him."

Jim Robertson looked up anxiously when I entered the small consult room inside the visitor waiting area. It was a comfortable room that allowed doctors to speak to families privately. I sat next to him on the couch and took a printed diagram of the heart and coronary arteries out of the pocket of my white lab coat.

"Mr. Robertson," I said after sitting next to him on the couch, "Doctor Madison found a severe blockage at the beginning of your wife's left coronary artery." I drew a black dot on the diagram. "The two main arteries beyond this blockage look okay and the right coronary artery is completely normal. The front of her heart—it's called the anterior wall—is not receiving enough blood, and this has weakened its pumping function."

I paused to let this sink in—he was tired and distraught and needed time to focus. He asked, "Could she die?"

I replied, "She's in shock. It's very serious. We need to operate right away." He said nothing. I continued," Dr. Eales is a very experienced heart surgeon. He's getting the operating room ready now. He will bypass her blockage. We need your permission to operate."

"What if you don't operate? Can't you treat her with drugs? What about the balloon I hear so much about?"

"Surgery is her best chance. Balloon angioplasty in situations like this has not proven very successful. In fact, it's quite risky."

"Well, I just talked to my daughter—she's in Chicago—she said you people have a good reputation. I guess you better go ahead."

He looked down at the floor for a few seconds, and then said, "You know, doc, she never had any chest pain. I thought people who had heart attacks had chest pain, or were short of breath, or—something. She didn't have anything except stomach pressure and diarrhea!"

If Dr. Nanette Wenger had been sitting there, she could have explained why we were missing coronary artery disease in women, and why many women had died as a result of our ignorance.

The mortality rate due to coronary artery disease for men steadily declined during the latter half of the 20th century. It did not change for women. Beginning in the mid-1980s, more women were dying each year of heart disease than men. A woman under 65 was twice as likely to die after a heart attack than a man. How could this be? I was taught that angina—heart pain—was relatively benign in women. I was also taught that women have far fewer heart attacks than men. My generation of cardiologists believed that coronary artery disease was largely a male problem. We held this tragically mistaken belief until Nanette Wenger and her colleagues got our attention and showed us how wrong we were.

When I attended Nanette Wenger's lectures, I always learned something new or acquired a fresh view of something old. She has written so many articles and book chapters during her 55 years as a physician and cardiologist that it is impossible to encapsulate the breadth of her writing in a paragraph. Nanette Wenger never fails to secure your interest with articles entitled: *Alice in Lipidland, Women and Coronary Heart Disease: Understudied, Underdiagnosed, and Untreated, You've Come a Long Way, Baby: Cardiovascular Health and Disease in Women*, and *Transforming Cardiovascular Disease Prevention in Women: Time for the Pygmalion Construct to End.*

The "Pygmalion Construct" refers to Sir George Bernard Shaw's play that became the musical "My Fair Lady." Henry Higgins, a professor of phonetics, wistfully chants, "Why can't a woman be more like a man?" When it came to cardiovascular disease, generations of physicians, including top cardiologists, believed women *were* like men. The squeezing, tight chest pain described by men who were having a heart attack was thought to be the typical symptom in women, too. Except it was not, and an untold number of women died because of this serious misconception.

Many women do experience the characteristic pain or discomfort associated with a heart attack or angina, but many do not, and Helen Robertson was one of them. Were it not for her husband's concern, we could have sent this woman home where she would have died.

Nanette Wenger changed this lethal paradigm with the same relentless determination that was characteristic of other modern medical pioneers. She was born in New York City in 1930 to parents who had immigrated to the United States from Russia. "You can do whatever you want to do," they told her. Neither parent was a physician; her father worked in Jewish resettlement organizations. Her mother, a talented artist, became a homemaker for her husband and two daughters.

Educated in public schools, Wenger graduated summa cum laude from Hunter College and briefly considered a career in constitutional law. However, medicine was a stronger attraction. In 1954, she obtained her medical degree from Harvard where she was one of ten women in her class. In those days, women students were still in a 10-year "probationary" period and not recognized in Harvard's Charter. Wenger and her female classmates even had to live off campus.

Following graduation, she trained in internal medicine and cardiology at Mt. Sinai Hospital in New York City. Dr. Charles K. Friedberg, one of the preeminent cardiologists of his time and author of the textbook, *Diseases of the Heart,* became Wenger's mentor. Nowhere in his third edition, published in 1966, did Friedberg mention gender differences in heart disease except for conditions associated with hormones and pregnancy. His trainee, Nanette Wenger, would change that. Presciently, Friedberg often introduced Wenger to his patients as the "physician who will likely guide the cardiac care of your children and grandchildren."

In 1959, Emory University recruited Wenger's husband, Julius, to head the gastroenterology program at the Veterans Administration Hospital in Atlanta. Nanette left Mt. Sinai and moved to Atlanta where female physicians were uncommon and married women rarely worked. She became Director of the Cardiology Clinics at Grady Memorial Hospital and embarked on a career that would have more bearing on the heart health of women and the elderly than anyone else in her generation.

Wenger combined leadership and scholarship with a single-minded, inclusive approach to herding the human butterflies that populate the medical and scientific communities. As she later wrote: "For many years the medical community viewed women's health with a bikini approach, focusing essentially on the breast and reproductive system. The rest of the woman was virtually ignored in considerations of health: the tacit assumption was that women and men reacted comparably to diseases and drugs."

It took 25 years but women's heart health finally emerged from the darkness in 1992 when Dr. Wenger chaired the National Institutes of Health's conference on heart disease in women. The following year she was the first author of a special article that appeared in the *New England Journal of Medicine* entitled "Cardiovascular Health and Disease in Women." In it, she and her co-authors wrote.

"Each year approximately 2.5 million U.S. women are hospitalized for cardiovascular illness, which also claims the lives of 500,000 women annually; half these deaths are due to coronary heart disease. Despite the magnitude of this problem and its adverse repercussions on the national public health, we have insufficient information about preventive strategies, diagnostic testing, responses to medical surgical therapies, and other aspects of cardiovascular illness in women. This lack of information is compounded by less frequent participation of women in research studies; the difference has been due in part to the exclusion of women of childbearing age and in part the exclusion of elderly women because of their frequent coexisting illnesses."

The result was a dramatic increase in awareness, plus a series of studies and clinical trials that have transformed cardiovascular care in women and debunked several myths. For example, menopausal hormonal therapy does not prevent cardiovascular disease; rather, it increases the risk of stroke. Second, recommendations for preventing, detecting, and treating coronary heart disease in women are based on studies of middle-aged men, obviously demonstrating major knowledge gaps and gender bias. Third, in contrast to men, aspirin does not prevent heart attacks in women under 65, but importantly reduces stroke.

In addition, there were these revelations: complications during pregnancy increase lifetime cardiovascular risk; women are particularly prone to small vessel (microvascular) coronary artery disease; common supplements—vitamins, beta-carotene—are ineffective preventive measures in women; and, women are at higher risk of death during heart attacks than men.

Helen Robertson arrived in the operating room where Frazier Eales and his open-heart team were waiting. The anesthesiologist gave her additional sedation, placed an endotracheal tube in her windpipe and connected it to a respirator. The intra-aortic balloon pump and levophed maintained her systolic blood pressure between 90 and 100. Eales quickly covered Helen with sterile drapes and opened her chest through the breastbone. He placed plastic cannulas in her right atrium and aorta, connected them to the heart-lung machine, and cooled her oxygen-deprived heart.

The first priority was to restore blood flow to her left anterior descending coronary artery that supplied the front (anterior) side of the left ventricle (main pumping chamber). He did this by freeing the left internal mammary artery from the underside of the sternum, cutting it, and suturing the cut end to the anterior descending coronary artery beyond the blockage.

Within 40 minutes of entering the operating room, blood flow was restored to the anterior wall of Helen's left ventricle. Almost immediately, Eales could see improvement in the muscle's color and movement. He then removed a section of saphenous vein from her leg and connected one end to the aorta and the other end to the circumflex coronary artery that supplied blood to the back (posterior wall) of her heart. It was 7:23 a.m. Sunday morning; a little more than 6 hours had passed since she had arrived in our emergency room.

I had more work for Madison and Eales. The heart attack patient from Hutchinson redeveloped chest pain. The EKG showed that his artery was likely blocked again with a clot. Madison performed emergency balloon angioplasty and opened the patient's thrombosed right coronary artery. Then a 48-year-old commercial airline pilot from Eau Claire, a town in western Wisconsin, arrived by air ambulance with a tear in his aorta just above the aortic valve. This aortic tear, known as a dissection, was life threatening. Eales took him immediately to the operating room and repaired it with a synthetic graft made of Dacron™.

Around 3 p.m., Helen Robertson was in the surgical intensive care unit when she developed rapid ventricular tachycardia. A nurse shocked her and I arrived at her bedside minutes later. Helen was sedated and unaware of what had happened. The respirator was controlling her breathing and the intra-aortic balloon pump was augmenting her blood pressure. However, the heart rhythm monitor above the bed showed frequent extra beats—premature ventricular contractions. An EKG revealed nothing new or unexpected. Her blood potassium and magnesium levels were within the normal range and her blood pH and oxygen saturation were satisfactory. I started lidocaine intravenously to suppress the extra beats.

The next morning, I returned at 6:30 a.m., and went directly to the surgical intensive care unit to check on Helen. During the night, she had several brief episodes of ventricular tachycardia but none were prolonged or required a shock. I told her nurse I would return after my morning clinic.

Ten minutes later I heard a Doctor Blue page for Helen's room in the surgical intensive care unit. By the time I ran through the skyway and down the stairs to the ICU, the Doctor Blue team had arrived and shocked Helen twice. For the moment, she was stable. I called the catheterization laboratory and said Mrs. Robertson needed an angiogram as soon as possible: we had to be sure her bypass grafts were functioning. Fifteen minutes later Helen was on her way to the lab and I sat in the family waiting room explaining the situation to her husband.

I watched as Dr. Richard Nelson did the angiogram. Both her internal mammary artery and saphenous vein bypasses were open. "Bob," Nelson said. They're beautiful." I thanked him and ordered amiodarone, a strong drug for treating ventricular tachycardia. Regrettably, in 1992, we did not have the intravenous form. Helen received the drug orally via a nasogastric tube placed through her nose, to her esophagus and into her stomach. I asked for another echocardiogram and headed to the clinic

Helen had no further episodes of ventricular tachycardia. Her heart continued to be irritable for a few days and then settled down. During the next few days, we removed the intra-aortic balloon pump and catheters and transferred Helen to a regular room. The cardiac rehabilitation specialist helped her walk the halls. She took multiple new drugs: aspirin, metoprolol, enalapril, lovastatin, and amiodarone. Amiodarone would be discontinued but the other drugs likely would likely be her regimen for life.

Helen Robertson was discharged from the hospital 13 days after her emergency coronary artery bypass surgery. I followed her in my clinic for the next 23 years, until I retired. Helen was one of my most conscientious patients: she lost weight, exercised daily, took all of her medications, and never missed an appointment. Her heart recovered reasonably well from the heart attack but over the years, despite the medications, her left ventricle gradually enlarged and reshaped itself into a less efficient ball. She remained active with minimal shortness of breath. When I last saw Helen, she and her husband were on their way to St. Louis to visit their daughter and grandchildren.

Nanette Wenger changed the face of cardiology. Her efforts, and those of her co-workers, contributed to the steady decline in cardiovascular disease mortality for women that began in 2000. Today, women are better represented in clinical trials, and medical school curricula and post-graduate training programs teach gender differences in cardiovascular diseases. Nanette Wenger helped her colleagues—male and female—to be better doctors.

CHAPTER 13

I drove to Douglas County Hospital in Alexandria, Minnesota on a cold gray day in February 2001 to see ten patients in the cardiology clinic. This visit was part of our outreach program that brought cardiology consultative care to communities outside the metropolitan area of Minneapolis-St. Paul. Patients, particularly the elderly and disabled, appreciated this service and the demand for it grew every year.

On this particular Monday morning, the 125-mile trip took longer than usual because snow coated Interstate 94. The road between Sauk Centre and Alexandria was especially treacherous because wind gusts off the prairie blew snow onto the highway and concealed sheets of ice. I counted four abandoned cars in a drainage ditch and a tractor-trailer that spun into the median just east of the Alexandria exit.

Douglas County Hospital opened in 1955 and it expanded at least four times to serve this growing resort community in northwest Minnesota. Most of its physicians were graduates of the University of Minnesota and they, like most of Minnesota's rural doctors, were hard working, knowledgeable, and conscientious. Many of the nurses graduated from the University of Minnesota or the College of St. Catherine.

In the lobby, a cheery Auxiliary volunteer greeted me. I sauntered to the north side of hospital where I shared a clinic office with a kidney specialist from St. Cloud. Charts for each of my patients were neatly arranged on my desk. The nurse told me that three patients were ready in their exam rooms.

The first two patients were follow-up visits: a middle-aged construction worker who had recovered nicely after coronary bypass surgery and an elderly woman with severe aortic stenosis, but no symptoms. The third patient, Orin Bergstrom, was a 16-year-old hockey player whose family physician found a heart murmur during a clinic visit for a fever and cough. The physician ordered an echocardiogram and scheduled Orin to see me.

John and Mary Bergstrom sat in the exam room with their son. The Bergstroms owned a farm north of Alexandria and Orin attended the local high school with his two younger sisters. He was a big boy, at least six feet three and he weighed a muscular 237 pounds. His fever and cough had resolved and he was looking forward to the state hockey tournament that would begin in March. Orin played goalie, and the college scouts were already showing interest.

I introduced myself, "Good morning, Orin. I'm Doctor Hauser, one of the heart doctors." Orin stood and shook my hand and introduced me to his parents. I was impressed with the young man's demeanor. His father, John, enclosed my hand in his; he could have crushed it in a second. Mary Bergstrom had blonde hair, a pretty face, and was still wearing her brown winter parka.

"My doctor," Orin began, "heard a heart murmur when I was in here for a cough. I had this heart test—an echocardiogram I think... and he wanted me to see you before the hockey tournament begins. I play goalie."

There was nothing alarming in Orin's medical history and he denied any symptoms suggestive of heart disease. His parents were healthy and both sets of grandparents were living. No relative had a heart condition, and none had died suddenly. Hopefully, I would find an innocent heart murmur and the echocardiogram would be normal.

His heart murmur was loud—grade 3 out of 6—and the intensity increased when I asked him to squeeze my fingers.

"Orin," I said, looking from him to his parents, "I heard the murmur. We should find out what's causing it. I'm going to ask the nurse to do an EKG while I go to the laboratory down the hall to review the echocardiogram."

Orin and his father nodded. His mother asked, "Do you think it could be serious?"

"The echocardiogram will be helpful," I replied. "We need a diagnosis. Sometimes these murmurs are of little concern. On the other hand, yes, it may be serious."

I reviewed the echocardiogram with Dr. Ron Verant, an internist who had developed special expertise in echocardiography. The echo was distinctly abnormal and characteristic of an inherited condition called hypertrophic cardiomyopathy. It is a relatively rare disorder, but it is the most common cause of sudden cardiac death in competitive athletes, particularly basketball and hockey players, like Orin Bergstrom.

I returned to the exam room and sat down with Orin and his parents.

I looked directly at Orin but made sure I had eye contact with both parents. "The echocardiogram shows that you have a thickening of you heart muscle. It is probably a condition called hypertrophic cardiomyopathy. We call it HCM for short. It tends to run in families but there is no one that we know of in your family who might have had this problem or died suddenly. Is that correct?"

Mary looked at her husband who shook his head. "No, we're third generation Norwegian, and no relatives has had a heart problem."

Orin, who had been silent, leaned forward in his chair and rested his elbows on his knees. "This could be serious, is that right, doctor?" he asked.

"Yes, it could be, Orin" I replied, "but let's not get ahead of ourselves. We need more tests, and I want you to see Doctor Barry Maron at the Minneapolis Heart Institute. Doctor Maron has spent all of his professional life studying this disease and he has become one of the world's experts." Then I said precisely what Orin did not want to hear, "You should stop any strenuous physical activity until we know more. That means no hockey…I'm sorry."

Orin asked the logical question, "Why?"

"Hypertrophic cardiomyopathy can cause sudden death, particularly during very strenuous exercise, and in young men like yourself. We will know your risk after the tests are completed in Minneapolis. You will have a stress test and MRI of your heart. Then you will meet with Dr. Maron, and he will make a recommendation."

I paused. The room was silent. The Bergstrom family was not prepared to hear what I had just told them. Continuing on I said, "One possibility is you may need an implantable defibrillator." I explained the ICD and how it was implanted.

Lastly, John Bergstrom asked, "What did that EKG show?"

"It's typical of hypertrophic cardiomyopathy," I replied. "I don't think there is much doubt about the diagnosis."

Hypertrophic cardiomyopathy (HCM) was the most complex, diverse, and unpredictable cardiac disorder that I encountered in my adult cardiology practice.

The disease is passed from generation to generation as a dominant trait and it is characterized by marked thickening of the heart muscle, particularly the ventricular septum—the wall between the lower pumping chambers.

HCM affects one in 500 or about 15 million people worldwide. I have seen HCM in teenagers, like Orin Bergstrom, and nonagenarians. It may be silent and innocuous, mildly symptomatic, or progressively debilitating due to angina and severe heart failure. The thickened muscle can obstruct blood flow, producing shortness of breath with activity, blackout spells, and chest pain. It may cause ventricular fibrillation or rapid ventricular tachycardia, and so is potentially lethal. HCM patients who die suddenly are frequently young and often their heart disease was never detected or diagnosed.

Dr. Barry J. Maron devoted his life to the study of HCM, a condition that was practically unknown until the 1960s when Dr. Eugene Braunwald and Dr. Andrew Glenn Morrow at the National Institutes of Health (NIH) described new treatments for the disease. Maron was born in 1941, the third child of immigrants from Belarus and Latvia. He grew up in West Los Angeles and graduated from Occidental College in 1963. While attending Tulane University School of Medicine he became interested in cardiology and completed his pediatric cardiology training at Johns Hopkins in 1972.

The academic environment at Hopkins stimulated Maron's natural curiosity and penchant for research. After joining the NIH, he used echocardiography to study every facet of HCM. During 21 years in the NIH cardiology branch, he authored hundreds of scientific papers and established an international network of physicians and scientists who had a special interest in HCM.

Drs. Fred Gobel and Bob Van Tassel recruited Maron to the Minneapolis Heart Institute Foundation (MHIF) in 1992 where he became the director of the Hypertrophic Cardiomyopathy Center. Generous community donors and a few grateful patients and their families funded the Center. During the next three decades, Maron evaluated and treated hundreds of patients from around the world. Each one underwent a series of sophisticated tests to establish the diagnosis.

Maron's principal contribution was his discovery of the risk factors that predict sudden cardiac death in HCM patients. With this knowledge, Maron and his colleagues have been able to quantify the value of the implantable defibrillator for preventing these awful events and thousands of patients—mostly young adults—have been saved. If sudden death can be prevented, most HCM patients will suffer little or no disability, and they will enjoy a normal life span.

Two weeks later Orin Bergstrom's parents and sisters accompanied him to the Hypertrophic Cardiomyopathy Center at the Minneapolis Heart Institute. Maron's nurse, Sue Casey, gathered more information, including details of the family's heart history. Then Orin had another echocardiogram to acquire specific views of his heart that Maron would want to see. This was followed by a treadmill exercise test with echocardiographic imaging during and immediately after exercise. Orin was in excellent physical condition, and ran on the treadmill at increasing speeds and elevations for 16 minutes.

Afterward I met with Maron and his team. Orin's echocardiogram showed marked thickening of his septum, but it did not obstruct his blood flow at rest or during exercise. During exercise, however, Orin had three brief episodes of rapid ventricular tachycardia (VT). This was very concerning. We showed the exercise EKGs to Dr. Adrian Almquist, a cardiac electrophysiologist, and he agreed that the rapid rhythm was VT.

Maron, Almquist, Sue Casey and myself sat in the small clinic conference room and discussed the recommendations we were going to make to the Bergstroms. There was no worrisome family history and Orin, at 16, was a star athlete on his high school's hockey team. Yet he had HCM and, based on Maron's research, and Orin's tests that day, this young star hockey player was at high risk for sudden cardiac death.

The only fail-safe, preventive measure was an implantable defibrillator, an ICD that Orin would have for the rest of his life. No one, especially a 16-year-old, wants a device implanted where it can be seen or felt. Every five or six years the battery must be replaced, and in time the wires can wear out and require another surgery. Orin could not participate in a contact sport like hockey where the defibrillator or wires might be damaged. He would have to sit on the sidelines with a machine inside his body, watching his teammates.

The three us of us agreed: Orin should have an implantable defibrillator. Maron, Sue Casey, and I walked down the hall to the exam room where the Bergstrom family waited. Almquist would see Orin later if the Bergstroms accepted our recommendation.

Maron entered the small windowless exam room first and introduced himself. I shook hands with Orin and his father and greeted his mother and two sisters. All of us sat on folding chairs.

"Let's begin with the good news," Maron said, looking directly at Orin. "Very good news, actually. Your heart is functioning well. The pump, the left ventricle, is squeezing normally and there is no significant obstruction to blood flow out of your heart. You do have hypertrophic cardiomyopathy, though. There is no question about that. It is a thickening of the muscle, but the thickening is not affecting your heart's pumping function, and the valves are perfectly normal."

Maron paused and asked, "Are you following me okay?" Orin replied, "Yes, sir." Maron looked to his parents who nodded in agreement.

"You indicated that was the good news," Mary Bergstrom said. "I assume there is, ah, not-so-good news?"

Maron had a yellow legal pad in his lap. He flipped a page and replied, "Orin's heart muscle is quite thick—about an inch—27 millimeters to be exact. That is more than we usually see. In addition, when Orin was exercising on the treadmill he had several short episodes of a rhythm called ventricular tachycardia. These were very fast heartbeats from the bottom part of Orin's heart—the main pumping chambers. The rate was more than two hundred beats per minute. If this rapid heart beating had gone on for more than a few seconds, Orin would have felt weak and, if it continued, he would blackout...."

"And could he die?" Mary Bergstrom interrupted. She looked anxiously at her son and then to me and back to Maron.

"That's possible, Mrs. Bergstrom," Maron responded.

"But I have never felt anything like that..." Orin said.

His sister, Amy, interrupted, "Yes, you have, Orin. Remember last summer when you almost fainted playing basketball. You had to hold on to the chain-link fence."

"It was just hot that day," Orin objected. "I was dehydrated."

"I was there, Orin, it wasn't that hot and you looked awful."

I asked Orin if he had any other spells like this, and whether his vision had been affected. He shook his head and said, "No, sir."

Maron continued. "So Orin, we need to talk about what this means." He paused, not wanting to appear hurried or unfeeling. He had done this so many times, and it was never routine, never easy. "There is a risk that you could die suddenly." All the Bergstroms stopped breathing, for seconds, then Maron said, "But there is a way to prevent it, and you can have a normal life."

John Bergstrom had farmed all of his life. Once he lost all of his hogs to brucellosis. Another year, one of the worst droughts in Minnesota history devastated his corn and soybean crops. His brother died when his tractor flipped and crushed him. Life held these setbacks and strong farm families dealt with them and moved on. John had always hoped Orin would take over the farm—it had been passed on to a Bergstrom since 1866.

"What can be done?" John asked.

"The implantable defibrillator," Maron replied. "It's a safety net, a back-up. It monitors the heart rhythm and delivers a shock only when it detects a life threatening rhythm, like ventricular tachycardia."

I stood, placed my finger below Orin's left collarbone and said, "We make an incision in your skin here, place a lead wire into the vein, and steer it into the right side of your heart using X-ray. Next, we connect the wire to the defibrillator that goes under your skin. Then we test it. You're asleep the entire time. It takes about an hour. You'll most likely go home the next day."

Orin leaned forward in his chair and said, "I won't be able to play hockey, will I?" It wasn't a question as much as a statement. Orin look down at his hands and then to his mother.

"Orin," Mary Bergstrom said, "it could save your life."

Orin looked at his mother and whispered, "I know. I've been reading about it on the Internet."

Adrian Almquist implanted Orin's AICD the following week. He used a new model defibrillator, a Prizm 2™, manufactured by Guidant that was smaller than previous models. The device was so small that it was invisible in Orin's large chest.

I met again with the family before Orin went home. We reviewed the follow-up schedule. All of the defibrillator checks would be done in Alexandria by our clinic staff, and Maron would see Orin annually. Eventually each sister would have an echocardiogram to determine if they had inherited hypertrophic cardiomyopathy: they did not.

A subset of HCM patients suffer chest pain, shortness of breath, and blackouts because the thickened muscle obstructs blood flow out of the heart. These symptoms are noticeable, particularly during exercise. Surgery to remove the muscle was devised by Dr. Andrew Glenn Morrow. He grew up in Indianapolis, Indiana, and graduated from Johns Hopkins University Medical School in 1946.

Morrow trained in surgery under Alfred Blalock at Johns Hopkins and studied thoracic surgery at Oxford in the United Kingdom. At the age of 30, Morrow became the Chief of Surgery at the National Heart Institute in Bethesda, Maryland. There he began a long and productive collaboration with Dr. Eugene Braunwald, a brilliant young cardiologist experienced in heart catheterization.

Together they conducted important basic and clinical research. Among their discoveries were the physiologic determinants of normal and abnormal heart function. Later Braunwald would say, "Rarely did a week pass when we did not observe or measure something that was new...We experienced the exhilaration that we imagined Lewis and Clark must have felt when they explored the great American wilderness early in the 19th century."

In 1958, Braunwald asked Morrow to operate on a man who was thought to have membranous tissue below the aortic valve that obstructed blood flow. Braunwald arrived at this conclusion because he had observed a pressure drop from the patient's left ventricle to his aorta during a heart catheterization.

After placing the patient on the heart-lung machine, however, Morrow found that no such membranous obstruction existed. Irritated that he had operated unnecessarily, Morrow closed the incision in the patient's heart, and repeated the same pressure measurements in the operating room that Braunwald had made prior to surgery. Surprisingly, he too found the same pressure drop. What could be going on?

Several additional patients had identical findings. All of these patients had marked thickening of their interventricular septum, the wall separating the left and right ventricles, the very same condition we now call hypertrophic cardiomyopathy—HCM. The thickened muscle created hydraulic forces that pushed and pulled one leaflet of the mitral valve against the septum, obstructing blood flow out of the heart.

Morrow conceived an open-heart surgical procedure called "myectomy" for these patients. This involved removing the thickened muscle from the septum. The Morrow operation helped thousands of patients, and it remains the treatment of choice for severe, symptomatic obstructive HCM. An alternative to surgical myectomy is chemical ablation, whereby alcohol is injected through a catheter into the septum and destroys a portion of the thick muscle; this approach does not require open-heart surgery but it may not be as safe or effective.

One day in 1960 Morrow asked Braunwald to listen to his heart. Morrow had been experiencing shortness of breath and lightheadedness. Braunwald placed his stethoscope on his colleague's chest and heard the typical murmur of HCM. How ironic that this 40-year-old surgeon had the very disease that he and Braunwald had elucidated so well.

For the next 20 years, Morrow had repeated blackout spells and shortness of breath. Often he had to stop and sit down midway between the parking lot and his office at the NIH. But he refused any diagnostic procedures or treatment. He died suddenly at home at age 60 of an embolic stroke, most likely caused by atrial fibrillation due to severe HCM.

Regrettably Morrow passed on his disease to two of his three children. Morrow's daughter, age 51, underwent successful heart transplantation for heart failure due to HCM. His son, at the age of 57, underwent a myectomy—the same surgical procedure that his father devised 50 years earlier.

In 2005, I was recovering from surgery when Barry Maron called me at home. "Bob," he said in a wispy voice, "Joshua Oukrup is dead." He paused. I groaned, unable to form words. Maron continued, "I got a call from a coroner in Utah. Apparently, Joshua and his girlfriend were biking there when Joshua collapsed. I think she tried CPR. "

In 2001 Joshua Oukrop was a 17-year-old student who had fainted during marching band practice. His father, Lee, and brother, Jacob, had HCM and both had implantable defibrillators. Joshua was tested for HCM at 12, but the echocardiogram showed no evidence of it. The HCM gene may not express itself until adolescence, so Joshua could well have had the disease in his body.

Maron and I saw Joshua and his father in the Hypertrophic Cardiomyopathy Clinic a few weeks after Joshua fainted. Joshua's echocardiogram that day revealed the same severe thickening as his brother Jacob. Given his symptom—fainting during exercise—Joshua was clearly at high risk for sudden cardiac death.

Joshua was very resistant to the idea of a defibrillator. Just like Mary Bergstrom's remark to her own son, Orin, Lee Oukrop also whispered, "Joshua, it could save your life".

Joshua received the same model defibrillator that Orin Bergstrom did earlier that same year, a Guidant Prizm 2™. He went on to teachers college and he was leading a normal, active life—snowboarding, hiking, biking—until he died suddenly in Moab, Utah, in March of 2005. The coroner removed the defibrillator from Joshua's body and returned it to Guidant. The company said the defibrillator had malfunctioned—it short-circuited—due to a defect in the device that engineers at Guidant had known about for several years. The company had decided *not* to inform patients or their physicians about the defect.

Maron and I met separately with Guidant officials and urged them to issue a recall, notifying every patient that this Guidant defibrillator model might fail. It seemed the only ethical action to take, but Guidant refused, offering the upside-down logic that doctors might over-react and replace defibrillators unnecessarily. The company ignored the simple truth: Patients have a right to make their own health care decisions independently, and they need to be fully informed. Why would a group of conflicted company executives think they could make life and death decisions for thousands of patients who had no idea their defibrillators could fail when they needed it most?

Maron and I sat in his small basement office in the Minneapolis Heart Institute and discussed what we should do. It was urgent. How many patients like Joshua Oukrup were out there? We did not know. By definition, every patient who received an implantable defibrillator had either survived an episode of sudden cardiac death or was at high risk for one. All of them were vulnerable—whether they had hypertrophic cardiomyopathy, coronary artery disease, heart failure or one of the other dozen deadly heart diseases. What were our obligations as physicians—and human beings?

"I know a reporter at the *New York Times*," Maron offered. I thought for a moment and said, "Call him."

A week later, on May 15, 2005, the *New York Times* published this article by reporter Barry Meier:

> "A medical device maker, the Guidant Corporation, did not tell doctors or patients for three years that a unit implanted in an estimated 24,000 people that is designed to shock a faltering heart contains a flaw that has caused a small number of those units to short-circuit and malfunction.
>
> "The matter has come to light after the death of a 21-year-old college student from Minnesota, Joshua Oukrop, with a genetic heart disease. Guidant acknowledges that his device, known as a defibrillator, short-circuited. The young man was in Moab, Utah, on a spring break bicycling trip in March with his girlfriend when he complained of fatigue. He then fell to the ground and died of cardiac arrest.
>
> "Guidant subsequently told his doctors that it was aware of 25 other cases in which the defibrillator, a Ventak Prizm 2™ Model 1861, had been affected by the same flaw. Guidant said it had changed its manufacturing processes three years ago to fix the problem. The physicians say that had they known earlier, they would have replaced the unit in their patient because he was at high risk of sudden death. His death is the only one known....
>
> "Joshua's father, Lee Oukrop, said that when his son was 17, he began fainting and falling down at marching band practice or while playing softball. The heart disease had previously been diagnosed in an older son, Jacob, so Mr. Oukrop took Joshua to see Dr. Maron in 2001. The physician determined that the teenager's condition was severe, and an implant was soon performed...

"Mr. Oukrop, a millwright who lives in Grand Rapids, Minn., a small town about 80 miles west of Duluth, said that Dr. Maron had said 'that this was the fix and that Josh could live with this.'

"'Whoever made this decision at Guidant, I pray he doesn't have a son who this happens to,' Mr. Oukrop said."

The day prior to the *Times* publication, Guidant abruptly issued a recall of the Ventak Prizm 2™ implantable defibrillator. This would be the first of multiple Guidant recalls during 2005. These disclosures revealed defects in tens of thousands of additional Guidant implantable defibrillators and cardiac pacemakers. It was as if the Oukrop tragedy had lanced a festering abscess.

In 2011, Guidant was convicted in U.S. Federal Court of criminal violations for its mishandling of the short-circuiting failures of three models of its implantable cardioverter defibrillators. The company was ordered to pay $296 million in fines. Guidant's executives, however, did well: Boston Scientific acquired the company in 2006 for $27.3 billion. No individual was held accountable for Joshua's death.

As a precaution, many of our patients, including Orin Bergstrom, had their Guidant Prizm 2™ defibrillators replaced.

Orin Bergstrom received a shock from his new Medtronic implantable defibrillator during the winter of 2006 while attending the University of Minnesota in Morris. He was shoveling snow around his Ford pick-up when he lost consciousness and collapsed on the street. Another student called 911. By the time paramedics arrived, Orin was conscious and sitting on the ground surrounded by a half dozen bystanders. He had suffered no ill effects, and had no recollection of anything prior to blacking out.

Orin was taken to the emergency room at Stevens Community Medical Center where his defibrillator was "interrogated" by a special computer provided by the defibrillator's manufacturer, Medtronic. It showed that Orin had lost consciousness due to a very fast (>220 beats per minute) ventricular tachycardia and that the defibrillator had promptly shocked him out of it. He was back in class the following day.

In 2013, John Bergstrom turned over the farm to Orin and moved to a cottage on Lake Darling near Alexandria. That same year, Orin had his defibrillator replaced when the battery ran down. He has received no further shocks. Orin and his wife, Melissa, have a son and twin daughters, who will be tested for HCM when they get older.

Barry Maron continued his research, authoring many articles, and chairing a biennial international summit on HCM that brought experts from around the world to Minneapolis for three days of lectures and panel discussions. Maron has received multiple awards from international professional societies. In 2014, the Minneapolis Heart Institute Foundation celebrated Barry Maron's contributions to medicine and mankind. At that event HCM pioneer and Harvard professor, Dr. Eugene Braunwald, offered this tribute:

> *"It is important to recognize that Dr. Maron stands head and shoulders above anyone else who has worked in hypertrophic cardiomyopathy…He is first and foremost a doctor, and he approaches science and medicine from a patient's perspective. He has a way of analyzing issues in terms of how they will affect patient care, how will they affect diagnosis, how will they affect prognosis, and most of all how will they affect selection of treatments."*

When I retired, Maron was still planning research projects. I could see him most mornings writing or editing manuscripts in one of several bagel shops west of Minneapolis.

CHAPTER 14

In the summer of 1996 Gerald Snow visited his internist, Dr. Bob Scott in Minneapolis. Gerald was 66 and recently retired from General Mills where he was an accountant for 37 years. Despite numerous attempts to quit, he continued to smoke a pack and a half of Marlboros™ daily. In fact, he resembled an aging, overweight Marlboro™ cowboy.

For weeks, he had experienced back pain that did not respond to a heating pad or ibuprofen. Occasionally the pain shot into his groin and upper abdomen. His wife finally prevailed, and he drove himself from their home in suburban Plymouth to Scott's downtown office.

Scott had seen Gerald four years earlier. At that time, he prescribed enalapril for hypertension, but Gerald stopped the drug on his own when he developed a dry cough.

Gerald's blood pressure was 205/105 in both arms and the odor of stale tobacco pervaded the small examining room. The examination was unremarkable until Scott palpated Gerald's generous abdomen: he felt a large pulsating mass: it was an abdominal aortic aneurysm that was probably rupturing. Scott called for an ambulance.

Thirty-five minutes later Gerald was in the emergency room of Abbott Northwestern Hospital. Scott had contacted Dr. Peter Alden, a vascular surgeon, who was waiting for Gerald. A CT scan showed a large abdominal aortic aneurysm that was leaking blood into the space between the aneurysm and Gerald's spine. The aneurysm was a soft spot in a garden hose that was dribbling water and poised to burst. Alden called the operating room supervisor and said his patient needed emergency surgery. Meanwhile Gerald was given a capsule of nifedipine to lower his blood pressure. He also had blood tests, a portable chest X-ray, and an EKG.

The EKG was abnormal. It showed that Gerald had had a heart attack at some time in the past. I got a call to examine Gerald in the emergency room. The nifedipine had begun to bring Gerald's blood pressure down. The EKG showed an old heart attack, but nothing acute. I spoke to the anesthesiologist and started esmolol, a short acting beta-blocker that would afford some cardiac protection during surgery. We would sort through the heart issues after the surgery.

In the operating room Peter Alden found precisely what the CT scan showed. He repaired the aortic aneurysm with a Gore-Tex™ vascular graft. Gerald was monitored overnight in the ICU and sent to a regular floor to continue his recovery. An echocardiogram—heart ultrasound—revealed an old heart attack on the underside of his heart; the left ventricle had been mildly affected and his ejection fraction was mildly reduced—40-45 percent (normal: 55-60 percent). I started him on aspirin, metoprolol (a beta-blocker) and lisinopril (an ACE inhibitor) for his heart and blood pressure, and simvastatin to bring his cholesterol down.

Around 5 a.m. on the third day after his surgery, Gerald called his nurse because he felt short of breath and heaviness in his chest. A chest X-ray showed early signs of heart failure and the EKG suggested a decrease in blood flow to the front and side of his heart. A blood test for troponin—an enzyme released from a damaged heart muscle—was mildly elevated.

I transferred Gerald to the coronary care unit and called Dr. Mike Mooney in the catheterization laboratory. Mooney was the director of the Minneapolis Heart Institute's coronary intervention program. I summarized Gerald's situation and asked if he could do an angiogram urgently. Mike agreed. I explained the plan to Gerald and called his wife.

The coronary angiogram revealed a near total blockage of Gerald's left anterior descending coronary artery. Gerald's entire left ventricle and his life were in jeopardy.

In 1980 Dr. Geoff Hartzler performed a routine angiogram on a patient who was suffering recurrent bouts of angina despite multiple medications. He found a severe 90 percent blockage in the right coronary artery and scheduled the patient for an angioplasty the following morning. Just before the procedure, the catheterization laboratory called Hartzler and told him the angioplasty was cancelled because the patient was having a heart attack. Apparently, the severely diseased right coronary artery had clotted, obstructing all blood flow.

At that time expert cardiologists believed that angioplasty was too risky if a patient was in the throes of an acute heart attack. Hartzler decided to defy the medical norm. Years later he recalled, "Just an hour before the patient was a candidate for angioplasty. What had occurred to negate that now?... I was maybe young, naïve, and aggressive but I brought him down to the lab and put a catheter through the occluded artery and inflated the balloon. It was the most amazing thing I had ever seen. The EKG came back to normal, and his pain went away. It was amazing! It was fantastic! The patient went home in three days." Hartzler had performed the world's first successful angioplasty on a patient suffering an acute myocardial infarction.

Geoff Hartzler was born in 1946 in Goshen, Indiana. His father was a Mennonite minister, who later worked in mental health, and his mother lived in an iron lung after contracting paralytic polio when Geoff was four- years-old. Rock music was Geoff's passion growing up. During his adult life, he continued to play bass guitar and even started his own band. He attended the University of Indiana School of Medicine and completed his internal medicine and cardiology training at the Mayo Clinic.

I first met Geoff Hartzler in the late 1970s. At that time, he was a young cardiac electrophysiologist at the Mayo Clinic, where he developed methods for diagnosing and treating tachycardias. He used rapid pacing to stop fast rhythms and implanted special pacemakers that patients could self-activate to terminate an abnormal rhythm. His treatment was innovative and aggressive, but that was typical of Hartzler's approach to medicine: he saw a problem and went after it. He did not spend a lot of time worrying about how his innovations would be perceived by his peers and supervisors. In many ways, Hartzler was the Walt Lillehei of cardiology.

After Andreas Gruentzig performed the first human coronary angioplasty, the Mayo Clinic developed a protocol to perform a series of 100 angioplasties in patient's legs before trying it in the heart. This was characteristic of the Mayo Clinic's deliberate approach to new therapies. However, before the series was completed, Hartzler was asked to do an angioplasty on a patient with a severe blockage in the proximal left anterior descending coronary artery. Hartzler tried to practice on a dog in the research laboratory, but the dog died before he could complete the procedure. Regardless, he declared, "We're ready!"

The following day he brought the patient to the Mayo catheterization laboratory. For two hours, he tried to get the angioplasty catheter across the severe blockage. A number of senior cardiologists were in the room to watch the procedure and they were getting restless. Finally, Hartzler maneuvered the angioplasty catheter into a good position across the blockage and inflated the balloon. The result was excellent. It was the Mayo Clinic's first coronary angioplasty.

Hartzler's pioneering spirit clashed with the Mayo Clinic's conservative culture. He needed freedom to grow at his pace, so he joined several former Mayo cardiologists at St. Luke's Hospital in Kansas City. There he became a luminary in interventional cardiology. He innovated novel techniques for treating coronary lesions that most observers thought would fail. Unlike most interventional cardiologists, including Andreas Gruentzig, Hartzler began doing angioplasty in multiple coronary arteries during a single procedure, and he attacked troublesome lesions that cardiologists had avoided in the past.

Geoff Hartzler's creative genius was complemented by his professional behavior. Four close colleagues wrote: "His skill in the laboratory was amazing, but his demeanor should be a lesson to all young interventional cardiologists. He was always thinking ahead, never used any derogatory language, never blamed others for complications, and always spoke personally to family members."

In 1983 I was lecturing at a cardiology program in Vail, Colorado, where Hartzler also was speaking. He described his approach to treating acute heart attacks with emergency angioplasty. There were 20 to 30 people in the audience. Hartzler asked for questions at the conclusion of his presentation. The negativity was intense. Several participants were highly critical, saying that it was dangerous and should be abandoned. A few correctly pointed out that more data were needed. Hartzler's response to one skeptic who questioned the rationale for opening an acutely blocked artery was unforgettable. Stroking his mustache and smiling in disbelief he said, "Gosh, I always thought that blood flow was a good thing."

Within a minute after finding Gerald Snow's blocked coronary artery, Mike Mooney swiftly slid an angioplasty catheter over a guidewire and through the clot. Then he inflated the high-pressure balloon with a handheld pump. Seconds later, he deflated the balloon and injected more dye to see the result. The blockage had been reduced to about 50 percent, but some of the plaque had shifted forward, partially blocking the opening of a large diagonal branch. Mooney inflated the balloon once again, this time with a higher pressure. Now the plaque was fully compressed. The left anterior descending artery was wide open.

Next, Mooney maneuvered the wire into the diagonal artery where the soft plaque had shifted. He advanced the angioplasty catheter and inflated the balloon, flattening the plaque. Another dye injection showed that blood was flowing freely through both arteries.

Then suddenly the wall of the left anterior descending artery collapsed. Gerald's EKG changed dramatically, showing all the signs of acute injury—a heart attack. The nurse watching the EKG and blood pressure monitor saw it first and she calmly, but forcibly told us to look at the monitor.

Mooney quickly injected dye into the left coronary artery: there was no blood flowing through the left anterior descending. The lining of the artery at the site of the angioplasty had been torn and a flap of tissue had plugged the artery as effectively as a clot, completely obstructing blood flow. This was classic *abrupt closure*, the dreaded complication that had plagued angioplasty from the beginning.

Abrupt closure during or after balloon inflation was a known risk and it occurred in three to six percent of angioplasty cases. This was why a cardiac surgeon and an operating room were always on standby and why angioplasty could not be done in hospitals without heart surgery during this era. The immediate challenge was to get the artery open and keep it open because the artery supplied blood to a large part of Gerald's heart.

Seconds later, Gerald's heart fibrillated. The circulating nurse charged the defibrillator next to the X-ray table, lifted the sterile sheet covering Gerald's chest, and applied the paddles. Mooney held onto the catheters and instruments and commanded, "Go!" The defibrillator's electric shock lifted Gerald slightly off the table, but it was successful: Gerald had a normal rhythm.

While they dealt with this emergency, other members of the catheterization team were anticipating what Mooney would do next. When he asked for a Palmaz-Schatz stent the technician had it ready. This device would save Gerald Snow's life.

Dr. Julio Palmaz was born in 1945 in La Plata, Argentina, also the birthplace of Dr. René Favaloro. Palmaz's parents were of Italian descent and lived modestly in Buenos Aires. They insisted that he learn English and taught him perseverance and entrepreneurship. Later he recalled that his mother was a very humble person, and she helped to support the family. He studied at the National University in La Plata, graduated from medical school in 1971, and practiced vascular radiology at the San Martin University Hospital.

By 1977, Palmaz was married and he moved his family to the United States to spend three years training in radiology at the University of California at Davis while pursuing academic research. His mentor, Dr. Stewart Reuter, an accomplished academic radiologist, encouraged him to publish: "You are already old," he warned him. "Start writing papers right away or you will get nowhere."

Reuter was President of the Society of Cardiovascular and Interventional Radiology and he urged Palmaz to attend the organization's annual meeting in New Orleans. "We have a great keynote speaker you must listen to," Reuter told him. It was Dr. Andreas Gruentzig. "Not only did I have the unique opportunity to hear about his recently developed angioplasty balloon," Palmaz said years later, "but he inspired me with the seminal idea of a balloon- expandable stent."

Gruentzig's detailed descriptions of angioplasty's complications, including abrupt closure, sparked Palmaz's imagination. He asked himself, "Why not put a scaffold in the vessel?" As he wrote up the idea, Palmaz added the critical enhancement, namely mounting the scaffold on a balloon, so that it could be deployed into the coronary artery. The balloon-expandable coronary stent was born, at least conceptually. The idea was disruptive and foundational because it would make angioplasty safer and more effective. In time, it would enable other groundbreaking therapeutic devices, including heart valves that could be implanted without major surgery.

Working in his California garage, Palmaz spent hundreds of hours building various prototypes of his scaffold with little success. He tried weaving and welding cylindrical nets but that did not work. One afternoon he found a piece of metal on the floor of his garage: it was a tube that masons used to apply plaster. The solid tube had slots that allowed it to *expand into a metal cage*. Here was another moment when a serendipitous observation spawned a great invention. Palmaz finally had the basic design for the first balloon expandable stent.

Palmaz didn't have the sophisticated tools required to build a stent worthy of animal testing. He approached several companies who turned him down. Then in 1983, Palmaz moved to San Antonio where Stewart Reuter had been named Chair of Radiology at the University of Texas Health Center. As Wangensteen had done for Lillehei at the University of Minnesota 25 years earlier, Reuter encouraged and supported Palmaz, who later wrote: "Flexible in his management but firm in his goals, he created a great academic environment in which the young faculty grew under his example."

Palmaz met Dr. Richard Schatz, a cardiologist from the Brooke Army Medical Center. Schatz had grown up in New York and graduated from Duke University Medical School in 1977. The two men began collaborating and they created a company with $250,000 from Philip Romano, the founder of Fuddruckers and the Macaroni Grill. Together, they experimented with many stent prototypes and implanted them in animals. Palmaz was awarded a patent in 1985, and he licensed his invention to Johnson & Johnson. Two years later Palmaz implanted his stent in the leg of a patient in Germany, and a patient in Brazil received the first Palmaz-Schatz coronary stent.

It took almost three years for the Food and Drug Administration to approve the Palmaz-Schatz™ coronary stent. The delays frustrated many, including the cardiologists who were participating in the stent's U.S. clinical trials. One of them was Dr. Paul Teirstein at Scripps Memorial Hospital in La Jolla, California, who cared for a very special patient in December 1991.

Mother Teresa of Calcutta, the 1979 winner of the Nobel Peace Prize, first suffered a heart attack in 1983 and she received a pacemaker in 1989 after a second heart attack. In 1991, while visiting one of her clinics in Tijuana, Mexico, she had another heart attack and developed symptoms of heart failure. Her cardiologist, Dr. Patricia Aubanal, recommended she be transferred to Scripps Memorial in La Jolla for coronary angiography. It was performed by Dr. Teirstein who found a significant narrowing in a large coronary artery and proceeded to perform an angioplasty. The dilation resulted in a tear in the wall of the artery that Teirstein treated successfully with implantation of the experimental Palmaz-Schatz stent.

Palmaz panicked when he was told that Mother Teresa had just received one of his stents. Palmaz feared that something might go wrong and he would have contributed to the demise of a woman who would later achieve sainthood. Mother Teresa, who had a long history of coronary artery disease, did well, however, and she lived four more years.

After seemingly endless regulatory delays, the Palmaz-Schatz™ stent was approved in 1994 for coronary applications.

The catheterization laboratory was cool and the lights had been turned down so that the high definition X-ray video monitors were more visible. Gerald Snow lay on the catheterization table. He was sedated and on a respirator. His left anterior descending coronary artery had closed a few minutes after Mike Mooney had inflated the angioplasty balloon. A major heart attack threatened Gerald's life and he was going into shock.

Mooney threaded the catheter containing the Palmaz-Schatz™ stent through Gerald's aorta. Within a minute, he had it positioned in the exact area where the severe blockage appeared on the first angiogram. Mooney inflated the balloon and expanded the stent, deploying it so that the stainless steel metal struts pressed firmly against the plaque and flap of tissue that caused the abrupt closure. Once the stent moved the flap aside, blood began flowing through the artery. The stent had done exactly what Palmaz and Schatz had designed it to do: the "scaffold" was in place, supporting the wall of the artery, preventing it from caving in and blocking blood flow.

Gerald's blood pressure rose to 110. He was no longer in shock and would not need the intra-aortic balloon pump or emergency coronary bypass surgery. I left the laboratory to speak with Gerald's wife and two sons. Using a diagram of the coronary arteries, I showed them the blockage where Mooney had performed angioplasty and inserted the Palmaz-Schatz™ stent.

Gerald Snow returned to the ICU for a day and remained in the hospital for seven additional days until his bowel recovered from the aneurysm surgery. He had dodged three bullets: the ruptured abdominal aortic aneurysm, a near fatal heart attack, and abrupt closure after balloon angioplasty. If these events had happened only five years earlier, Gerald would have needed emergency bypass surgery and would have been fortunate to survive; and, if he did survive, his heart likely would have sustained significant damage.

The medical community rapidly adopted the Palmaz-Schatz™ stent. While Palmaz thought it would be used in 20 percent of angioplasty procedures cardiologists began implanting stents in most of their patients who needed coronary angioplasty. By 1999, 85 percent of patients undergoing coronary angioplasty received a stent. Some observers called it "stent fever" and Johnson & Johnson struggled to manufacture the stent fast enough to meet the demand. Soon, other companies offered their versions of a coronary stent and, by the new millennium, multiple stent models were available and their manufacturers were battling for market share.

Coronary stents had problems, however. One was stent thrombosis when a blood clot formed in the stent, acutely blocking blood flow, and causing a heart attack. To prevent this, most cardiologists placed our patients on strong blood thinners, including warfarin and aspirin. Consequently, some patients bled into their groins where the femoral artery had been punctured. Others bled into their stomachs or bowels, or most tragically into their brains. The safe zone between too much blood thinner and too little was quite narrow, and it was very slim for patients who had known bleeding tendencies.

Eventually deploying the stent with high balloon inflation pressures mostly solved the stent thrombosis problem. This maneuver pressed the stent more firmly against the inner wall of the coronary artery, eliminating spaces where clots could form and propagate. We were able to eliminate warfarin, and instead treat our patients with aspirin and ticlopidine, two drugs that inhibit platelets and prevent the formation of blood clots. In time, clopidogrel (Plavix®), a safer and more effective antiplatelet drug, replaced ticlopidine.

The second, far more common problem was a phenomenon called "in-stent restenosis," a condition in which tissue grows into the stent and blocks blood flow. It was just as troublesome as a blockage caused by coronary artery disease, and the quest for a solution is a story in itself.

Sixty-one-year-old Isaac Taylor had driven a truck since he was in the Army Reserve. He once drove for the Montfort meatpacking company in Colorado, which prided itself on delivering fresh meat anywhere on time. This meant that Montfort trucks had to get from point A to point B fast. Other truckers began referring to the left passing lane on the Interstate as the "Montfort Lane." In the late 1970s, Isaac quit Montfort after accumulating so many speeding tickets that he risked losing his license.

I saw Isaac at the Lakeview Clinic in Waconia, Minnesota, in the winter of 1997. His internist, Dr. Jim Lehman, was a very astute clinician. For the past ten days, Isaac had been experiencing central chest pressure whenever he did any physical work, especially in a cold wind. It went away as soon as he stopped working, or escaped the wind and cold in his truck. Given his cigarette smoking and pre-diabetes condition, Isaac was a prime candidate for coronary artery disease. Based on his symptoms, Lehman diagnosed new onset angina pectoris, and treated him with aspirin, atenolol (a beta-blocker), and sublingual nitroglycerin tablets that he could place under his tongue to relieve his angina.

Isaac was a big man with a big belly and he sported a ragged gray-streaked beard. He lived in the nearby town of Norwood Young America with his wife, and he had switched to driving local delivery trucks rather than long haul, 18-wheelers. He had felt no further angina since Lehman started the drugs.

"I haven't had a cigarette since Doc Lehman told me to quit yesterday," he said proudly. I congratulated him and asked if his wife smoked. Fortunately, she was a non-smoker, because patients like Isaac had difficulty quitting if someone in the home was always lighting up.

I placed my stethoscope on his chest and noticed he had many random and extra heartbeats. His blood pressure was slightly elevated. I sent him for an EKG. The EKG showed multiple premature ventricular contractions (PVCs).

One option was to continue the medications and perform a nuclear stress test to determine the severity and extent of Isaac's coronary artery disease. If the test suggested mild to moderate disease affecting a small region of his heart, then continued treatment with medications would be reasonable. However, I sensed that Isaac had a serious problem and recommended a coronary angiogram.

"Do you do that here in Waconia?" Isaac asked. "No, we'll do the angiogram in Minneapolis at Abbott Northwestern Hospital. We may do angioplasty at the same time if there is a serious blockage. That's the balloon…"

"I know about angioplasty," Isaac interrupted. "My neighbor had it in Arizona and the next thing he knew he was having emergency heart surgery. I think they call it bypass. He did okay."

"Certainly that can happen," I replied, "the artery can shut down after the balloon is inflated. We now have metal stents, a little spring-like device that we insert in the coronary artery to keep it open."

Two days later, Isaac had his angiogram at Abbott Northwestern Hospital. Dr. Jim Madison called me to review the films.

When I arrived in the film viewing room, Madison said, "I sent Mr. Taylor to the recovery room while we decide what to do."

Madison placed Isaac's angiogram film on a special viewing machine and forwarded it to the pictures of Isaac's left anterior descending and diagonal coronary arteries. Pointing to the left anterior descending, Madison said, "He has a 90 percent stenosis (blockage) here and another 90 percent stenosis in this large diagonal branch. Nothing else."

"How is his left ventricle?" I asked. Madison fast-forwarded to the left ventriculogram. We watched a large volume of X-ray dye enter the left ventricle. "The anterior wall is a little sluggish," Madison said, "but the ejection fraction calculates at 50 percent—not too bad."

So Isaac had severe two-vessel coronary artery disease, but his pumping function was good. We thought both arteries should be treated with the goal of restoring normal blood flow. The two treatment options were angioplasty with or without stents, or coronary artery bypass surgery. Madison thought both blockages were suitable for angioplasty and stenting. The two arteries—the left anterior descending and diagonal—were free of disease beyond the blockages and were fine for bypass surgery. What to do?

I walked over to the recovery room where Isaac was awake on a gurney. He could not sit up because Madison left the sheath in his femoral artery. Isaac asked that his wife be present. "She knows more about these things than I do," he said. One of the volunteers escorted her from the waiting room. She was a pleasant woman, overweight like her husband, with short, brown, curly hair and rosy cheeks. She stood at my side as I drew a picture of Isaac's coronary arteries.

"Mister Taylor, you have two severe blockages here and here," I said, pointing to my diagram. "They are causing your chest discomfort and they supply the muscle of your main pumping chamber. The good news is there is no scar tissue that we can see." I paused, waiting for questions. They had none.

"I think we should try to improve the blood flow, and there are two options," I said. "One is coronary artery bypass—heart surgery. The surgeon should be able to bypass both arteries quite well. He would most likely use the mammary artery under your breastbone as one bypass, and a section of vein from your leg for the other bypass. The second possibility is angioplasty, and I think Doctor Madison would most likely place a stent here and here." Again I pointed to the diagram.

Mrs. Taylor had questions about both procedures. How long would Isaac be laid-up? When could he go back to work? Would the stents last? What were the risks? There was about a 30 percent chance that the angioplasty or stent would eventually fail due to restenosis and the procedure would have to be redone in the next year or two. The surgical mortality for bypass surgery was less than five percent, but there were other complications related to any major surgery. The recovery time was short—several days—for angioplasty, and four to eight weeks for bypass surgery.

Isaac listened and did not say a word, until the end. "Doc," he said. "I need to get back to my job as soon as possible or I'll lose it. The wife doesn't work and I have no disability. We're pretty much living on my check week to week." That settled it. I called Madison and asked him to proceed with angioplasty that afternoon.

It took Madison less than an hour to insert two Palmaz-Schatz™ stents into Isaac's left anterior descending and diagonal coronary arteries. The two 90 percent blockages were reduced to zero. In their place were tiny metal tubes composed of a lattice-work of 316L stainless steel. Each was imbedded into the lining of the artery, a mixture of normal and diseased tissue.

From the moment the stents engaged his tissue, Isaac's body reacted to the presence of a foreign object. A million years of evolution had equipped Isaac with the tools required to repair scrapes and scratches, penetrating traumas, broken bones, and other physical insults. Like an army going to war, his body mobilized millions of cells and chemical substances, and transported them to the sites where the stents were holding his coronary arteries open. Before he left the hospital and returned home to Norwood Young America, Gerald's stents were coated with platelets and fibrin that in turn stimulated the overgrowth of smooth muscle cells. With time, these "neointimal" cells multiplied, unchecked, layer upon layer until Gerald's stents were clogged like sludge in a drainpipe. This was in-stent restenosis.

I received a call from Dr. Lehman five and half months after Isaac Taylor received his stents. Isaac was in his clinic complaining of the same chest discomfort he had before the implantation of his stents. It was all too familiar: a patient who had received bare metal stents within the past year was back with recurrent symptoms.

The following day Isaac had his second angiogram. Both stents were 90 percent blocked due to the proliferation of tissue within the stent. The options were bypass surgery, try angioplasty and re-stenting (place a stent within the stent), or perform local radiation therapy with the goal of suppressing regrowth of tissue within the stent.

Once again, Isaac resisted bypass surgery. I recommended radiation therapy (called brachytherapy) rather than simply opt for another angioplasty or stent. Dr. Wes Pedersen performed the brachytherapy the following day. First, he inserted new bare metal stents within the previously placed stents in the left anterior descending and diagonal coronary arteries. He deployed the stents with high pressure balloon inflations until there were no residual blockages. Then Pedersen placed a wire containing a radiation source, Iridium-192, across each stent. A precise, timed radiation dose was delivered from the radiation source to the artery surrounding each stent. Hopefully the radiation would suppress the proliferation of tissue that caused Isaac's first stents to plug-up. He was discharged on dual anti-platelet drugs, namely aspirin and ticlopidine.

The radiation treatment worked for Isaac, but seven years later he became sweaty, nauseated, and short of breath while chopping wood behind his house. He had retired from trucking. His cholesterol and diabetes were under satisfactory control on simvastatin and insulin, and did not smoke. Forty minutes later, Isaac was in the Ridgeview Medical Center's emergency room where his EKG and blood tests suggested a small heart attack. His symptoms improved with oxygen and morphine but he began to have chest heaviness. I spoke with the emergency room physician, Dr. David Larsen, and we decided he needed an urgent coronary angiogram.

Isaac had lost weight and shaved his beard. By the time he arrived in the catheterization laboratory Isaac was no longer in pain. I sat behind the leaded window and watched Yale Wang perform Isaac's angiogram, expecting to see a problem involving one of his previous stents. Instead, those stents looked fine, but he had a new stenosis in the middle of his right coronary artery, which was 99 percent blocked. The muscle supplied by the artery was barely moving because it blood flow was compromised. Isaac was close to having a major heart attack.

Providentially, Isaac would benefit from a new type of stent that the FDA had approved the year before, in 2003. Like the Palmaz-Schatz™ stent, it was manufactured by Johnson & Johnson and branded the Cypher™. By any measure, the Cypher™ stent had become an out-of-the-park home run.

Easter Island, also known as Rapa Nui, is perhaps the most isolated inhabited land mass on earth. Located in the Pacific Ocean 2,250 miles northeast of Chile, it is famous for the finely carved ancient statues that are featured on travel brochures. In the mid-20th century, pharmaceutical manufacturers scoured remote regions of the planet looking for novel antibiotics. The process involved collecting and culturing soil samples and isolating organisms and their byproducts. In 1965, a group of Canadian scientists collected a soil sample from the remote Vai Atare region of Easter Island. A strain of the bacterium, *Streptomyces hygroscopicus,* was isolated from this sample, and it produced a soluble crystalline material that was named sirolimus.

Sirolimus, also known as rapamycin, had antifungal and potent immunosuppressive properties. It was first marketed in the 1990s as Rapamune® for the prevention of kidney transplant rejection. It also inhibited the very kind of cell proliferation that clogged coronary bare metal stents like the ones Isaac Taylor received. Sirolimus had another important attribute: it prevented blood platelets from massing together and forming clots.

The next step was the development of a drug delivery polymer that would coat the stent's inner wall. Sirolimus was then combined with the polymer so that it could be delivered slowly—eluted—to the artery surrounding the stent over days and weeks. In animals, these sirolimus-coated stents vastly reduced the proliferation of cells, preventing tissue growth into the stent. Would this beneficial effect translate to humans?

The Cypher™ sirolimus-coated stents were compared to bare metal stents in several international clinical trials and the results were stunning. In one trial, known as RAVEL, patients who received the Cypher™ sirolimus-coated stent had no recurrent blockages, while 23 percent of the patients who received the bare metal stent developed restenosis. In a second study, named SIRIUS, involving a thousand patients, the Cypher™ stent had a very low restenosis rate of 3.2 percent versus a rate of 35 percent for the bare metal stent.

These results led to regulatory approval in Europe and the United States. The Cypher™ sirolimus stent would end the awful era of frequent stent failures caused by restenosis. A few patients would still experience restenosis but physicians could be more confident when recommending angioplasty and stenting instead of coronary artery bypass surgery. For me, this advance ranked in the top ten during my career. That soil sample from Easter Island proved to be a godsend for many of my patients and tens of thousands of others.

Dr. Yale Wang placed a Cypher™ stent in Isaac's right coronary artery. When he was done, there was no residual narrowing. The following morning, Isaac's nurse on Station 44 called me because he was complaining of chest pain. I ordered an EKG and walked over to the hospital from my office in the Minneapolis Heart Institute. On the way, Lorna Finseth, one of the veteran cardiology nurse clinicians, joined me. Mrs. Taylor stood anxiously at Isaac's bedside. Before I could say a word, she asked, "Now what? Is he going to need surgery?"

"I don't think so," I replied, "but we need to figure out what's going on."

The nurse handed me the new EKG, and said, "I gave him one nitro but it didn't help."

I compared the EKG to one from the previous day after the stent was placed: it looked good—there was no change.

"Mister Taylor," I said, "tell me about the pain. Is it like the pain yesterday?"

Isaac pointed to the middle of his chest. "It's kinda sharp, Doc. Hurts when I breathe. It's different from yesterday."

I gently pressed the spot. "Do you feel this?" I asked. Isaac shook his head. I sat him up and listened to his heart and lungs. I checked his groin where Yale Wang had inserted the catheter yesterday, and palpated his legs and calves. Nothing.

"I don't think the pain is coming from your heart," I said. "I'm going to give you Tylenol® and keep you here for another day."

Isaac's pain resolved with the Tylenol® and he left the hospital the next day. I saw him a few years later. His wife had developed dementia and he was spending most of his time caring for her. "My heart's doing good, Doc," Isaac said. "It's the rest of me that's slowing down. I just need to stay healthy so I can take care of the wife…you know what I'm sayin»?

Indeed, I did.

The first patient to undergo coronary angioplasty, Dolph Bachmann, became somewhat of a celebrity, primarily because he appeared on Swiss television as a professional card game instructor and country music expert. He quit smoking but resisted taking any medication, preferring lifestyle changes and stress reduction (he remarried).

Bachman experienced chest pain in 2000, twenty-three years after Andreas Gruentzig performed his angioplasty. Dr. Bernhard Meier performed a coronary angiogram at a hospital in in Zurich. The site of Bachman's 1977 angioplasty was perfect—no blockage whatsoever—and no significant plaque was present elsewhere in his coronary arteries.

Yet Bachmann's chest pain recurred, and another coronary angiogram was done five months later. A narrowing of borderline significance was found close to the angioplasty site. Even though blood flow appeared to be normal, Bachmann insisted that it be stented. Drug eluting stents were not available at that time, so he received a bare metal stent that was implanted in the region of the 1977 angioplasty. He did well for three months but then returned with worsening angina. An angiogram showed severe in-stent restenosis. In a very short time tissue had proliferated inside the stent and caused a severe blockage.

Balloon angioplasty reduced the blockage within the stent to nearly zero, and Bachman did well for 14 years. In 2014, the now seventy-five-year-old Bachman redeveloped angina, and another angiogram showed a new lesion near the previously placed stent. This time a drug-eluting stent was positioned inside the previous stent, covering the new blockage and the portion of the artery that was originally treated with balloon angioplasty.

While he had been resistant to medication, Bachman finally agreed to stay on a statin (Crestor®) and a platelet inhibitor (Effient®). In the summer of 2016, Bachman was doing well nearly 39 years after Gruentzig dilated his left anterior descending coronary artery with a homemade angioplasty balloon.

Dolph Bachmann rode the wave of progress in the treatment of severe coronary artery disease. Like millions of other patients, he avoided the surgeon's knife and suffered no disability. Dr. Andreas Gruentzig died while angioplasty was still in its infancy. If he returned today, he would applaud what has happened to his innovation, and doubtless devise new techniques to improve it.

During the 20 years after the Palmaz-Schatz™ stent was approved, a host of clinical trials clarified the role of coronary stents in various patient populations. We learned that diabetics with complex coronary artery disease often did better with coronary bypass surgery than with multiple stents. New generations of stents were introduced that used different drugs to prevent restenosis. Clinical studies gauged the relative effectiveness of each new drug-eluting stent. While some appeared better than others, the real world differences were usually slight. What these studies proved time and again was that drug-eluting stents, compared to bare metal stents, reduced the need for repeat coronary intervention, be it stenting or coronary artery bypass.

By 2015 coronary angioplasty and stenting were routine procedures that yielded excellent outcomes in hundreds of medical centers around the world. No longer did we avoid stenting of the left main coronary artery or complex cases that required multiple stents. Emergency angioplasty for heart attacks was so successful that most communities had systems in place to facilitate rapid transfer of heart attack patients to hospitals capable of performing the procedure. Cardiologists were developing new ways to open coronary arteries that had been totally blocked for years.

In the new millennium, however, quality improvement and systems of care outpaced technology developments. We knew how to get an artery open and keep it open. After 2000 we began to focus on opening arteries faster and making life-saving interventions accessible to everyone regardless of their geographic proximity to a heart center.

CHAPTER 15

It had been an intense month in the hospital. Critically ill patients arrived from all over the state and western Wisconsin. Most had come to the Minneapolis Heart Institute® by ground ambulance, but many came by helicopter. We were short of intensive care beds and nursing administration had resorted to bringing critical care nurses in from as far away as Missouri and Ohio. The on-call teams in the catheterization laboratory worked every night, and some nurses and technicians had not had a day off for weeks. The on-call cardiologists rarely slept, and the practice asked its physicians to delay their vacations.

Yet the mood was decidedly upbeat in 2003, and for good reason. We were doing something new that was, for many of us, the best thing we had ever done in our careers. The nursing staff and the dozens of technicians and hospital administrators shared our enthusiasm. All of us pulled together to care for patients in a new way.

The game changer was our Level One acute myocardial infarction angioplasty program. Level One eliminated the barriers and delays that stood between a patient having a heart attack and the angioplasty balloon that would open his or her blocked artery. It was the brainchild of one of our cardiologists, Dr. Tim Henry, and Dr. David Larson, an emergency room physician from Waconia, Minnesota. Henry and Larsen were inspired by clinical trials in Denmark that demonstrated the safety and effectiveness of rapidly transporting heart attack patients from community hospitals to heart centers for emergency angioplasty. This was just one of many contributions the Danes have made to improve cardiovascular care. Drs. Henry and Larsen decided to introduce the Danish approach for treating heart attacks to Minnesota.

Barb Unger managed Level One. She was a veteran nurse with high energy and organizational skills who worked for the Minneapolis Heart Institute Foundation. It took a full year to implement but, by late 2003, Level One was transforming heart attack care in our region. It improved nearly every measurable outcome: mortality, complications, functional recovery, and the number of days spent in the hospital. The incidence of shock and number of hospital deaths were cut in half, and far fewer patients left the hospital with severely scarred and dysfunctional hearts.

Level One provided physicians around the state with a hotline number to call when a patient arrived in their emergency room with symptoms of a heart attack. No waiting, no callbacks, just one number and the Level One emergency system went into action. All of the participating emergency rooms used a standard treatment protocol. This protocol reduced confusion and variability, and simplified communication. Moreover, the program's implementation required no new technology or capital improvements, no additional employees or salaries, and the results were measurable. It was classic quality improvement, and the effects were visible and tangible immediately.

The message on my pager said a patient, Paul Miller, was being brought in by a Minneapolis emergency medical team that activated the Level One system. The ambulance was seven to ten minutes out. Mr. Miller's condition was deteriorating, so I went to the ambulance entrance and waited. It was about 10:30 a.m.

The ambulance rear doors flew open as the rig came to a stop. Two EMTs quickly unloaded the gurney holding the patient. Miller looked about 50. He was barely conscious and his skin was bluish gray. He was dying.

An EMT handed me the EKG they had recorded at Miller's workplace in downtown Minneapolis. It showed a large acute inferior-lateral myocardial infarction. In all probability, his right coronary artery was 100 percent blocked. I called the catheterization laboratory to tell them we were coming straight up on the emergency elevator. The nurse said the team was ready in Room 7.

Hospital security was waiting at the elevator. We pushed the gurney in and punched the button for the third floor. The doors had just closed when Miller's heart fibrillated. He already had defibrillation electrodes positioned on his chest, so in seconds we shocked him back to a normal rhythm. As the elevator doors opened, he fibrillated again. This time two shocks failed, so I started chest compressions

(CPR). Barb Unger was waiting for us. She grabbed the front end of the gurney and pulled it down the corridor to Room 7.

Dr. Jay Traverse and his team were gowned and gloved with all their angioplasty instruments and drugs ready to go. Traverse was an experienced interventional cardiologist who had trained at the University of Minnesota. I continued the chest compressions until a staff member took over. A nurse anesthetist came into the room, slipped a tube into Miller's trachea, and ventilated him with an anesthesia bag.

Traverse quickly gained access to the right femoral artery and inserted a Judkins coronary angiogram catheter. He advanced the catheter to the opening of the right coronary artery and injected dye. As expected, the X-ray screen showed a blood clot completely blocking Miller's artery. Next Traverse slipped a guidewire through the clot, followed by an angioplasty catheter. He quickly inflated the balloon and disrupted the clot.

Blood began flowing to Mr. Miller's oxygen-starved muscle. His heart was still in ventricular fibrillation and we were doing CPR. We shocked him again. This time the shock successfully restored an organized rhythm interspersed with extra beats. He had already been given intravenous amiodarone, an antiarrhythmic drug and, within minutes, his rhythm settled into a steady cadence. His blood pressure improved.

Getting the artery open fast and restoring blood flow was the key. Otherwise the heart muscle will die. Anything that delayed the re-establishment of blood flow was a waste of time and sacrificed heart muscle. Miller's artery was open in less than 90 minutes after he first experienced chest pain in his Minneapolis office. He left the hospital four days later with a heart that was pumping normally.

What would have happened if Paul Miller had his attack a year before? The ambulance might have taken him to the nearest hospital emergency room, even though that hospital was not equipped to perform emergency angioplasty. On arrival, Mr. Miller would have fibrillated again, and again—just as he had in our elevator. As I had seen too often, time—and heart muscle—would be lost while doctors treated the ventricular fibrillation with shocks and drugs and CPR when the only effective solution was getting the blocked artery open. Critical care too often was provided on an *ad hoc* basis, a throwback to an era when we did not have the knowledge or tools to restore blood flow. Level One became a system of care that would change how all cardiovascular emergencies were managed.

When I graduated from medical school in 1968, 20 to 30 percent of people suffering heart attacks died before or shortly after they arrived at the hospital. For those who survived, the most we could do was put patients to bed, give them stool softeners—and pray. Even after coronary care units were introduced in the 1960s, heart attack mortality rates, although lower, still remained in the double digits. Thrombolytic therapy further reduced the death rate but many patients did not receive these clot dissolving drugs in time to salvage heart muscle. Other patients, particularly the elderly, did not receive thrombolytics at all because doctors feared they might bleed into their brains. Those who survived often developed heart failure or they were at risk for sudden cardiac death. Drugs and the implantable defibrillator helped these patients, but they were palliative and costly treatments.

Geoff Hartzler was the first to advocate emergency angioplasty for heart attacks, and eventually the data supported his approach. Level One dramatically reduced the time it took to open the artery, and further made it possible for patients living outside a metropolitan area to access angioplasty quickly at any hour of the day or night. Far fewer patients went into shock, so much so that coronary care unit nurses in our hospital worried that they would lose their skills for managing critically ill patients.

During its first 10 years, the Level One program at the Minneapolis Heart Institute treated nearly 4,000 heart attack victims from Minnesota and Wisconsin. The hospital mortality rate for all Level One patients was just five percent, a number so low that I never believed I would see it my lifetime. As important was the preservation of heart function. This meant that many fewer patients developed heart failure. It meant also that they could enjoy full lives, and they would not require devices like implantable defibrillators and buckets of drugs.

Level One was an initiative that translated into lives saved and quality of life preserved. This is why the brutal, relentless workload did not bother us, and why it was the best thing that we had ever done as physicians. Soon the Level One approach would benefit patients who suffered a cardiac arrest outside the hospital. These patients rarely survived with an intact brain. Level One and Dr. Michael Mooney changed this dire outlook.

CHAPTER 16

Miriam Santos was a 38-year-old registered nurse who worked the afternoon shift on a surgical unit at Abbott Northwestern Hospital. She and her husband, Jose, had met and married in Nashville, Tennessee, while both attended Vanderbilt University. They moved to Minneapolis in 2004 when Jose, a biomedical engineer, joined Medtronic, the cardiac pacemaker company founded by Earl Bakken. The Santos' purchased their three-bedroom home in Golden Valley near the peak of the housing boom, and their two sons, Jose Jr., and Carl attended school at Meadowbrook Elementary.

In the summer of 2008, Miriam was preparing her lunch in the kitchen when she heard an unusual sound from the family room. She found her 40-year-old husband unconscious on the floor. Bright red blood trickled across his brow. He had fallen and his head struck the coffee table. Miriam shouted, "Jose, what's wrong? What happened?" He did not respond. He was not moving or breathing and she could not find a pulse.

Jose was a big man. Miriam struggled to roll him onto his back. She opened his mouth and started CPR. Twice she shouted for her sons playing in the back yard but they did not hear. After several minutes, Miriam stopped chest compressions, ran to the kitchen, grabbed her cell phone, and dialed 911. The operator answered after a single ring. "My husband is down," she said breathless. "He's not breathing and there is no pulse. Please send an ambulance!"

Miriam continued to alternate chest compressions with mouth-to-mouth breathing. Jose's body was flaccid, his eyes partly open and staring. She began to sob. "Please God, help my husband." Minutes passed. Her shoulders began to ache. She was short of breath and her muscles were tiring with the effort. Finally, Miriam heard the siren, at first distant, then a piercing crescendo as the ambulance turned into their street and pulled into the driveway. She rushed to the front door, opened it, and hurried back to her dying husband.

Three members of the emergency team entered the living room carrying equipment. Miriam was thrusting downward on her husband's chest with clenched hands. "I found him 15 minutes ago," she gasped. "I'm a nurse...." One of the EMTs said, "I'll take over here." He moved Miriam aside. The second EMT tore open Jose's shirt and placed EKG electrodes on his chest. The portable defibrillator monitor showed ventricular fibrillation. "I'm charging!" the EMT shouted as he placed the paddles on Jose's chest.

The shock failed. The first EMT resumed chest compressions while the defibrillator was charged again. "Clear!" The second shock triggered a slow rhythm. "I have a pulse!" the third EMT exclaimed. Gradually Jose's pulse rate increased. The EKG showed a normal rhythm, and no signs of a heart attack. Jose's blood pressure was 90 to 100, but he was not moving. Miriam shouted into his ear, "Jose, Jose, can you hear me!" He did not move. No response. Nothing.

The first EMT placed an airway in Jose's mouth and ventilated him with a facemask.

"We'll take him to Methodist Hospital," the first EMT said to Miriam as he placed an oxygen mask on Jose.

"No! No! I want him to go to Abbott," she said firmly. "I'm a nurse there. Absolutely, I want him to go to Abbott!" She fought back the sobs. Her sons had heard the ambulance and were now standing in the entry hall. "Boys," Miriam said, "your father's had an accident. He needs to go to the hospital. Get in the car. Now!"

The third EMT called the emergency room at Abbott Northwestern Hospital and spoke to one of the physicians. The EMT listened, hung up the phone, and asked, "Mrs. Santos, the doctor at Abbott wants us to pack his head and neck in ice. Do you know anything about the hypothermia protocol?" Miriam did. "Yes, I heard about it." She went to the kitchen and came back with three large clear plastic bags filled with ice.

Jose Santos was one of nearly 300,000 Americans who suffered a cardiac arrest outside of a hospital in 2008. Statistically, he had a one chance in ten of surviving and, if he lived, he would almost certainly have significant and permanent brain damage. However, Jose was lucky: his wife started CPR within minutes of his collapse, and an emergency medical team defibrillated him shortly thereafter. Nevertheless, his brain was deprived of oxygen for many minutes. How well his brain recovered from this severe insult would determine Jose's ability to return to work, and enjoy the kind of life we all desire.

In 2006, Dr. Michael Mooney at the Minneapolis Heart Institute™ designed and implemented a Level One approach to treating patients like Jose who suffered a cardiac arrest. The program was named "Cool It" and, as the name suggests, the principal treatment was lowering the victim's body temperature as quickly as possible. The medical term is *therapeutic hypothermia,* and it is beneficial because it lowers the brain's metabolism and blocks the damaging effects of chemicals that are produced when the heart is not pumping and no blood is flowing.

Based on the results of favorable clinical trials in Europe and Australia, the American Heart Association in 2003 recommended that therapeutic hypothermia could improve brain function recovery in patients who suffer cardiac arrest due to ventricular fibrillation. However, as Mooney observed, hypothermia was not being used routinely, and cooling was not even started until patients arrived in the intensive care unit, if at all. This illustrated a fundamental weakness in emergency care. Even in medically progressive communities, practices varied widely. At a minimum, there were significant delays, and victims living in rural communities suffered most due to the time lost during their transfer to facilities capable of providing therapeutic hypothermia. Lack of organization and focus was the problem.

Mooney worked with Barb Unger to use the Level One emergency heart attack system's infrastructure to establish a regional therapeutic hypothermia treatment program called Cool It.

Before this innovation (Cool It), we had less interaction with families of patients who died of cardiac arrest because half of the patients died at home or never made it to our hospital. Now that emergency medical systems were highly organized, many more patients reached us. Patients whose hearts were pumping blood after CPR and defibrillation were most likely to benefit from Cool It. If their circulation did not return after treatment, then further aggressive measures were unlikely to result in a good outcome. We began to see spectacular "saves": patients who recovered against all odds. These "victories"—I cannot think of a better word—energized the staff. Mooney and Unger organized courses to teach other providers and health systems how to build Cool It programs in their communities.

Jose was comatose when he arrived in our intensive care unit. His pupils did not react to light, because he had sustained a major insult to the reflex centers of his brain. A respirator controlled his breathing. The nurses had the cooling system ready and applied it to Jose within minutes. They put water-based gel pads on his torso and his thighs. By circulating cold water through the pads, Jose's body temperature was lowered to 91.4° F. After 24 hours of cooling, Jose would be slowly rewarmed to a normal 98.6° F.

I discussed Jose's management with Dr. Bill Parham, the critical care specialist who would manage him in the intensive care unit. Miriam Santos was at her husband's bedside when I entered the room.

"Hi Mrs. Santos," I said. "I'm Doctor Hauser, one of the heart doctors."

Miriam looked up. "Yes, I know who you are. I see you occasionally on my floor." She was a small woman, dressed in jeans and a too-large purple and gold Minnesota Vikings sweatshirt. She had dark brown hair braided into a ponytail and she wore no make-up.

We reviewed Jose's medical history. He snored heavily and Miriam thought he had sleep apnea. He stopped at Caribou Coffee every morning on his drive to work and had a double espresso. After that, he switched to Mountain Dew. Jose neither smoked nor used alcohol. Shortly after he was born, Jose had surgery for pyloric stenosis, a narrowing in the opening from his stomach to the intestine. As a teenager, he played competitive football and ran track. Jose had joined the YMCA and worked out on weekends. He had never fainted or complained of symptoms suggestive of heart disease. Both of his parents were living and healthy in their late fifties. One uncle on his mother's side had a pacemaker, but he lived in California and no one had seen him for years.

"What do you think?" Miriam asked after I examined her husband.

"His heart sounds fine, and his EKG is basically normal," I replied. "The blood tests show low potassium, which isn't unusual in this circumstance. The troponin (heart enzyme) is mildly elevated, again not unexpected given the CPR and defibrillation. We will do an echocardiogram—an ultrasound of his heart—when the cooling pads are removed."

I sat down on a folding chair next to her. "Of course the question is always how well his brain will recover."

Looking at Jose she sighed, "This is so unexpected. Thank God, I was home. Otherwise he would have died." Her voice trailed off, and then she asked, "What's next?"

"We'll keep the cooling going for 24 hours, and then allow him to warm up," I began. "Doctor Parham will manage him while he is in this unit. Neurology will be consulted. We'll decide on what heart tests he will need after the echocardiogram. Jose is 40 and has no risk factors for coronary artery disease, but we should consider all the possible causes for a cardiac arrest."

"What are they?" she asked.

"I think it is more likely an inherited condition or myocarditis—an inflammation of the heart muscle."

Miriam grasped her husband's hand. The tube connecting him to the respirator was in his throat. EKG electrodes on his chest were attached to a cable from the monitor above the bed. Three intravenous pumps delivered fluids and drugs in precise quantities through veins in both his arms. Blue cooling pads surrounded his torso and thighs. A nasogastric tube passed through a nostril into his throat and stomach; it was draining small quantities of yellow-white gastric fluid. Jose's eyes were closed.

"When will we know if he's going to wake-up?" She turned to me, scrutinizing my expression as I spoke.

"Late tomorrow or the next day. Difficult to predict." I waited, and then asked, "Where are your sons?"

"They're in the waiting room. My mother is flying up from Nashville. She should be here this evening and will pick up the boys. I'm going to stay with Jose."

I placed my hand on her shoulder. "I'll ask the head nurse to reserve the family conference room for you tonight. You can get some sleep on the couch."

I stood up but found it difficult to leave. "Anything I can do?" Miriam shook her head. I took a card out of my coat pocket and wrote down my cell phone number. I handed it to her and said, "Call me, whenever, if you have questions or just want to talk." She nodded and took the card.

Within two hours, Jose Santos' body temperature was lowered to 91.4 °F. His metabolic rate decreased to 50 percent of normal, meaning that his body was consuming less oxygen. The respirator was adjusted to prevent him from exposure to excess oxygen, which could be toxic to his brain. As it cooled, Jose's body shifted to metabolizing more fat, making his blood slightly more acidic. His pancreas secreted less insulin, causing a rise in blood glucose; he needed insulin injections.

Reduced body temperature slows and interrupts the destructive processes that cause cells to die, especially in the brain. The cooling also blunts some of the harmful inflammatory responses that occur when a heart isn't beating. The pressure inside the brain decreases because at cooler temperatures, less fluid (edema) accumulates in the tissues. These factors combine to mitigate cellular damage and improve the chances of complete neurologic recovery.

Equally important, cooling also prevents fever. Even a mild fever can triple the risk of a bad outcome.

Jose received drugs, including magnesium and propofol, to prevent shivering that would raise his body temperature and blunt the favorable effects of cooling. Shivering can increase oxygen consumption and metabolic rate, counteracting the benefits of hypothermia.

Miriam noticed that Jose's heart rate slowed as his body temperature dropped. She astutely observed some effects on the EKG as well. These were the known and expected results of cooling and did not require specific treatment, except that certain drugs were avoided because they could cause dangerous rhythms such as ventricular fibrillation.

The next day, 24 hours after Jose had been cooled, Bill Parham slowly began the rewarming process. It would take about eight hours. He discontinued the drugs for sedation and shivering when Jose's body temperature returned to normal around midnight.

This began the most trying time for Miriam and her family. Would Jose wake-up? Would he regain full brain function? Would he be neurologically impaired, requiring prolonged rehabilitation, and possibly institutionalization?

Jose's mother and father flew in from Nashville and sat with Miriam at the bedside. The three of them were there when I came by the following morning at 7:30 a.m. The wall-mounted television displayed a muted network show. Rivulets of rain streamed down the large window overlooking 26th street. Mother, father and wife sat on folding chairs, not speaking, staring at the motionless Jose.

The head of Jose's bed was elevated 45 degrees, and the ventilator noiselessly delivered breaths at 14 times a minute. The EKG monitor showed a normal rhythm and the oxygen saturation, measured by a sensor on his finger, was 98 percent. The calibrated plastic bag hanging at the foot of his bed held about half liter of clear yellow urine.

I had spoken to Jose's nurse before entering the room. He had shown no spontaneous activity but coughed whenever she suctioned the tube in his throat. His pupils were equal in size, and constricting when she opened his eyelids. These were good signs.

"Good morning," I said and stepped around the bed where Jose's parents were sitting. "I'm Doctor Hauser—the heart doctor." Carl Santos was nearly bald and wore a well-tailored brown suit and gold tie. Nancy Santos had blonde hair that spread onto her shoulders; she was immaculately groomed in a white silk blouse, gray pearl necklace, and black jacket and slacks. They were in their fifties and had the look of people who exercise regularly.

Miriam, still in her Vikings sweatshirt and jeans, was bedraggled. I sensed that she and Jose's parents were not close. Turning to Miriam, I said, "Everything—rhythm, blood pressure, oxygen—look good."

"We're waiting for the sedation to wear off," Miriam said matter-of-factly.

"Yes," I said, "and he's reacting when the nurse suctions his mouth and endotracheal tube." The gel pads had been removed. I listened to Jose's heart—no murmur or unusual sounds. His lungs were clear—no rattles or wheezes. I gently pressed on his abdomen; it was soft and my prodding produced no reaction. The morning EKG showed that Jose was textbook normal.

I looked at Miriam and then to his parents. "So far, so good. Now we wait. I'll be back later this afternoon. The echocardiogram should be done by then."

"Doctor Hauser," Carl Santos said softly, "what if my son does not wake up? What if he stays in a coma?" He paused. "I suppose I'm asking…." His voice trailed off.

"Will he be a vegetable? That is what my husband wants to know." Mrs. Santos began to weep. The tears flowed and she covered her face with her hands. Miriam got up from her chair and knelt by her mother-in-law. They hugged each other, perhaps for the first time, like this.

My pager beeped. I had an emergency call from an outside hospital. It was a Level One heart attack.

I placed my hand gently on Mrs. Santos' shoulder and looked at her husband. "Let's see what the day brings. I understand your concern. There's reason to be optimistic."

"Thank you, doctor," Carl Santos said, looking at his son. "We'll be here."

Miriam said to me, "You have to answer your page. We're fine."

Later that morning, I received a text message from Jose's nurse. His echocardiogram—the ultrasound of his heart—was done and available for review. I took the elevator down to the second floor of the Heart Hospital and walked into the large room where three of my partners sat at computer-based reading stations. Displayed on large screens in front of them were digital ultrasound video images of hearts that had been studied during the previous 24 hours.

Dr. Richard Bae was reading Jose Santos' echo. I sat down next to him and summarized Jose's medical history. "What do you think?" I asked. Both of us looked at the images of Jose's beating heart displayed in black and white on the high definition monitor. Occasionally a flash of bright red or blue appeared near a valve; these were color Doppler waveforms that reflected the velocity of blood traveling through his heart.

"His heart looks pretty good," Bae said. "Left ventricular function is normal, no valve problems, and the right side looks okay." Using the computer mouse, he shuffled the digital images on the screen and focused on the tip of the left ventricle. "I don't see the left ventricular apex very well but it may be thickened. I can't rule out atypical hypertrophic cardiomyopathy or non-compaction (a rare fetal developmental disorder that affects the heart)."

I said, "He'll need a cardiac MRI (magnetic resonance imaging)."

"Yes. Exactly" Bae agreed. "Let me know what you find."

I thanked him and left for the catheterization laboratory where the Level One acute heart attack patient was arriving from New Ulm, a charming town 90 miles southwest of Minneapolis. The helicopter had just landed on the roof and I could smell the fumes of its exhaust in the elevator.

As the door opened, I received a text message on my pager from Jose Santos' nurse. It read simply, "He is awake." I whispered to myself, "Thank you, God."

The patient from New Ulm was a 56-year-old homemaker who had been the picture of health all of her life. The previous weekend she and her husband were dancing a polka when she got lightheaded and sweaty. She refused to go to the emergency room and instead drove home. This morning she was helping her son put up hay in the barn when she got nauseated and complained of chest pain.

Her son dialed 911 from his cell phone, and an hour later she was in a helicopter on her way to our hospital. The EKG, faxed to us from the New Ulm emergency room, showed signs of a heart attack involving the underside (inferior wall) of her left ventricle. Her name was Geraldine "Gerry" Stumpf.

By the time I arrived Dr. Nick Burke was already injecting dye into Gerry's right coronary artery. The dye flowed down the vessel, showing no clot or obstruction. Burke injected the artery twice more and recorded images at different angles. There was no blockage but the tip of her right coronary artery was narrowed, like a river abruptly becoming a stream. The artery could be in spasm. Burke injected nitroglycerin directly into the artery but the narrowing did not change, indicating that spasm was less likely. Next, he injected dye into the left coronary artery; it contained no clot or plaque and all of the vessels were normal in size. Finally, Burke performed a ventriculogram—dye injection into the left ventricle. This revealed a weak area in the underside of the ventricle, just where the EKG indicated the heart attack would be.

I reviewed the blood tests from New Ulm. The troponin (an enzyme released from damaged heart muscle) was mildly elevated, confirming there had been heart muscle damage. Gerry had a heart attack, but the angiogram revealed no culprit, no cause, except that she had no plaque and thus did not have atherosclerotic coronary artery disease. The only remarkable finding was the narrowing that we saw at the end of the right coronary artery. We did not have an explanation, and treatment without a diagnosis was like driving down a winding road at night without headlights.

Gerry was lying on the X-ray table. Nick Burke was explaining what he found. I introduced myself and said, "The good news is we found no blockage. We will do some additional tests to find out what caused this."

"What could it be?" she asked. "I've been healthy all of my life. Nobody in the family has heart trouble."

"There are several possibilities, Mrs. Stumpf," I said. "Sometimes the artery goes into spasm, or there could be a blood clot that formed in the artery, or came from somewhere else in your body, and dissolved by the time you got here. How long did you have the chest pain?"

"They gave me nitroglycerin in the ambulance, and the pain was gone by the time we got to the hospital. My husband carries nitroglycerin tablets. He had a stent put in at this hospital last year. I think you did it. You look familiar."

I pressed on, "It could have been spasm that caused your pain and your heart attack. By the time we did the angiogram, the spasm could have resolved. Another possibility is inflammation. We simply do not know. We will do an MRI of your heart tomorrow. You'll stay overnight in intensive care where we can monitor you closely."

She looked at me, somewhat apologetically, and said, "The polka contest finals are this Saturday. It's the first time Howard and I have ever made it to the finals. Do you think I will be able to do it?"

Polka was still a big deal in New Ulm, although it was nothing like the glory days of the 1950s when many New Ulm polka bands toured the country. "I don't think that would be a good idea. Your heart will need time to heal," I replied.

I returned to the intensive care unit early that afternoon. My first stop was Jose Santos's room. What a change. Parham had taken him off the respirator and removed the tube from his throat. Jose was sitting up, talking to Miriam and his parents who were standing around his bed. He was slightly hoarse. His two sons and mother-in-law were also in the room. There were flowers from his company on the bedside table, and two pink "Get Well" helium-filled balloons tethered to the foot of his bed.

Miriam introduced me, "Honey, this is Doctor Hauser, the cardiologist who's looking after you." We shook hands.

"How do you feel?" I asked.

Jose placed his right hand on his head and replied, "Like I've been hit by a truck!" He coughed and laughed. "I'm okay, a little woozy, not sure what day it is. Glad to see my Mom and Dad, Angela, and the boys." His speech was perfect and he gestured appropriately with his hands. There were no evident neurologic deficits.

Being the biomedical engineer that he was, Jose wanted to know the details of therapeutic hypothermia. I explained the rationale and described the equipment. He then asked the key question, "Why did this happen to me, Doctor Hauser? I was feeling fine, and then I went out. I don't remember a thing."

"How were you feeling that morning? Anything unusual? Heart racing? Extra beats? Palpitations?" I asked.

"Absolutely okay. Felt great. I was getting ready for a business trip to Europe. The last thing I remember is going downstairs to get my passport in the study." He looked at Miriam and back to me.

Miriam asked, "What did his echocardiogram show?"

"It looked okay," I replied, "except for one area we could not see very well. It's at the tip of the left ventricle—the main pumping chamber—there may be some thickening. But we can't be sure. We'll do an MRI to get a better picture."

"What if there is some thickening? What does that mean?" Miriam persisted.

I sat on the edge of Jose's bed and directed my answer to him. "There are two possibilities. One is an unusual condition called *apical hypertrophic cardiomyopathy* and the second is *left ventricular non-compaction*. Both are inherited and both could have caused the rapid rhythm—the ventricular fibrillation or tachycardia—that caused your cardiac arrest."

Understandably, everyone in the room was trying to digest what I had said. I went on to explain hypertrophic cardiomyopathy. Left ventricular non-compaction was a rare fetal developmental disorder in which the heart muscle does not mature, retaining some its embryonic characteristics.

I continued, "You will also have a CT coronary angiogram. We'll give you dye into your vein and take a high-resolution X-ray scan of your coronary arteries. I doubt that you have coronary artery disease, but we need to rule out other coronary abnormalities that may have triggered your ventricular fibrillation. You may recall the basketball player Pete Maravich. He died suddenly at 40. He was born with an abnormal coronary artery. "

Jose asked, "Will I need an implantable defibrillator?"

I had anticipated his question. "I think so. One of our electrophysiologists will see you, of course, but I think no matter what we find, you will need a defibrillator implanted before you go home."

I paused and looked at each family member. Finally, Carl Santos said, "Thank you, Doctor, it's very clear. I have no questions."

Jose said, "I know Doctor Katsiyiannis. My company is doing a project with him. Could he implant the ICD?"

Bill Katsiyiannis was one of our senior electrophysiologists. I replied, "I'll see if he's available."

The following morning I was paged by the intensive care unit. Gerry Stumpf had an episode of chest pain at 6 a.m. and the nurse gave her a nitroglycerin tablet. But the chest pain persisted and spread to both arms. Twenty minutes later, I was at her bedside. Gerry looked comfortable. She had received morphine and her discomfort had nearly resolved. Her EKG was unchanged. I called the cardiology diagnostics laboratory and ordered an emergency CT angiogram.

Soon Gerry was in the CT scanner, an X-ray machine that moves around the body and takes high resolution pictures of the heart and coronary arteries. X-ray dye was injected into Gerry's blood stream through a vein in her left arm. A digital X-ray movie was made of the dye traveling through her heart, lungs, and coronary arteries. The movie was stored on a computer whose special software processed the images and transferred them to a computer workstation for interpretation.

Cardiologist Dr. Bjorn Flygenring reviewed the CT angiogram and within minutes he had the diagnosis. Gerry Stumpf had a rare, life-threatening condition called *spontaneous coronary artery dissection*, known by its abbreviation, *SCAD*.

Usually the dissection begins when a clot forms in the wall of the artery and spreads along its entire length, compressing the artery's lumen (channel), blocking blood flow, and causing a heart attack. Why the clot forms is a mystery.

I was in the intensive care unit when my cell phone rang. It was Flygenring. "Bob," he said, "Mrs. Stumpf has a big problem. There are four coronary dissections—in her right, left main, left anterior descending, and circumflex coronary arteries. You need to look at this."

Just when you think you have seen everything, a unique case or new disease appears. This is one reason cardiology is so stimulating. I was lucky to work with a cadre of exceptionally talented and experienced people. Flygenring was one of them: he grew up in Iceland and trained in cardiology in the United States. He and I joined the Minneapolis Heart Institute full-time in 1992, and we worked well together.

When I entered the darkened CT reading room, Flygenring said, "These are incredible images. I've never seen anything like this."

I pulled up a chair and focused on the images Flygenring manipulated with the computer's software. There, on the large flat-screen monitor, we could see that four of Gerry Stumpf's coronary arteries were compressed and distorted by blood that encased and constricted them, so much so that normal blood flow was impossible.

On a second computer, we loaded images from the invasive coronary angiogram done the previous day. It was now clear that the narrowed end of the right coronary seen on that angiogram was a spontaneous dissection and not a spasm. During the night three new coronary dissections had developed, resulting in her chest pain a 6 a.m. Her situation was precarious. Already she had had four small heat attacks. Another dissection could be fatal. I picked up the phone and dialed the cardiac surgery office.

Spontaneous coronary artery dissection is rare—or it is rarely recognized. Like many other cardiac conditions, so-called "rare" diseases were being observed with increasing frequency because new imaging technology allowed us to see anatomic structures in greater detail than ever before. Imagine the difference between the grainy black and white television screens of the 1960s and the high-definition, multi-pixel digital pictures we have in the 21st century. Advanced imaging was opening up new frontiers of knowledge and enhancing our ability to make the correct diagnosis. This recent advance would save Gerry Stumpf's life.

Later that day, Dr. Tom Flavin took Gerry to the operating room and placed her on the heart-lung machine. He used the left internal mammary artery under the breastbone to bypass her left anterior descending coronary artery. Next, he removed the saphenous vein from her leg and cut it into sections to bypass the circumflex and right coronary arteries.

Gerry recovered from surgery and she returned to her home in New Ulm after a week in the hospital. Six months later a CT angiogram showed that Gerry's four coronary artery dissections had healed. An echocardiogram revealed that the pumping function of her left ventricle was nearly normal

The following year Gerry and her husband, Howard, made it to the polka finals, and came in second.

The CT coronary angiogram revealed Jose's normal coronary arteries that arose as they should from above the aortic valve. From the CT scan, he was taken to the adjacent MRI laboratory where Dr. John Lesser would oversee the test and interpret the images. Lesser developed the Minneapolis Heart Institute's advanced cardiac imaging program that included MRI and CT angiography. He was and is a gifted teacher and an internationally recognized leader in cardiac imaging.

Jose Santos joked with the technicians as they readied him for his MRI. They placed special EKG electrodes on his skin so the MRI was synchronized with his heartbeat, resulting in crisp images. They connected his intravenous line to a remotely controlled power injector that sent a contrast agent, gadolinium, through his bloodstream to his heart where it caused any scar tissue to appear white. Next, Jose was positioned on the table that would move him in and out of the tunnel formed by the magnetic coils.

I sat in the control room with Lesser. Through a thick window, we could see Jose lying flat in the scanner. Jana Lindberg, the lead technician, turned on the MRI, activating the coils and generating a strong 1.5 Tesla magnetic field. Jose could hear loud banging sounds as the electrical pulses caused the coils to vibrate.

Inside his chest, the magnetic forces caused hydrogen atoms to change direction and resonate with special radiofrequency pulses that would differentiate the various tissues that comprise the heart. Different pulses produced images of blood, fat, and muscle until a picture of the heart appeared on the monitor. Sequences of pictures became a motion picture, revealing the four chambers of Jose's heart beating in exquisite detail. Lindberg then triggered the injector, sending gadolinium to his heart muscle. Jose's heart muscle was not stained by the gadolinium, meaning there was no scar tissue.

The MRI images vividly captured the disease that had nearly taken Jose's life. He had left ventricular non-compaction. During fetal development, the inside of his left ventricle consisted of a sponge-like network of muscle fibers called trabeculations. Normally this collection of fibers is compacted—pressed—into a smooth inner wall called the endocardium. When fibers are not compacted, the sponge-like tissue persists as a bizarre patchwork of muscle, forming recesses in the heart and creating a catalyst for life-threatening rhythms like ventricular fibrillation. This is what happened to Jose.

We rarely diagnosed left ventricular non-compaction in living patients until the advent of cardiac MRI. Like hypertrophic cardiomyopathy, non-compaction may be silent and never cause symptoms or complications. For patients like Jose, it can be lethal and it may be inherited and passed on to future generations. Fortunately, neither of Jose's sons had the disease.

Dr. Katsiyiannis implanted a defibrillator in Jose the day after the cardiac MRI. Jose returned to work and subsequently left Medtronic to join a start-up company developing a urology device. He has not needed a shock from the defibrillator. At the time of my retirement, the Minneapolis Heart Institute was caring for more than 150 patients with left ventricular non-compaction cardiomyopathy, many of whom had implanted defibrillators.

Eventually Mike Mooney would report that more than half of patients admitted under the Cool It program survived, and nearly all of them had positive neurologic outcomes. This was a major advance, and it was published in the journal of the American Heart Association. Prior to this, only one in ten cardiac arrest victims survived, and those that did were often severely disabled. The Level

One heart attack and Cool It programs complemented each other, preserving heart muscle and brain tissue by delivering the best care as fast as possible 24 hours a day, every day.

After practicing cardiology all these years, I thought there was nothing that could truly dumbfound me. I was mistaken. One of my partners, Dr. Scott Sharkey, and a patient, Lois Hagen, would show me how insular I had become.

CHAPTER 17

My pager said another Level One heart attack patient was on the way by helicopter from Grantsburg, Wisconsin. She was a 59-year-old widow who developed chest pain and shortness of breath while arguing with her son. She was given nitroglycerin in the local emergency room. Her blood pressure dropped but it was improving with intravenous saline. The EKG was abnormal and her heart enzyme—troponin—was elevated, indicating heart muscle damage.

Forty minutes later, I heard the helicopter landing on the roof of Abbott-Northwestern Hospital. I headed for the catheterization laboratory and arrived at the same time as the patient. Her name was Maude Thorsen and she appeared much older than the age listed on her records. She was tearful and the nurse was trying to comfort her.

I obtained a quick history. Her chest pain and shortness of breath began that morning when her 30-year-old son became angry when she would not give him money. "He can't keep a job," she said, "and he sits around the house all day drinking beer. Then he goes out at night with his buddies." Mrs. Thorsen was a widow with no history of heart disease. She smoked two packs of cigarettes a day, and had not seen a doctor in years because she could not afford it.

One of my partners, Dr. Jay Traverse, performed her angiogram. Her coronary arteries were normal; in fact, they were surprisingly pristine—no plaque and no calcium. Traverse then injected a bolus of dye into her left ventricle. This revealed a markedly abnormal chamber that was enlarged and shaped like an urn. Mrs. Thorsen had classic *takotsubo cardiomyopathy*, so named by a Japanese physician because the left ventricle in this condition is shaped like the ceramic pot that Asian fisherman use for trapping octopus.

In 2005, another of my partners, Dr. Scott Sharkey, described a series of patients who also had takotsubo cardiomyopathy. It had been renamed *stress cardiomyopathy* because it was uniquely related to emotional or physical stress. Sharkey delved into the case histories of patients in our practice who had takotsubo cardiomyopathy.

He found that many of these victims were typically post-menopausal women who had experienced profound emotional distress, such as an unexpected death in the family, domestic abuse, or financial loss. Other patients had a physical rather than emotional illness that seemed to trigger the cardiomyopathy.

The evident connection between emotional stress and a serious heart condition evoked the term "broken heart syndrome," a condition long suspected but unproven until new imaging technologies like MRI allowed Sharkey and others to connect the dots.

Maude Thorsen's "broken heart" appeared to be the daily stress of dealing with her son. We treated her with stress reduction therapy and a beta-blocker to blunt the effects of adrenalin-like substances on her heart. She recovered in the hospital and was ready to return home after five days.

On the day of her discharge, I met with her son privately and told him that his behavior had contributed to his mother's illness. He broke down, crying, saying he had a drinking problem and needed help. I paged one of the hospital's social workers; she arranged a clinic appointment near his home. A month later, I saw Mrs. Thorsen in the Cambridge Clinic: she was better and her son had been drug and alcohol free for three weeks. This, too, was part of her treatment.

By 2010, Sharkey had identified 130 stress (takotsubo) cardiomyopathy patients who had been treated in our hospital. All but a few were women. One of them was another of my patients, a sixty-three-year-old woman, who had been severely beaten by her husband. He had served a 10-year jail sentence for the assault and was about to be released. She was admitted to the hospital with chest pain, terrified that her former husband would find and kill her—a threat he had made at his trial. Her cardiac MRI confirmed stress cardiomyopathy, and I treated her with a beta-blocker. I had never observed such fear in anyone, and years later I can still see her face and recall the very room she occupied on Station 44. She received police protection and her heart recovered with the help of medications. Her ex-husband never appeared, evidently concluding that 10 years in prison was enough.

Lois Hagen grew up in a large Catholic family in Pennsylvania, just east of Pittsburgh, where her father taught math at the local high school and coached the track team. Her mother was the school nurse when she was not having babies. Lois had three older brothers and three younger sisters. The seven children occupied two bedrooms in a gray stucco house on a dead-end street in a neighborhood that sprouted after World War I. Lois's earliest memories were playing kick the can and touch football with her brothers. She was delighted when her sisters were born and she could play dolls and dress-up.

When Lois entered high school in the fall of 1970 her oldest brother, Paul, was a helicopter pilot flying combat missions with the 1st Air Cavalry in Vietnam. Every evening the family watched the CBS anchor, Walter Cronkite, describe the latest battle and its casualties. "I don't know how my parents endured the year my brother was flying combat missions in Vietnam," Lois later recalled. "My father sort of withdrew, and mom just kept very busy all the time. Thankfully Paul came home, healthy, and happy to be out of the Army."

Lois entered Notre Dame in 1974. Her goal was to be a clinical psychologist. Lois won a small scholarship for her senior science project that described the statistical challenges in assessing Pavlovian conditioning. Her work was so sophisticated that her high school teacher needed the help of a graduate student at the University of Pittsburgh to understand and grade the project.

Lois' mother developed breast cancer in January 1975, and underwent bilateral radical mastectomies, the favored treatment at the time. Lois was midway through her first year in college when, on Valentine's Day, her mother suffered a massive pulmonary embolus—a blood clot to the lung. A surgeon at the Medical Center attempted to remove the clot, but she died in the operating room.

The family was devastated, especially Lois's three young sisters. Over her father's objections, Lois left Notre Dame, transferring to Duquesne University in downtown Pittsburgh where she could commute from home. Her sisters, in the 7th, 9th, and 11th grades, were comforted by the presence of 19-year-old Lois who did what she knew her mother would have expected her to do. Overnight Lois began to think like a parent—a mother—rather than a sister.

For the next six years, Lois looked after her sisters. Denise, the youngest, graduated from high school in 1980 and left home for nursing school. The other sisters were working and part-time students at a local community college; they shared an apartment in the city. All three boys had careers and families of their own. Her father, who had become increasingly withdrawn, was otherwise healthy and a year away from retirement. Lois felt her mother would be pleased with what she had done for the family.

At 24, Lois became restless. She needed ten credits to graduate with a liberal arts degree. After the first year at Duquesne she decided to forego clinical psychology and focus on statistics, an attractive discipline because she found math and data stimulating, and she could work alone. The advent of personal computers had liberated statisticians from the restrictions imposed by institutional mainframe computers. Individuals like Lois could write their own programs and crunch megabytes of data. She saved money and purchased an IBM desktop.

Quite suddenly, though, Lois felt that she had to get away from Pittsburgh. In many ways, the previous six years had stolen her youth. She rarely dated, had no close friends except her sisters, and her brief time in South Bend was her only worldly experience. She was not resentful but a voice within screamed, "Let me out of here!"

Lois became a flight attendant for Northwest Airlines. She moved to Minneapolis and shared an apartment with three of her co-workers. After a year of flying domestic routes, she qualified for international assignments and was soon spending weeks away, primarily in the Asia-Pacific but also in Europe and the Middle East. During her time off, she completed her undergraduate degree and became a part-time graduate student in statistics at the University of Minnesota.

In February of 1986, Lois was on a layover in Tokyo when she received a telegram from her oldest brother, Paul. He wrote that their father had committed suicide. Her father had turned into a recluse after becoming the sole occupant of the house. Moreover, his retirement from teaching and coaching had removed any need for social interaction. On Valentine's Day, their father placed the barrel of a 38-caliber pistol in his mouth and pulled the trigger. After not hearing from his father for a week, Paul drove to the family home and discovered his body in the bathroom. It was exactly eleven years since his wife's death.

The next day Lois did not work during the return flight to Minneapolis. Rather, she sat in the last row of the Boeing 747, in a window seat, where there was near-total isolation. At first, she experienced guilt, a bitter bite of conscience. Lois had not seen her father for six months; she had spent Christmas in Colorado with friends, and she had not spoken to him by telephone for many weeks. "It was thoughtless of me," she said to herself. "If I had been there, or spoken to him, I may have seen the warning signs…if, if, if."

Then shame engulfed her. It was no longer a matter of guilt, but rather a sense that something was terribly wrong with her as a person. The emotion was devastating and she felt defective, naked, exposed to the world as an uncaring child, witlessly pursuing social thrills and self-satisfaction. Surely, the passengers around her, she imagined, sensed her failings. Later she recalled, "I wanted to lock myself in the toilet for the rest of the flight." Instead, she remained in her seat, staring out the window, absently watching the Pacific Ocean 38,000 feet below.

Her chest discomfort started insidiously. Lois became aware of a tightness, a pressure, a nagging fullness that brought acid to her throat and alarmed her. She could feel her pores spout tiny droplets of cold perspiration, sweat that crawled into her clothing and caused her to draw the thin red polyester Northwest Airlines blanket tightly around her. "Am I having a heart attack?" she wondered. "No, of course not. I am too young and healthy." Yet the discomfort persisted, waxing and waning, a cycle of anxiety and relief. "Should I call one of the flight attendants?" she asked herself. The call button was within easy reach above her. "No, that would draw attention to myself. Perhaps this is what I deserve."

The mammoth airplane droned onward, mile after mile on its eastward passage. Lois's chest comfort subsided somewhere over northern Canada. After nearly 6,000 miles and 12 hours, the 747 landed in Minneapolis and taxied to its gate at the international terminal.

Lois was the last passenger to leave the airplane. She made small talk with several of the flight attendants. They were aware of her father's death and expressed their sympathies. The chest discomfort returned as she struggled up the jet way with her carry-on luggage.

She passed quickly through the crewmember lane in the immigration hall and took the shuttle bus to the Northwest employee parking lot. Thankfully, her five-year-old, 3-series BMW started despite the near zero temperatures it had been exposed to for five days. As she drove north on Interstate 35W the aching in her chest left and did not return. The following day Lois flew to Pittsburgh for her father's funeral.

I met Lois Hagen 28 years later in February 2014 when she was transferred to the Minneapolis Heart Institute by helicopter. Her husband, Marc, had driven her to the Cambridge Medical Center that morning after she complained of chest pain. "I had this once before," she told the emergency room physician in Cambridge. "It was on a flight from Tokyo when I was with Northwest. My father had just died, and I guess I was upset."

The physician nodded and took the EKG off the clipboard at the foot of the gurney. "Your EKG isn't entirely normal, but there are no definite signs of a heart attack." He said. "We'll wait for the blood test results. They should be back soon."

"Doctor, my pain is pretty much gone," Lois said. "Do I have to stay? I have a lot of projects right now."

"I think it would be wise to wait for the blood tests," he replied.

Lois asked Marc to hand her the iPhone from the handbag she had packed hastily at home. She called her assistant and told her where she was and to cancel her morning appointments. Half a dozen emails needed replies.

The monitor above Lois's gurney displayed one lead of the EKG and digital readings of her blood pressure and heart rate. Each heartbeat triggered a muted beep from the monitor. Lois watched the emergency room staff through the sliding glass door. The doctor sat in front of a computer screen. A nurse behind him filled a syringe with clear liquid from a glass vial. Every few minutes, the clerk spoke briefly on the telephone.

A half hour passed. Marc left to get coffee from the cafeteria. Lois, impatient, checked her emails again. Nothing. She scanned the calendar, reviewing her schedule for the next few days. Tomorrow was Valentine's Day. She and Marc planned a quiet dinner at home. As he did every year, Marc would have two dozen roses delivered to her office. Then he would bring home a heart-shaped red Valentine box full of gourmet chocolate candy.

Inside Lois's heart, two organic chemicals, epinephrine and norepinephrine, were accumulating in and around the muscle cells of her left ventricle. Epinephrine came from the adrenal glands positioned atop her kidneys, while norepinephrine was largely produced by the nervous system, including the hypothalamus in her brain and the sympathetic nervous system throughout her body. These chemicals, called catecholamines, normally cause a rise in heart rate and blood pressure, particularly during exercise, but also in response to emotional stress. When present in excessive amounts, these chemicals can be toxic, killing muscle cells and interfering with normal blood flow through the smaller branches of the coronary arteries. They may cause the arteries to spasm and shut down, obstructing the artery as effectively as a blood clot.

In some women who have passed through menopause and lack the vascular protection of estrogen, the toxic effects of epinephrine may be amplified by a factor of two or three, especially when the arteries are in spasm. As she lay on the gurney in the emergency room, the biochemical cauldron in Lois's chest simmered and then boiled over. The tip of her left ventricle stopped contracting. Indeed, the entire front side of her heart ballooned, abruptly cutting its pumping capacity in half. Lois's blood pressure plummeted, and her heart rate took off like a rocket in an exaggerated attempt to provide the life-sustaining oxygen that her body needed to stay alive.

When Marc returned from the cafeteria, he was alarmed to see Lois surrounded by nurses and the emergency room physician. A nurse intercepted him, said Lois was in shock, and that an air ambulance would take her from Cambridge to Abbott Northwestern Hospital.

Within twenty minutes, the blue and white helicopter landed on the pad next to the emergency room at the Cambridge hospital. Lois's blood pressure had stabilized on intravenous Levophed®, a drug that constricted her blood vessels. She was pale and barely conscious. Marc followed the gurney as the air ambulance crew pushed it to the landing pad and loaded her into the helicopter. "We'll get her there in twenty minutes max, "the pilot told Marc. "You can't go with us. That's the rule. Sorry." Marc headed for the parking lot; the forty-nine-mile drive south to the hospital would take just under an hour.

Lois' blood test in Cambridge indicated that she was having a heart attack. The troponin was quite elevated, suggesting that the attack had been going on for more than a few hours. The picture was not typical. This was a woman with no coronary risk factors. I read her electronic chart on the computer in my office. It revealed nothing more than routine annual preventive care in Cambridge. Her cholesterol and blood glucose levels had always been normal.

The catheterization laboratory was ready for Lois. Dr. Ivan Chavez was gowned and gloved and the intra-aortic balloon pump team was in the room. I had paged another of my partners, Dr. Kasia Hryniewicz, who was on-call for the Shock Team at the Minneapolis Heart Institute. I described Lois's situation. Hryniewicz said she would tell her eight-member team that mechanical extracorporeal membrane oxygenator (ECMO) support might be needed.

When I graduated from medical school in 1968, shock caused by all forms of heart disease—called cardiogenic shock—usually led to death despite intensive treatment. Many of us thought that the intra-aortic balloon pump would alter this terrible prognosis for heart attack victims, but studies had shown that the intra-aortic balloon pump did not improve a patient's chance of surviving. For this reason, our attention shifted to devices that actually pumped and oxygenated blood, allowing time for the heart to heal and recover. The ECMO was one such device.

I entered the catheterization laboratory just as Chavez was sliding the coronary catheter up Lois's aorta from her leg. He connected the catheter to a pressure transducer: her systolic blood pressure was still low on a moderately high dose of Levophed®. The tip of the catheter engaged the opening of the left coronary artery. X-ray dye injections in three different views revealed a large, dominant left coronary, which was wide open and free of plaque. Her small right coronary artery was also normal. Chavez exchanged the coronary catheter for a catheter that he inserted into her left ventricle via the femoral artery.

All of us watched the X-ray screen as dye was injected into her left ventricle through the catheter. The dark contrast filled the left ventricle's cavity and sharply outlined its inner walls. There, before us, was the classic picture of takotsubo stress cardiomyopathy. The front end of Lois's ventricle was shaped like a balloon, barely moving, while the backside was constricted, as though it was being clutched in a powerful fist. It was similar to the shape of Maude Thorsen's heart, but the dysfunction was much worse.

"This is the worst case of stress cardiomyopathy I've ever seen," Chavez said. "The EF (ejection fraction, or proportion of blood ejected with each beat) can't be more than ten percent."

"Right," I replied. "I have the Shock Team on standby. I'll call Kasia."

"Yes, absolutely," Chavez said. He turned to the circulating nurse "Let's get the ECMO equipment ready while I insert a Swan-Ganz™ catheter." This catheter would allow us to monitor the pressures and flows through the right side of Lois's heart.

The Shock Team arrived, led by Hryniewicz and Dr. Ben Sun, a cardiac surgeon who specialized in ECMO and mechanical artificial hearts. They reviewed the angiogram and laboratory data. One key measurement was Lois's blood lactate level; it was critically high, indicating that her body needed oxygen. Without aggressive treatment, she would die.

"We should go ahead with ECMO," Hryniewicz said. "What do you think, Ben?"

"I think we should do it here, now, and not waste time taking her to the operating room." Sun replied.

The Shock Team set about their individual tasks. Meanwhile an anesthesiologist further sedated Lois and slipped an endotracheal tube into her throat: she would be on a respirator to reduce the energy she expended to breathe.

I sat at the monitoring desk behind the clear leaded glass window and watched as Chavez and Sun dilated the femoral artery and vein and inserted large plastic cannulas (tubes) that would connect Lois's circulation to the ECMO pump and oxygenator. The perfusionist assembled the small, portable Centrimag™ blood pump and the Quadrox-D™ oxygenator. The Centrimag™ was a centrifugal pump with a magnetically levitated impeller designed to move blood forward, while the Quadrox-D™ oxygenator used hollow fiber membranes to exchange oxygen and carbon dioxide. I was familiar with the oxygenator technology, having tested it in patients during heart-lung bypass for the NIH's Artificial Heart Program in 1972. It was highly efficient and easy to use.

A message on my iPhone said that Lois's husband had arrived and was in the waiting room. I called the receptionist and asked that he be shown to one of the private family's rooms where I would meet with him.

As I would later learn, Lois had married Marc Hagen in 1994 after she had finished her doctorate in statistics at the University of Minnesota. He owned a building in Fridley where Lois rented a small office to begin her statistics consulting business. Marc was divorced and had custody of his two small children who were just beginning grade school. They dated for nearly a year before their church wedding in Pittsburgh, where Lois's oldest brother, Paul, gave the bride away.

I opened the door to the small family room next to the catheterization laboratory. Marc Hagen rose from his chair and shook my hand. He was stocky with sandy hair and an easy smile.

"Hello, Mr. Hagen," I said, and gestured for him to sit down. I pulled up a folding chair and sat across from him. "I'm the cardiologist who will be looking after your wife. We just finished the angiogram and found that her coronary arteries are normal. There is no sign of a blockage that would cause a heart attack. The problem is with her pump. It's called the left ventricle. It is enlarged and very weak, and not pumping enough blood to maintain her blood pressure. She is in shock. We have a team in the laboratory that is placing her on a type of heart-lung machine."

I paused, waiting for him to absorb what I had told him. Then continued, "The shape of her heart suggests that she has been under a lot of stress. We have seen this in other women her age. It's called stress cardiomyopathy. It usually occurs in women under considerable emotional strain." Again I paused and asked. "Has there been a death in the family? Are there any problems that aren't resolved, that may be causing anxiety? Anything?"

"No, nothing," Marc replied. "She's been working hard, but she always works hard. She is very successful."

The door to the family room opened and a young man and woman entered. "Hi, Dad," the woman said, "how's Lois?" Marc introduced me to his daughter and son, Kris and John. I summarized what we found and outlined how we were treating their stepmother.

I left the Hagen family and returned to the catheterization laboratory where Chavez and Sun had finished connecting Lois to the pump and oxygenator. The perfusionist was adjusting the pump's flow rate. Kasia Hryniewicz sat in front of the computer, typing a note and entering orders. "She looks better, Bob," Hryniewicz said. "We'll get her up to one of the critical care rooms on 4100. I'll try to wean her off the Levophed®—it can't be good for her heart."

I thanked her and called the receptionist to direct the Hagen family to the waiting room in the intensive care unit on Station 4100. I also sent a text message to Scott Sharkey, asking him to review Lois's chart and give me his thoughts. This was the time to tap everyone's brain.

Forty-eight hours after being placed on the ECMO pump and oxygenator, Lois's heart showed definite signs of recovery. An echocardiogram revealed that her left ventricle was beginning to contract more vigorously and the ballooning was less prominent. Kasia Hryniewicz began to wean her from ECMO. The breathing tube was removed from Lois's throat and she was able to speak. At first, we were concerned about kidney failure, but she began to produce urine and blood tests indicated her kidneys were recovering from the ill-effects of low blood flow.

Three days after Lois was admitted to the hospital in shock, she was taken to the operating room where Ben Sun removed the cannulas from her femoral artery and vein. She was transferred to a cardiology floor where she continued to recover and I had the opportunity to speak with her privately for the first time.

Lois was an attractive woman. She had shoulder-length dark brown hair, brown eyes, and full lips below a delicate straight nose. I thought she looked around 50 years old. When I entered her room, she was sitting up with the head of the hospital bed elevated. There was a MacBook Air on her lap and a sheath of papers at her side.

"Good morning, Mrs. Hagen," I said, taking her hand in mine. "I'm Dr. Hauser, one of the cardiologists looking after you. How do you feel?"

Lois smiled and removed her reading glasses. "Like I've been run over by a truck, Dr. Hauser," she replied. "You may not remember me but I met you at the Cambridge Clinic when I brought a neighbor in to see you last year."

"You do look familiar," I said. "I hope your neighbor is doing well."

"He's better. You sent him down here, and someone—I thought it was you—put in three stents."

"It wasn't me, but I'm glad to hear that he is doing okay." I waited a few seconds and shifted the conversation. "You had quite a spell last week. I would like to know more about what was going on before your attack."

There was a knock at the door. It was Anne Hendrickson, the cardiology physician's assistant who worked with me in the hospital. I introduced her to Lois. Hendrickson remained standing while I unfolded a chair and sat down.

"What happened to me in Cambridge?" Lois asked.

"You went into shock in the emergency room, and they flew you here in a helicopter."

"Why did I go into shock? Did I have a heart attack?""

"You did, but not the typical kind. It wasn't a blockage. You have a condition called stress cardiomyopathy. We think it is due to an excess of chemicals like adrenalin that accumulate and cause the heart to enlarge and weaken. This condition affects people differently. Some have a mild case, others—like you—a more severe case. Nearly everyone recovers."

Lois closed the laptop and scooted higher up in bed. Her eyes shifted from me to Hendrickson and said, "Anyone who works has stress. I guess I'm no different than other people…" She turned back to me and asked, "Is it important to know?"

"Stress reduction is part of the treatment. Knowing the triggers could help."

My iPhone beeped, announcing a message. I was being called urgently to the catheterization laboratory to review an angiogram. I excused myself and was gone about thirty minutes. When I returned Anne Hendrickson was sitting outside Lois's room entering orders into the computer.

"What do you think?" I asked her.

"When I was about to leave the room," she replied softly, "Mrs. Hagen very calmly whispered, 'Everything bad happens in February.' I asked her what she meant and she said, 'My mother died in February, my father committed suicide in February, and I lost my only baby in February.' And then she began to cry."

Guilt is one thing, but shame is another. Shame is a powerful emotion that can affect women more than men. Unlike guilt that can be mitigated, shame endures and intensifies, inducing destructive feelings and behaviors that incubate and periodically surface. Shame is a psychological cancer that the sufferer strives to conceal, driving it inward until it erupts under pressure and becomes manifest in anger or illness. Guilt can be repaired and neutralized; shame is corrosive and resists healing.

I re-entered Lois's room. She sat on the edge of the bed with her back to the door, staring out the window at the snow-covered playground across the street. I walked around the foot of the bed and saw that her eyes were red with tears. She was clutching a balled-up facial tissue.

Lois, looked down at her hands, and asked, "Did Anne tell you about my Februarys?"

I replied simply, "Yes, she did."

"I told her that I lost my baby. That wasn't exactly the truth. I had an abortion, a late-term abortion at 21 weeks. I had an ultrasound that showed the baby had a brain malformation—I can't pronounce it, but it is spelled h-o-l-o-p-r-o-e-n-c-e-p-h-a-l-y.

"Marc and I met with a pediatrician who was familiar with the condition. We decided the right thing was to have the abortion even though we're Catholic." She paused and dabbed her eyes with the tissue. "It was February 20, 1995. Nineteen years ago."

"Have you spoken to anyone about this?" I asked.

"No," she replied, "not even with my husband after the abortion. And I have never confessed my sin to a priest. It is as though it never happened. Except, for me. I haven't been able to forget or forgive myself. Every February I live the abortion again. For some reason this year was the most difficult."

For more than 40 years, one after another of my patients have asked if stress could cause or contribute to their heart problems. My usual answer was "yes", because there are multiple examples of life's stressors causing heart attacks and sudden death. Natural disasters, such as earthquakes, and war and terror attacks are well known triggers. Anger that is personal or work-related also can precipitate cardiac events, and it does so in a way that differs from physical exertion.

Treating anger and prescribing stress reduction techniques, such as yoga or meditation, have become as much a part of managing heart patients as drugs and devices. The Penny George Institute for Health and Healing in Minnesota and other similar programs are striving to integrate conventional and alternative therapies in order to treat the entire person. This holistic approach has been particularly successful for mitigating the toxic consequences of fear, shame, and hostility on the body. As medicine becomes increasingly specialized, physicians must be mindful of the essential truth that they must treat the whole person, not one or two organs, or a single disease.

Lois Hagen was an extreme case of the mind-body axis gone haywire. Lois's heart recovered completely. With the help of a psychiatrist and her priest, she made it through the following February, including Valentine's Day, without difficulty. Eventually we will understand the molecular mechanisms behind stress cardiomyopathy and identify those who may be prone to it.

CHAPTER 18

The 90-minute drive from our home in Long Lake to Willmar in western Minnesota was typical for a Monday morning in June 2013. The 77-mile route still passed through many farm communities: Delano, Montrose, Waverly, Howard Lake, Cokato, Dassel, Litchfield, Grove City, and Atwater. I had patients in each of these towns. Unfortunately, I was familiar with a few of the local sheriffs, who rigorously enforced the 30 mph speed limits through their communities.

Willmar was a city of 20,000 people, mostly Scandinavians, with a growing number of immigrants from Latin American and Northeast Africa who worked in agriculture and the poultry industry. For 20 years, I saw patients at the Lakeland Family Practice Medical Center and Rice Memorial Hospital. Dr. Lyle Munneke, a native of South Dakota, started the practice in 1976. He was a good doctor, kind to his patients, and devoted to the community. He retired in 2002 and passed away five years later. I missed discussing patients with him.

This June morning I would see nine patients in the clinic. One of them was Margaret "Peggy" Lindquist, a 92-year-old "farm girl" I had followed for five years. Peggy had severe aortic stenosis and we had treated her valve twice before with a technique called balloon valvuloplasty. This non-surgical procedure involved placing a large balloon mounted on a catheter across the aortic valve and inflating it with high pressures to break up the scar tissue that immobilized the valve's leaflets. Both of Peggy's valvuloplasties were performed by Dr. Wesley Pedersen at the Minneapolis heart Institute. They were successful and she gained immediate relief from her chest pain and shortness of breath. Her last valvuloplasty, in 2011, was complicated by acute kidney failure that resolved without dialysis.

I was chagrined to see Peggy on portable oxygen. She looked frail. Her granddaughter, Amy Johnson, who lived in Clara City, southwest of Willmar, accompanied her.

"Hi, Mrs. Lindquist," I said, entering the small exam room.

Peggy's usually perky voice was soft and hoarse. She spoke slowly. "Hello, Doctor Hauser," She paused. "I bet you never wanted to see me again…." Her words trailed off. She looked pleadingly at her granddaughter.

"Grandma was here in the hospital last week," Amy said. "She got short of breath in the middle of the night and they brought her in by ambulance from my parents' house. They kept her for three days and got a lot of water off her lungs. They did an echo and said her valve is bad again. So here we are."

Aortic stenosis is a progressive disease that begins with scarring of the valve followed by calcification. The normal aortic valve has three leaflets. About one to two percent of people are born with two leaflets, called a bicuspid valve. Nearly all bicuspid aortic valves eventually become severely narrowed—stenotic—and activity brings on symptoms: chest pain, shortness of breath, severe lightheadedness or blackouts.

A normal aortic valve may develop stenosis and calcification with aging, particularly in men and people with high blood pressure or diabetes. When the narrowing becomes severe, patients experience the same symptoms as those who have bicuspid aortic stenosis. Once a patient develops symptoms, there is a 40 percent chance that he or she will die within a year, and most patients will pass away within five years.

The Starr-Edwards™ ball-in-cage valve, initially implanted in the early 1960s, was the first artificial valve used routinely for severe aortic stenosis. While revolutionary, it had drawbacks, including its size, flow characteristics, and tendency to form clots. Surgeons were also aware that some hearts were too small to accommodate the bulky Starr-Edwards prosthesis. High doses of the oral blood thinner, warfarin, prevented the valve from clotting, but too often this resulted in bleeding elsewhere in the body, including the brain and gut. Blood flow through a Starr-Edwards valve in some patients was not much better than it had been through the diseased valve itself.

In 1963, Vincent Gott, who trained with Walt Lillehei, built the first valve with leaflets rather than a ball. Gott and engineer Ronald Daggett at the University of Wisconsin fashioned the two leaflets from Teflon™. Blood flow through the valve was better compared to the ball-in-cage Starr-Edwards valve. However, despite anticoagulation with warfarin, clots formed on the valve and it was abandoned after being implanted in 500 patients.

One year later in 1964, Walt Lillehei and Dr. Bhagavant Kalke, a surgical resident from Mumbai, built another version of a two leaflet valve. A dam near Kalke's native village in India inspired this bileaflet valve's design. The Lillehei-Kalke valve performed well in animal experiments but it was abandoned after being implanted in only one patient. Lillehei had decided to pursue a different valve design: this was the Lillehei-Kastor tilting disc valve that eventually was implanted in 55,000 patients.

During the 1960s and 1970s a plethora of artificial valve models emerged. Many were variations of the ball-in-cage design while others used a disc to control and direct blood flow. While a valve's design was important, the materials used to construct the valve were critical. Stainless steel and titanium were common metals in many early valves, but surgeons searched for a material that was both durable and resistant to clot formation, called *thromboresistance*. Such a material was found in an unlikely place, the nuclear fuel industry.

Jack Bokros, a Gulf Atomic metallurgist who graduated from the University of Wisconsin, used pyrolytic carbon to encapsulate nuclear fuel rods. Pyrolytic carbon is manmade by super-heating hydrocarbon and allowing the graphite to crystallize. Bokros read of Gott and Daggett's valve work and sent them samples. The pair quickly concluded that pyrolytic carbon was the ideal material: it was hard, smooth, and thromboresistant. In 1968, pyrolytic carbon was first used in an aortic ball-valve designed by Dr. Michael DeBakey in Houston.

By the early 1970s, the scientific pieces were in place to combine the superior flow characteristics of a bileaflet valve and the material benefits of pyrolytic carbon. This effort was led by Dr. Demetre Nicoloff.

Demetre "Nick" Nicoloff grew up in a small town west of Cleveland, Ohio. In 1957 he received his medical degree from Ohio State where he was mentored by Dr. Robert Zollinger, a prominent academic surgeon and friend of Dr. Owen Wangensteen at the University of Minnesota. Subsequently Nicoloff trained under

Wangensteen and became his protégé, acting as Chief Resident and Director of the Research Laboratory. When Wangensteen became disabled by illness, Nicoloff cared for his patients while earning doctorates in both surgery and physiology. After Wangensteen retired in 1966, Nicoloff began his training in heart surgery at the University of Minnesota.

In 1972, Nicoloff was approached by Zion "Chris" Possis, a mechanical engineer, who had an idea for a valve. As Dr. Albert Starr did with Lowell Edwards, Nicoloff met often with Possis and they designed a bileaflet valve that Possis patented. Together they approached Manny Villafana who suggested the valve be made entirely of pyrolytic carbon. The result was the St. Jude heart valve, so named because Villafana had prayed to St. Jude when his young son was ill; his prayers were answered and his son recovered. St. Jude Medical Inc. was formed with private money and a royalty-based license for the Possis valve patent.

On October 3, 1977, Nicoloff and surgical resident Dr. Robert Emory implanted the first St. Jude valve in 67-year-old Helen Heikkinen from Angora, Minnesota. Mrs. Heikkinen had severe symptomatic aortic stenosis. The surgery was successful, and Mrs. Heikkinen lived another eleven years.

During the next five years St. Jude Medical struggled to achieve Food and Drug Administration (FDA) approval for its new valve. FDA regulatory oversight of medical devices was new, and every medical device manufacturer was experiencing the first wave of bureaucratic delays that continue to bedevil the industry today. St. Jude Medical had to raise more money in order to survive while it awaited FDA approval. Finally, in 1982, the FDA notified St. Jude Medical that it could sell its valves in the United States.

By 2002, more than one million St. Jude Medical mechanical valves had been implanted worldwide. In that year, Nicoloff and Emory, who were practicing at the Minneapolis Heart Institute, reported their experience with these valves. Of the 4,480 St. Jude mechanical valves they implanted, only one valve failed mechanically during an average implant time of seven years (the longest was 25 years). This Minnesota-designed valve became the most successful mechanical heart valve ever produced, and it remains in use today.

Despite early optimism that pyrolytic carbon would eliminate the need for long-term blood thinners like warfarin, this highly desirable goal was not achieved. Most patients who received St. Jude and other pyrolytic carbon valves continued to be anticoagulated and, over time, about one in every five patients taking warfarin had bleeding complications. This amplified interest in biologic valves constructed of tissue that would not require blood thinners.

The quest for a biologic tissue heart valve began in the 1960s. Dr. Donald Ross, a South African by birth, trained in chest surgery at Guy's Hospital in London. His British research team found that most human aortic valves removed at autopsy could be freeze-dried and preserved. Ross called these valves homografts because they came from humans and would be used in humans.

Ross implanted them in patients with the belief that these cadaver-derived homograft aortic valves would be viable and regenerate themselves. They did not. The recipients' immune systems rejected the foreign tissue. After four to five years, the aortic homograft valves began to leak and some patients died or needed a second valve operation. Ross had to abandon homograft aortic valves. The search for a durable biologic valve shifted from London to Paris.

Dr. Alain Carpentier was born in Toulouse, France, in 1933. His father was a civil engineer and the family moved about the country following construction projects. They lived in Algeria for four years during World War II because the elder Carpentier would not build airfields for the German Army.

At age eight, Carpentier developed peritonitis and a surgeon, who happened to be visiting his village, saved his life. This inspired Carpentier to become a surgeon and, after graduating from the University of Paris, he trained under Dr. Charles Dubost, a prominent French cardiovascular surgeon who performed the world's first successful repair of an abdominal aortic aneurysm in 1951. Dubost, like many outstanding mentors, not only supported Carpentier with resources, but also gave him the freedom to pursue his scientific ideas.

In the early 1960s, Carpentier began performing heart surgery at Hospital Broussais on rue Didot in southwest Paris. Early in his career, Carpentier implanted

Starr-Edwards valves in two patients. Both later became partially paralyzed by strokes because clots formed on their artificial valves and traveled to their brains. These tragedies affected Carpentier deeply. Later he said, "When you are a young surgeon and you have completed a successful valve replacement operation and then the patient has hemiplegia [partial paralysis] from an embolic event [blood clot] related to the valve, it is a very emotional and discouraging event."

Carpentier focused his research on developing a biologic valve made of tissue that would reduce the risk of blood clots and avoid the need for lifelong blood thinners like warfarin. He tried harvesting valves from pigs because French law made it difficult to retrieve valves from human cadavers.

The adjective *porcine* describes pig valves. Carpentier knew that a porcine valve, like any foreign protein, would be rejected by the body's immune system unless it was first treated with a chemical that made it less antigenic, i.e. less likely to stimulate the production of antibodies that would attack the valve. The first porcine valve was pretreated with a mercurochrome-formalin solution. Carpentier and Dr. Jean-Paul Binet performed the surgery in Paris in 1965, marking the first time a valve from a different species—a heterograft—was implanted in a human. Within several years, however, these mercurochrome-formalin-treated porcine valves began to degenerate. Carpentier went in search of a better chemical preservative.

Heart surgeon Carpentier became a chemist. He returned to the Faculty of Science in Paris to improve his knowledge by enrolling in a Ph.D. program. He investigated a variety of chemicals and concentrated on aldehydes, which are organic compounds. Aldehydes, Carpentier knew, were also used to tan shoes. After evaluating 50 aldehydes, he found one—glutaraldehyde—that not only made the pig valve sterile and less antigenic, but also tougher by strengthening chemical bonds within the tissue. Curiously, glutaraldehyde was used to tan the soft white leather for baby shoes.

By 1968, Dubost and Carpentier began implanting glutaraldehyde-preserved porcine valves in patients. The valves were mounted on a Teflon™ coated metallic frame with a cloth sewing ring to facilitate suturing. Because the valve was a combination of tissue and materials, Carpentier called it a *bioprosthesis,* a term still in use. After the implant, the patients' own cells grew over the frame, further reducing the possibility of clot formation. They would not need anticoagulant drugs.

These valves performed well but Carpentier did not know how durable they would be. He chose not to commercialize his valves until they had been implanted for three years.

One year after Carpentier's first glutaraldehyde-preserved porcine valve implant, Dr. Albert Starr visited him in Paris. Starr was so impressed with the new porcine valve that he asked Carpentier to visit Edwards Laboratories in southern California. Albert Starr was remarkably unselfish because Carpentier's valve could compete with Starr's own mechanical valve. Carpentier collaborated with Edwards Laboratories and produced the Carpentier-Edwards glutaraldehyde porcine valve, which became available for implant in 1971.

Porcine valves performed well for five to ten years, but then they began to malfunction. Some leaked, resulting in regurgitation, and others calcified and obstructed blood flow. Few failures caused emergencies, but many porcine valves had to be replaced, requiring repeat open-heart surgery. The central issue with tissue valves was durability. If only a tissue valve could last the average patient's lifetime, it would be preferable to a mechanical prosthetic valve requiring life-long anticoagulation.

Some patients were so averse to taking warfarin that they opted for the tissue valve anyway, knowing that they may face another heart surgery later in life. In most cases though, porcine valves were reserved for elderly patients, and patients who were likely to bleed and could not tolerate blood thinners. It was not until after 2005 that manufacturers found better preservatives and new materials for fabricating tissue valves. These 21st century models performed well. By the time I retired in 2015, 80 percent of valve replacements were tissue valves and most of these used bovine tissue from the sac (pericardium) around a cow's heart.

Regardless of what kind of valve was chosen, a patient still required open-heart surgery for valve replacement. For many, particularly the elderly like Peggy Lindquist, open-heart surgery was simply too risky. We needed ways to treat valves effectively without placing elderly or debilitated patients on the heart-lung machine. Despite all the advances in heart-lung bypass, the risk of open-heart surgery still escalated with age and other health problems.

At 87, the three leaflets of Peggy Lindquist's aortic valve were severely calcified. They were so rigid that they could barely open. The left ventricle had to squeeze hard in order to produce the force required to eject blood through the valve's narrow opening. The blood flow from her heart to her body was low at rest, and woefully inadequate during physical activity.

As the years went by, Peggy's heart muscle thickened and became stiffer. When she climbed the stairs to her bedroom or carried groceries, it was like a twelve cylinder BMW engine being fed fuel barely sufficient to power a lawnmower.

When I first saw Peggy in 2008, she steadfastly refused valve replacement heart surgery, saying, "I'm too old. I'm afraid of a stroke." Two months later, she was gripped by chest pain with any activity. I saw her again in the Willmar clinic, and she agreed to undergo a procedure called balloon aortic valvuloplasty or simply BAV.

Historically, the elderly have been treated far less aggressively than young and middle age patients. This occurred, in part, because we believed that older patients were more likely to be injured by bold treatments such as thrombolytic drugs (clot busters), heart surgery, and angioplasty. Yet as new technologies evolved, we learned that the elderly often benefited more from aggressive therapies than any other age group. The challenge of symptomatic aortic stenosis in the elderly was to find a less invasive solution.

Dr. Alain Cribier, a French cardiologist, performed the first balloon aortic valvuloplasty in 1985. It was reserved primarily for patients who were not candidates for surgical aortic valve replacement because they were too old or their surgical risk was too high. A catheter with a large balloon on its tip was inserted into an artery or vein and advanced to the heart until the balloon was positioned across the diseased aortic valve. The balloon was inflated several times with progressively higher pressures. As the balloon expanded, the scar tissue and calcium deposits were disrupted—split—allowing the valve's leaflets to open more freely. This increased the valve opening, so more blood flowed, especially during activity.

Valvuloplasty, however, fell into disfavor because the initial benefits did not last: scar tissue returned often within months, accompanied by the same symptoms.

The transient benefits did not seem to justify the risks.

However, by 2000, we saw a growing population of very elderly patients with severe, symptomatic aortic stenosis who were too frail for surgical valve replacement. Others, like Peggy Lindquist, were opposed to the operation because they feared the complications of open-heart surgery. Some patients were content to accept their fate, but many more wanted to live and sought relief from their suffering.

We felt the same helplessness that our predecessors experienced until open-heart surgery rescued so many patients from the death sentences of congenital and valvular heart disease. Pain and suffering is pain and suffering, regardless of age.

Dr. Wesley Pedersen at the Minneapolis Heart Institute was drawn to the challenge of treating aortic stenosis in the elderly and in patients too infirm to tolerate traditional valve replacement. Beginning in 2003, Pedersen began performing aortic valvuloplasty in these patients. By 2007, he and his colleagues had treated 103 patients, 30 percent over 90 years of age. All of them suffered chest pain or shortness of breath with minimal activity, and some had blackouts. A few were in shock or near death due to heart failure. It would be difficult to find a more desperately ill group of patients.

Nearly all of them improved following valvuloplasty. Even the 90-year-olds had a low mortality rate and benefited from a 30 percent improvement in the opening of their aortic valves. In time, as expected, the scar tissue returned, once again restricting blood flow through their valves. Often a second or third valvuloplasty was necessary, but eventually most patients succumbed to their heart disease. Even so, a majority of the group gained years of life worth living. Their doctors finally had a way to help them: valvuloplasty relieved their pain and suffering, at least for a while.

The results of aortic valvuloplasty improved as Pedersen and his team gained experience and refined the techniques. Patients often had coronary angioplasty and a stent placed at the time of valvuloplasty. Pedersen designed a novel balloon, shaped like an hourglass that had fewer drawbacks than traditional cylindrical balloons.

Still, valvuloplasty remained a largely palliative procedure. For a few patients, it allowed the heart and body to recover sufficiently so that open-heart surgery and valve replacement could occur safely. Even with improvements, valvuloplasty did not offer the permanent relief that patients needed. Pedersen and his colleagues around the world recognized that valvuloplasty was a treatment in need of a destination. In other words, a definitive therapy was needed, and this would require replacing the valve without open-heart surgery.

In 2002, a 57-year-old man entered the Charles Nicolle Hospital in Rouen, France, a port city on the river Seine northwest of Paris. He had severe aortic stenosis, chronic inflammation of his pancreas, a history of lung cancer, and severe atherosclerosis affecting the circulation in his legs (peripheral vascular disease). He was in shock, and his lips and fingers were purple from poor circulation and lack of oxygen. His right leg was mottled because it was not receiving enough blood flow. Emergency valvuloplasty stabilized and improved his condition. However, his symptoms returned in a few days and again he went into shock. His cardiologist, Dr. Alain Cribier, had pioneered aortic valvuloplasty and had performed more than 1000 procedures. He knew better than anyone that valvuloplasty was a temporizing measure, a bridge without a destination.

Born in Paris in 1945, Cribier had attended medical school there before moving to Rouen in 1983 where he became the director of the catheterization laboratory. Realizing the limitations of valvuloplasty, he imagined mounting a tissue heart valve on a balloon-expandable stent and deploying it in the diseased aortic valve. He approached several major medical device companies and they told him it would not work. Undeterred, Cribier and several associates formed a small private company—Percutaneous Valve Technologies (PVT)—based in the United States and Israel. By 2002, Cribier had a device ready for human implantation.

When his 57-year-old patient again went into shock, Cribier knew that it would be senseless to attempt another valvuloplasty. The only option, born in desperation, was to insert his invention, the PVT valve. The valve had performed well in sheep but this would be the first human use. He sought approval from his hospital ethics committee. The patient was dying, and permission was quickly granted.

The valve's three leaflets were made with bovine (cow) pericardium, the tough sac that surrounds the heart. The leaflets were mounted on a stainless steel expandable stent and the entire unit was placed over a deflated balloon at the end of a large catheter that was 0.9 inches in diameter.

The patient's blood pressure was 70 when Cribier started the procedure. The left ventricular ejection fraction was 10 percent, barely compatible with life (normal is 55 percent or higher). Due to severe peripheral artery disease, Cribier inserted the thick catheter and valve into a leg vein and advanced it to the right side of the heart and left atrium, into the left ventricle, and across the diseased aortic valve. Just maneuvering the catheter into position was a masterful feat.

Cribier viewed the densely calcified valve on the fluoroscopy screen. The lumps of dark calcium served as landmarks for positioning the new valve. It was vital that the valve not obstruct the openings of the coronary arteries. Once satisfied with the location, Cribier rapidly inflated the balloon, expanding the stent so that it engaged the surrounding tissue. The metal stent holding the bovine pericardial valve pressed against the scarred valve leaflets and aortic annulus, a thick structure that is part of the heart's fibrous skeleton.

As Cribier deployed the new valve, his patient's heart stopped beating—for 20 seconds -- an eternity when a life is in your hands. Then slowly, steadily, the heart awoke and began to beat. Blood began flowing across the new aortic valve. The patient's blood pressure rose to 120. The large pressure difference across the diseased valve was gone. There was no obstruction to blood flow. The proportion of blood ejected by the left ventricle with each beat doubled. The patient was no longer in shock, and the symptoms and signs of heart failure began to improve.

For the first time, an aortic valve had been replaced without opening the chest and placing the patient on a heart-lung machine. Cribier and his team demonstrated that it was feasible to insert a new valve with a catheter. Best of all, the new valve functioned as well as a surgically implanted valve.

By 2013 Pedersen and the interventional group at the Minneapolis Heart Institute were routinely implanting aortic valves with catheters. The procedure is called transcatheter aortic valve replacement or simply TAVR. Edwards Lifesciences (the company Lowell Edwards started to make the Starr-Edwards valve) had purchased PVT, the company Cribier founded, in 2003, for $125 million. During the next ten years, the original Cribier device was improved, as well as the methods to deliver and insert the valve into the heart.

The Edwards TAVR valve model, branded SAPIEN™, was evaluated in clinical trials. The first trial showed that fewer patients, whose risk of surgery was prohibitive, died if they underwent SAPIEN™ valve implantation than if they were treated medically with or without valvuloplasty. The second trial, called PARTNER, revealed that high-risk patients did as well with a SAPIEN™ valve as similar patients did with valves implanted by open-heat surgery.

With this knowledge, I raised the possibility of TAVR with Peggy Lindquist. "Mrs. Lindquist," I said, "we have a valve that can be implanted in your heart without surgery. It is done with a catheter and the procedure is similar to valvuloplasty, except that we will insert a new valve."

Peggy and her daughter were intrigued by the possibility, and I went on to describe the SAPIEN™ valve and how it would be deployed in Peggy's heart. Then we discussed the risks, and for Peggy the most worrisome was a disabling stroke.

"There is a risk of stroke," I said. "It's around four percent during the first month. It could be higher for you because of your age." I paused, waiting.

Peggy looked at her granddaughter. "What do you think, Amy?"

"It's up to you, Grandma," Amy replied. "It sounds like a reasonable thing to do. You're not getting better." Amy turned to me and asked, "What about her kidneys? We had trouble last time."

"That's right, "I replied, looking straight at Peggy. "The kidneys could fail again, particularly if we need to use X-ray dye."

"How much longer do I have if I don't do this?" Peggy asked.

"Maybe a year, possibly less. A few patients live longer than we expect."

I paused, then said as gently as I could, "Some patients—particularly when they get to a certain stage in life—just want to let nature take its course. There's nothing wrong with that, Peggy. It's your decision. A lot depends on how aggressive you want to be. This procedure has been successful, it is FDA approved for patients like you, but there are risks. There will always be risks."

"You don't have to make up your mind now," I continued. "You can think about it, meet with Dr. Pedersen in Minneapolis, or call me…whatever is most comfortable for you. If you don't want the valve we could try valvuloplasty again."

Peggy smiled and sighed. "You know, Dr. Hauser," she said, "I've had a good life. In many ways, I've been blessed. My husband has been gone for a long time now. Nobody lives forever. I feel pretty comfortable now that I've got this oxygen. I'm sleeping much better." She reached out, took her granddaughters hand, and held my eyes with a reflective gaze. "Doctor Hauser, do the best you can with the medicine. I just want to stay home…with my family."

"I understand," I said, leaning forward, touching her hand. "We can always talk again."

I prescribed more diuretics and filled out a form for the oxygen deliveries to her home.

Peggy had to use the restroom before the drive back to Clara City. I asked the nurse to help her. After she left the exam room, her granddaughter said to me, "Doctor Hauser, I think the family will be relieved. I know Grandma is."

Peggy Lindquist died in her sleep on Thanksgiving Day, five months after our visit in Willmar. Her granddaughter sent me a nice note and enclosed a picture of Peggy and her family taken at her 93rd birthday party in early October, about a month before she died. She held her great granddaughter, Margaret. Both were smiling.

There was a time in my career when I would have felt defeated: my patient died when maybe, just maybe, she could have been saved by a novel procedure. Was I too forthright with my description of the risks? Should I have applied more pressure? I think not. Peggy made her decision, as every patient has a right to do, independently, fully informed, and I helped her in that process. Peggy reached a point in her life, as most of us will, when she wished to place herself in the hands of God completely, without reservation. As I viewed the picture of Peggy and her great granddaughter, surrounded by her family, any sense of defeat or disappointment vanished.

By the end of 2015, transcatheter aortic valve replacement (TAVR) was a common procedure at qualified medical centers in the United States, Europe, and Asia. The procedure required teamwork. No longer did cardiologists and surgeons work in isolation. TAVR was a multidisciplinary undertaking, requiring advanced imaging as well as the skills unique to surgeons and cardiologists. Each individual case was planned in advance by a group of specialists who met to review the needs and physical characteristics of every patient.

The first patients who were FDA approved for TAVR were at high risk for open-heart surgery. Clinical trials had shown that TAVR was as good as surgical valve replacement in these patients. In 2016, a study of moderate surgical risk patients also showed that TAVR was as good as surgical valve replacement, and a study was ongoing to assess the safety and efficacy of TAVR in low risk patients.

During my career, I witnessed the first aortic valve replacements with the Starr-Edwards prosthesis, and the dawn of an era when most patients with severe aortic valve disease were treated much less invasively with a valve delivered by a catheter. Could this happen with the mitral valve as well?

CHAPTER 19

Ted Foster was an impressive physical specimen and his wife, Jeni, could have been a model for Vogue.

In 2012, at the age of 42 years, Ted Foster awoke at 3 a.m. with rapid heart beating. His pulse was very irregular and, when he stood up, he felt lightheaded and mildly short of breath. He sat back on the bed, awakening Jeni.

"What's wrong, Ted?" she asked in her Flemish accented English.

"My heart is pounding… fast. It woke me up," he replied.

Jeni threw off the covers and grasped Ted's wrist. She palpated his radial pulse. "You're going very fast. It's very irregular. We should go to the hospital."

"I have a flight to Detroit this morning. Very important meeting…."

"Don't be ridiculous. You are not going to get on an airplane."

Forty-five minutes later Ted Foster was in the emergency room of Abbott Northwestern Hospital. His electrocardiogram showed atrial fibrillation at a rate of 170 to 180 beats per minute. The emergency room physician heard a loud murmur and paged the on-call cardiologist, Dr. David Hurrell.

After examining Foster, Hurrell ordered intravenous diltiazem, a medication to slow his heart rate, and heparin, an anticoagulant. The results of Ted's 2007 echocardiogram were not available in the electronic medical record. Hurrell, hearing the prominent mitral regurgitation murmur, ordered a repeat echocardiogram, and admitted Foster to Station 5200, a cardiology unit.

The mitral valve is a marvelously complex and elegant structure. Its two leaflets—anterior and posterior—separate the left atrium from the left ventricle, so that freshly oxygenated blood from the lungs travels in one direction—forward. Normally, each leaflet is thin, pliable, and translucent. When the left ventricle contracts, blood is propelled through the aortic valve because the mitral leaflets align with each other, edge-to-edge, forming a barrier that prevents blood from leaking—regurgitating—backward. Unlike the aortic valve, the mitral leaflets must withstand the high pressures generated by the left ventricle when it contracts over 100,000 times a day.

At the juncture of the atrium and the ventricle is a flexible, ovoid structure, called the annulus. The annulus has muscular and fibrous elements to which the mitral leaflets are attached. Two conical bundles of muscle fibers are mounted in the left ventricle, like animated organic stalagmites. These are the papillary muscles that give rise to an arbor composed of tough tendons—chordae tendinae—that insert themselves on the ventricular side of each leaflet. As the ventricle contracts, so do the papillary muscles, tightening the chordae, thereby restraining the leaflets, preventing them from losing their orientation to each other and flopping back into the left atrium.

The mitral valve apparatus is a physiologic quartet—leaflets, annulus, chordae, and papillary muscles—whose performance can be corrupted by diseases like rheumatic fever, tissue degeneration, and cardiomyopathies (enlarged hearts).

When the mitral valve is leaking severely, a large volume of blood is "recycled" through the left side of the heart, heightening the work that the heart must perform. It is like climbing a tall dune in soft sand—for every three steps up, one slides two steps down. The ascent is three times the work. The same principle applies to severe mitral regurgitation. Eventually the heart's compensatory mechanisms fail, and patients experience fatigue, shortness of breath, water retention, and an inability to perform routine tasks—all symptoms of heart failure. As the heart decompensates, rhythms like atrial fibrillation often appear, further reducing the heart's ability to function efficiently. This condition may occur abruptly, but it usually takes years to evolve.

Mitral regurgitation may be caused by a multitude of diseases, some of them present at birth, others that are acquired during adulthood. Four out of five adults will have a little mitral regurgitation, but this does not mean that they have heart disease. A person can live a long and active life with mild mitral regurgitation. When the volume overload of severe mitral regurgitation occurs, the left ventricle begins to enlarge, the heart muscle weakens, and the pressures inside the lungs rise and cause congestion. If left untreated, severe mitral regurgitation and its consequences lead to progressive heart failure and disability.

A star athlete at his high school in Brainerd, Minnesota, Ted Foster's sports were hockey and tennis. He was twice runner-up in the state high school singles tennis tournament. Foster attended Carleton College in Northfield, Minnesota, where he majored in history and political science and graduated cum laude in 1989. After backpacking through Europe for two months he entered the Carlson School of Management at the University of Minnesota and received his MBA in 1991. 3M hired Ted as a marketing associate in its health care division.

He became a passionate tri-athlete—swimming, biking, and running. He was tall, lean, and his blonde hair was closely cropped for practical reasons rather than style. In 1994 he finished well enough in Chicago's Mrs. T's Triathlon to qualify for the Ironman competition in Hawaii where he finished, respectably, in the middle of the pack after a 2.4-mile swim, a 112-mile bike ride and a 26.2-mile marathon.

For the next five years, Ted was consumed with work and physical training. In 2000, he earned a promotion to 3M's offices outside Brussels, Belgium. There he met Jeni Ector, a dentist, at a 3M professional education event and soon married her. In 2005, after the birth of their second daughter, Ted returned to Minnesota with another 3M promotion and the family purchased a home in Kenwood, an upscale neighborhood of Minneapolis.

In 2007, a routine physical examination with Ted's internist revealed a heart murmur. An echocardiogram showed mitral valve prolapse, also known as a floppy valve, and moderate mitral regurgitation. His main pumping chamber, the left ventricle, was normal. The internist told Ted that he had a degenerative condition affecting his mitral valve and suggested a cardiology consultation. Ted, who never felt better in his life, declined. He was working to qualify for another Ironman. Ted decided not to worry his wife and did not tell her of the murmur or the results of the echocardiogram.

I entered Ted Foster's room around 9 a.m. on the morning of his admission to the hospital in May of 2012. The echocardiography technician—a highly trained sonographer—was already there and she had just acquired the last of the multiple ultrasonic pictures of Ted's heart. Anne Hendrickson, a cardiology physician's assistant, was also present, gathering information, answering questions, and discussing the plan for the day. She introduced me to the Fosters.

I asked the technician to show me the latest digitized videos of Ted's echocardiogram. The images were excellent and the color Doppler signals flashed the telltale signs of a severely leaking mitral valve. The billowing posterior leaflet flailed about in the turbulent blood flow like a loose sail in a storm. The result was a torrential jet of blood traveling in the wrong direction, reversing flow from the lungs, and creating a kaleidoscope of reds, yellows, and blues portraying a malfunctioning valve apparatus.

With each beat, Ted's overburdened left ventricle filled with blood only to have a large quantity of it regurgitate back to the left atrium. Also visible was a faint string-like structure that flipped in and out of view: it was a ruptured chordae tendineae that normally supported the mitral valve's leaflets

When I asked Ted, "Have you ever had a heart problem?" my question created quite a stir. He told me about the echocardiogram in 2007. Jeni Foster's jaw dropped and she exclaimed, "You didn't tell me about that!" I looked at Anne Hendrikson and waited while Ted Foster did his best to assuage his spouse's outrage.

Finally, I interrupted, "Let's talk about what needs to be done. Mr. Foster, you have atrial fibrillation, almost certainly due to a very leaky mitral valve. We need to assess the severity of the leak and determine if your main pump is being affected." I paused, and then asked, "Have you noticed, during your workouts, that anything has changed. Any unexpected symptoms—shortness of breath, chest discomfort, dizziness, less endurance?"

"No", he replied firmly

"Have you had any of these symptoms any other time? Any change in your sleep habits or appetite?"

Again, he replied, "No, never."

Being a competitive athlete myself, I thought he most likely kept track of his training times—how long it took for him to run a mile, bike ten miles, and swim 200 yards, for example.

"What about your splits?" I probed.

He appeared thoughtful, rubbed his jaw and said, "Not what they used to be. Particularly this spring." He glanced at his wife.

"I think he is more tired after his workouts," she said. "Yes, he is definitely different than he was last year. I really didn't think too much about it. He travels frequently and brings a lot of work home. Lately he has not played as much with our daughters."

The characteristic picture of an otherwise healthy man being affected by severe mitral regurgitation was emerging. It was impossible to know just when the chordae tendineae ruptured but it was likely recent. Ted would need heart surgery to repair or, if that was not feasible, implant a new valve. The goals were straightforward: preserve heart function, provide a reasonable quality of life, and prevent atrial fibrillation and other arrhythmias.

Surgical repair was the preferred treatment for Ted's mitral valve disease. The surgeon would reconstruct the valve, restoring it to normal function without replacing its leaflets. Studies had shown that repair by experienced surgeons was superior to valve replacement because it preserved the valve's natural apparatus and had fewer complications.

Dr. Alain Carpentier, the same heart surgeon who invented the glutaraldehyde porcine bioprosthetic valve, also pioneered this surgery. In 1983, he described his technique for repairing the mitral valve in a memorable address at the annual meeting of the American Association for Thoracic Surgery. Appropriately, it was entitled "The French Connection."

In his systematic way Carpentier described how he evolved methods for fixing diseased and malfunctioning mitral valves. The valve's annulus is the anatomic tissue structure that serves as the fulcrum for the leaflets. Early on it was apparent that the size and shape of the annulus had to be restored and stabilized in order to repair the valve successfully. To accomplish this, Carpentier developed a prosthetic annular ring that could be sutured around the leaflets. In the illustration below, the mitral valve's front (anterior) leaflet is torn. To repair it, an annuloplasty ring is inserted before the leaflet is repaired with sutures. Carpentier developed a variety of annuloplasty rings and so did other surgeons.

Each repair was tailored to the specific valve problem. The primary goal was to restore function, and do so in a way that would be long lasting, i.e. durable and capable of withstanding the high pressures to which the mitral valve is exposed with every heart beat.

In the early afternoon Ted Foster was brought down to the echocardiography laboratory on the second floor of the Minneapolis Heart Institute. Dr. Jim Daniel gave him intravenous sedation and slipped a probe down his esophagus in order to acquire high definition ultrasound images of the malfunctioning mitral valve. The procedure is called a transesophageal echocardiogram or simply, TEE.

The pictures revealed, in exquisite detail, the flailing posterior mitral valve leaflet that, with each contraction, flopped back into the left atrium accompanied by a torrent of blood traveling in the wrong direction. Daniel recorded multiple images of the mitral valve to be certain that there was no evidence of infection or other variables that might affect Forster's treatment.

Daniel called me after he finished the TEE. "Bobby", he said, "Mr. Foster has severe mitral regurgitation due to a flail [floppy] posterior mitral leaflet. Everything else looks good. No shunts (holes). No clots. No infection. Looks like a good candidate for repair." I thanked him, and he added, "By the way, he is back in sinus rhythm." Jim Daniel was one of the original founders of our cardiology group and an outstanding diagnostician. I hung up the phone and called Dr. Vibhu Kshettry, a heart surgeon who was highly skilled in mitral valve repair.

Kshettry was born into a medical family in India and practiced cardiovascular surgery at the University of Minnesota before joining the Minneapolis Heart Institute. He traveled frequently to Ethiopia and India where he operated on children with rheumatic valvular heart disease. These valves were so damaged by the rheumatic inflammatory process that most surgeons would not even attempt to repair them.

However, Kshettry recognized that implanting mechanical valves in these young patients was impractical because they would have to take blood thinners for the rest of their lives. In these medically underserved and remote communities, the safe administration of a drug like warfarin was not feasible. Moreover, a teenager who received a tissue heart valve would need reoperation when it wore out in 10 or 20 years, a difficult proposition in countries where access to health care was severely limited. Kshettry figured out how to repair these rheumatic valves—a tribute to his skill and desire to help these desperate children.

Kshettry called me back on Station 5200. "Vib," I said, "I have a 42-year-old guy who needs his mitral valve repaired. He came in last night in heart failure and

Jim Daniel just finished the TEE. Can you see him today?"

Kshettry said, characteristically, "Sure. Sure. Has he had an angiogram? What room is he in?"

I replied, "He'll have a CT coronary angiogram in the morning. He's in room 5218." The phone clicked, and he was gone. Kshettry, a delight socially, never made small talk in the hospital.

Ted Foster's CT coronary angiogram revealed no plaque, and the arteries and aorta were normal. Kshettry met with Ted and Jeni in the afternoon and described what he proposed to do. First, he would open Ted's chest through an incision in his sternum and place him on the heart-lung machine. Next he would expose the mitral valve through an incision in the atrium and repair it with a special ring placed around the valve. In addition, he would remove any excess tissue from the valve's posterior leaflet. The surgery would take about three hours.

Kshettry described what would happen if the valve repair turned out not to be feasible. In that case, he said, valve replacement would be necessary. Ted Foster did not want to be on warfarin all of his life, so he opted for a tissue valve. Ted knew he would need another open-heart surgery if the tissue valve wore out.

The following morning, the anesthesiologist, Dr. Rajarao Dwarakanath, introduced himself and explained what Ted Foster could expect during the next few hours. Then he and a nurse anesthetist guided Ted's gurney down the hall toward the operating room. On the way, Dwarakanath injected propofol into the intravenous line in Ted's arm. As they pushed the gurney into the operating room, Ted Foster was in a deep sleep.

The surgery took just under two hours. After exposing the mitral valve through an incision between the atria, Kshettry carefully measured the valve and chose a Carpentier-Edwards ring specifically designed and sized for degenerative valves like Foster's. Then he placed sutures through the Carpentier-Edwards ring and the annulus of the mitral valve so that the ring was both secure and did not distort the annulus. Once the ring was in place, he took a scalpel and removed an elliptical segment of excess tissue from the posterior leaflet. The thin chord that had torn loose from the posterior leaflet was no longer needed and it was removed. Lastly, he sutured together the free edges of the posterior leaflet where he had made the incision. Before closing the atrium Kshettry injected saline around the valve to assess it for leaks: there were none. A transesophageal echocardiogram confirmed that the repair was complete.

Forty minutes later Ted Foster was in the surgical intensive care unit to begin his recovery. Around 5 p.m., when he was fully awake, the endotracheal tube was removed from Ted's throat, and he was breathing on his own. The next 12 hours were uneventful, except for a short burst of atrial fibrillation around midnight that required no treatment. The following morning he was transferred out of the intensive care unit to H4039, a private room in the Heart Hospital. The temporary tubes that Kshettry had placed in his chest to prevent blood or fluid from accumulating were removed by one of the surgical nurses. By the 4th postoperative day he was eating, walking the halls, and becoming increasingly restless for discharge. At 5 p.m., Jeni arrived to take Ted home.

Three months after his surgery, Ted Foster resumed training. In 2014, he traveled to the Big Island of Hawaii where he and Jeni were spectators at the 38th Ironman World Championship. "I think I could have made it back to the Ironman myself," Ted told me, "but we have twin boys now and there's no time for anything else."

I thought open-heart mitral valve repair would be the last major advance in the treatment of mitral regurgitation in my professional lifetime. I was mistaken. Like aortic stenosis, there were many patients with mitral valve regurgitation who were too fragile to survive open-heart valve repair or replacement. This group included the very elderly and patients who had weak hearts or other conditions that made open-heart surgery risky.

A number of gadgets were conceived for repairing the mitral valve without surgery. Some of them worked reasonably well in animals but failed in humans. Others remained on the drawing board, unfunded, and destined for obscurity. Yet one idea seemed to hold promise because it was based on a surgical technique developed by an Italian surgeon, Dr. Ottavio Alfieri.

In 1991 Alfieri took a very sick patient with severe, symptomatic mitral regurgitation to the operating room. He wanted to keep the surgery as simple and quick as possible, so he placed several stitches through the edges of the anterior and posterior leaflets of the mitral valve. This simple maneuver—known ever since as the "Alfieri stitch"—drew the edges of the two mitral leaflets together and reduced the degree of mitral regurgitation from severe to moderate. The stitching method reduced the area of the mitral valve opening by about a half. Most patients treated with an Alfieri stitch improved symptomatically, and many did reasonably well for years.

The Alfieri technique was never widely adopted because surgeons preferred Carpentier's approach. However, the "Alfieri stitch" laid the groundwork for a catheter-based device that clips the edges of the mitral valve together. This device called the MitraClip™ was developed in 1998 and first implanted in a patient in 2003. The clip is V-shaped and mounted on a catheter. It enters the body through the femoral vein into the right side of the heart and passes through the wall between the right and left atria and on to the left ventricle. Using fluoroscopy and transesophageal echo for visualization, the clip is opened, aligned with the middle of the two leaflets, and closed until it grasps their edges like a staple. As was true with the Alfieri stitch, the MitraClip reduces the leakage from severe to moderate or less.

The MitraClip™ system was studied extensively in patients under the direction of Dr. Ted Feldman, an interventional cardiologist at Evanston Hospital north of Chicago. Dr. Wes Pedersen lead the study of the MitraClip™ at Abbott Northwestern Hospital. In 2011, Feldman published a landmark article in the *New England Journal of Medicine* showing that the MitraClip™ was safer than mitral valve repair or replacement and resulted in similar outcomes: improved symptoms and a reduction in the size of the left ventricle. The Food and Drug Administration approved it for sale in the United States in 2013.

Betty Vaughn was an 87-year-old widow who lived in Independence, Minnesota, a farm community 24 miles west of Minneapolis. Betty looked forward to her bridge club, and especially their New Year's Eve party. However, Betty had severe mitral regurgitation, and in the winter of 2014 she began to have fatigue and shortness of breath. She decided to skip the New Year's Eve bridge party and stay home by the fire.

"Years ago," she told me, "my doctor said 'live with it.' It was not living—it was existing. I liked the fact that I was independent. I asked very little of my kids. I thought my symptoms would go away—then one day I found myself lying on the steps. I knew something had to be done."

Betty visited Dr. Paul Sorajja at the Minneapolis Heart Institute. Sorajja was an interventional cardiologist and Director of the Minneapolis Heart Institute's center for treating valvular heart disease. Born in Detroit, Michigan, he trained and practiced at the Mayo Clinic, where he pioneered non-invasive methods for treating a variety of heart valve disorders.

Sorajja told Mrs. Vaughn that it would be possible to reduce the amount of her mitral regurgitation with a new device, called the MitraClip™. "Open-heart surgery was not recommended for Mrs. Vaughn because of her age and the risk of the operation," Soraja said. Dr. Saeid Farivar, a cardiac surgeon, evaluated her and agreed that the MitraClip™ -- rather than open-heart surgery -- was the best choice.

On the day of the procedure, Sorajja inserted the catheter into Mrs. Vaughn's heart from the femoral vein in her right leg. Dr. Desmond Jay, a cardiologist and echo cardiographer, passed an ultrasound probe through her mouth and into her esophagus. Jay would visualize the mitral valve as Sorajja deployed the MitraClip™ from the catheter.

Once the tip of the MitraClip™ catheter was in Mrs. Vaughn's left atrium, Soraja guided it forward between the two leaflets of the mitral valve and into the left ventricle. He unfolded the two arms of the MitraClip's V-shaped clip. With the clip's arms spread outward, Sorajja drew them backward to engage the mid-sections of the two leaflets. Once each arm was in the proper position, he closed them, effectively clipping together the edges of the two leaflets. The result was a vast decrease in the amount of blood regurgitating backward into her left atrium. The entire procedure took one hour.

Betty Vaughn went home the following day. Her symptoms improved immediately. "I'm living now," she said later. "I'm doing almost everything I want. I'm going anywhere I want. I'm doing yard work and driving. I'm not perfect but If it had not been for this I would be in a nursing home...or worse. I feel very fortunate."

Would the MitraClip™ be the final chapter in the 60-year quest for treating mitral valve regurgitation? No, of course not, because many diseased mitral valves are not suitable for "clipping". These are the valves whose leaflets are too damaged or distorted to be clipped. Additionally, the leaflets may be scarred or calcified, confounding attempts to grasp them.

Just as in 1960, when Starr and Edwards changed everything with their invention of the first artificial mitral valve, the new frontier in the 21st century was a fully functioning mitral valve that could be implanted in a beating heart through an incision no longer than your thumb.

Once again a Minnesota company lead the way. Tendyne was a small start-up company in Roseville that developed the first-in-man mitral valve to be inserted without open-heart surgery. The Tendyne valve was a masterpiece of medical engineering. It had three leaflets fashioned out of porcine pericardium that were sewn into an elastic frame of nitinol, an alloy of nickel and titanium. Nitinol was discovered in the 1950s during the development of nose cones for intercontinental ballistic missiles; it is superelastic and has shape memory—properties that are ideal for medical devices that are inserted through small holes and then unfold in the heart.

The first patient treated with a Tendyne valve was a 68-year-old woman whose heart was so weak she could not undergo traditional mitral valve replacement using the heart-lung machine. She received a Tendyne valve in 2014 at the Royal Brompton Hospital in London.

A few months later, in April of 2015, Wes Pedersen, together with Drs. Sorajja, Saeid Farivar, and Richard Bae implanted the first Tendyne transcatheter mitral valve in the United States at the Minneapolis Heart Institute. The Tendyne valve was folded onto a special delivery catheter inserted into the left ventricle through a small incision in the left side of the chest. Guided by X-ray fluoroscopy and 3-dimensional ultrasound, Pedersen and his team advanced the catheter through the mitral valve where the nitinol frame was deployed, releasing the three porcine pericardial leaflets. An anchoring wire secured the valve to the heart. The entire procedure required about an hour, and the patient went home in a few days.

In the near future, aortic, mitral, and tricuspid valves will be repaired or replaced routinely with catheters or minimally invasive surgery. No longer will it be necessary to open the chest, connect the patient to a heart-lung machine, and stop the heart as Ted Foster's surgery required in 2012. Patients will have their replacement valves custom-made based on highly detailed images acquired with CT scanners and MRI machines.

What would the early pioneers like Lillehei, Favaloro, and Gruentzig say about these new techniques? I suspect they would wonder why it took so long!

CHAPTER 20

I was the junior medical resident on duty in the emergency room of Cincinnati General Hospital in the spring of 1970. Around 9 a.m., an ambulance brought in a middle- aged African-American man, Clifford Jones, who had collapsed at home. "He was awake when we got there," the ambulance attendant said, "but his heart rate was about 180. It's still about 180."
Quickly we connected Clifford to an EKG machine. It showed an ugly, rapid, irregular heart rhythm that looked life threatening. He was conscious, however, breathing comfortably, and his blood pressure was 100 over 60. The senior medical resident, my supervisor, told me to give him lidocaine, an intravenous drug for treating ventricular tachycardia. "This looks like VT," the resident said, "we need to stop it. Now."

I gave him 100 mg of lidocaine through the intravenous line and watched the monitor. Nothing happened. Clifford's rhythm was unchanged. A few minutes later the senior resident came back and decided we should shock him. "It's too risky to sedate him. Just shock him. We should get him out of this rhythm."

I wheeled the big American Optical defibrillator into the room. "Oh shit, man," Clifford cried, "you're not going to do that again! It happens every time I come in here! It doesn't work! And it hurts like hell!" I left to tell the senior resident what Clifford said. "Shock him," he replied. "We'll ask cardiology to see him later."

I shocked Clifford with 200 joules of electrical energy synchronized to his heartbeat. He was awake, and his shout of pain echoed throughout the emergency room. It was awful. However, the rhythm changed. His rate dropped to about 110 beats a minute and he was in sinus rhythm, the normal rhythm for his heart. I went out to the charting area and began writing orders for Clifford's admission to the hospital.

I did not know it then but Clifford was my introduction to a new cardiology specialty, clinical electrophysiology, the diagnosis and treatment of heart rhythm disorders.

The heart is an intricately coordinated pump consisting of four muscular chambers that must contract in harmony in order to maintain a smooth, consistent flow of blood. To do this, a network of specialized tissue produces and conducts electrical signals to the heart's cells so that each one squeezes—contracts—at precisely the right moment. The pulses of electrical energy originate in the heart's native pacemaker, a cluster of unique cells, called the sinus node, located at the top of the right atrium. Normally each pulse, each heartbeat begins in the sinus node and spreads outward, through thousands of fibers, first to the left atrium and then onward to the right and left ventricles.

The pulse of electricity that begins in the right atrium makes its way to the ventricles via a single, critical pathway consisting of the atrioventricular node, the His bundle, and the right and left bundle branches. The bundle branches deliver pulses to their final destination via thousands of delicate Purkinje fibers, so named for the Czech anatomist who described them in 1837.

The atrioventricular node—called the AV node—is highly specialized tissue and acts as a gate, or traffic cop, allowing only a certain number of beats per minute to travel from the atrium to the ventricles. If too many beats arrive at the AV node, some are blocked, i.e. the gate shuts. The AV node is a protective, fail-safe mechanism that prevents the ventricles from beating too fast and fibrillating.

The heart's normal rhythm begins in the sinus node, and is called sinus rhythm. A rhythm that begins elsewhere in the heart is known by its anatomic origin—atrial, ventricular, or atrioventricular—and they are considered *arrhythmias* because they are not normal. Bradycardia is a slow rhythm, typically less than 50 beats per minute. Tachycardia is a fast rhythm, technically more than 100 beats a minute, but usually faster, about 150-180 beats a minute. Sinus tachycardia is usually (but not always) normal because it occurs when the body needs more blood. The other fast rhythm is fibrillation, when the chambers—atria or ventricles—are beating rapidly, as high as an uncoordinated 300 to 400 times a minute. Fibrillation is always abnormal; ventricular fibrillation is lethal.

Twenty minutes after I shocked Clifford into a normal rhythm the nurse came out of his room to tell me the rapid rhythm was back. By this time the medical records department had delivered Clifford's old records. Indeed, he had been in our emergency room multiple times over the past five years. Further, he was under the care of Dr. Ralph Scott, a cardiologist at the University of Cincinnati, who was treating him for "paroxysmal atrial fibrillation and Wolff-Parkinson-White syndrome (WPW)."

I called Dr. Scott. One hour later, he arrived in the emergency room and reviewed the EKGs. Then he gave an impromptu lecture on atrial fibrillation in patients who had the Wolff-Parkinson-White syndrome. "Everyone thinks its ventricular tachycardia," Scott said. "It's not. It's the WPW that makes it look like ventricular tachycardia. Give him 300 milligrams of quinidine sulfate by mouth every four hours. He should convert to sinus rhythm after the second or third dose, and the WPW will go away. Call me if he does not convert. Otherwise I'll see him in the hospital tomorrow morning."

Just as Scott had predicted, Clifford converted from atrial fibrillation to sinus rhythm after the second dose of quinidine sulfate. Before he went home, I apologized for the painful shock I had given him. He gave me a surprised looked and said, "Well that's a first," and walked out.

Cardiology was a single specialty for decades, but in the late 1960s cardiologists began to focus on specific areas within their specialty, such as heart catheterization, coronary care, and echocardiography. Electrophysiology emerged from electrocardiography—the study of EKGs—and basic science discoveries that elucidated the electrical properties of the heart. A generation of clinical electrophysiologists was born out of these disciplines, and they laid the foundation for giant leaps forward in the diagnosis and treatment of abnormal heart rhythms.

My emergency room patient, Clifford Jones, had Wolff-Parkinson-White syndrome -- one of the first rhythm disturbances to be unraveled and successfully treated by the first generation of clinical electrophysiologists. Willem Einthoven, a professor of physiology at the University of Leiden, developed the electrocardiogram

(EKG) in 1892. The EKG was a giant step forward, allowing physicians to diagnose many forms of heart disease, including arrhythmias.

From the surface of the body, Einthoven recorded the electrical signals that occur with each heartbeat and named them P, Q, R, S, and T, designations that have never changed. The P-wave represents electrical depolarization—or change in electrical charge—that occurs in the cells of the atria as the pulse spreads outward from the sinus node. The QRS is produced when the electrical charges of the cells within the ventricles change and *depolarize*. The T-wave represents the process of cellular recovery or *repolarization*. The P-wave corresponds to the contraction of the atria, and the QRS signal is correlated to ventricular contraction.

The heart's finely tuned electrical system can be upended by anything that alters or disrupts the conduction system or muddles the rhythmic function of the sinus node. In 1893, an Englishman, Albert Kent, found a rare (1 to 3 in 1000 hearts) extra connection between the atria and ventricle. This connection, now called the *Bundle of Kent*, is capable of rapidly conducting pulses between the atria and ventricles in *both* directions. It is an *accessory pathway* that can bypass the AV node. The accessory pathway circumvents the normal protective mechanisms that minimize how rapidly pulses can travel between the upper and lower chambers of the heart. This Bundle of Kent was responsible for Clifford Jones' very fast WPW tachycardia.

WPW is a congenital abnormality originally described by Dr. Louis Wolff, the son of Lithuanian immigrants, who graduated from Harvard Medical School in 1922. Wolff worked with Dr. Paul Dudley White at the Massachusetts General Hospital. White was a major force in the establishment of the American Heart Association and the National Institutes of Health.

One day in 1928, White saw a young man with a rapid rhythm occurring sporadically that was becoming more troublesome. The young man's EKG was quite unusual and White sent it to Wolff who directed the electrocardiography department at the Beth Israel Hospital in Boston. The EKG was unique because there were two different QRS signals. One QRS was shaped normally with sharp upward and downward slopes, but the second QRS had a slurred, rather than sharp, upward slope and it began very soon after the P-wave from the atria. During a trip to London, White showed the EKGs to Dr. John Parkinson who had collected seven similar cases in London. Together, Drs. Wolff, Parkinson, and White published their findings in 1930.

But the three physicians did not know *why* these EKGs were abnormal. What was the *mechanism*? What was the meaning of the slurred sloping QRS? There was a great deal of debate and speculation. Then two Philadelphia physicians, Drs. Charles Wolferth and Francis Wood, brilliantly deduced what was happening.

They hypothesized that patients like this young man had an extra electrical connection—a second, or accessory pathway—between the atrium and ventricle. This extra connection was in fact the Bundle of Kent. When a heartbeat traveled over the Bundle of Kent it caused the beginning of the QRS to be slurred because it stimulated a portion of the ventricles *early*. If the heartbeat traveled only through the AV node, the ventricles were stimulated at the *same time* and so the QRS was normal. Why then were these patients with differently shaped QRS complexes prone to rapid heart beating, i.e. tachycardia?

Wolferth and Wood correctly identified the tachycardia's mechanism. They theorized that the tachycardia was started by a beat that traveled down one of the two pathways (Bundle of Kent or AV node) and rapidly back up the other, forming a loop, like a racetrack. The heartbeat continued around and around the loop, repeatedly stimulating the atria and ventricles and causing a fast tachycardia that persisted until something interrupted the loop or the tissue became exhausted, like a tiger chasing its tail.

Yet my patient, Clifford Jones, did not have an endless looping tachycardia. His problem was caused by atrial fibrillation. When the atria fibrillate they throw off signals at a frequency exceeding 300 beats per minute. The Bundle of Kent can conduct these beats faster than the AV node and produce a very fast, life-threatening tachycardia. When I saw Clifford Jones in 1970, the only treatment was to prevent his atrial fibrillation with a drug, i.e. quinidine sulfate.

As more patients were identified, it became clear that the rapid heart beating associated with WPW was a serious problem for many patients. WPW could cause sudden death or disable otherwise healthy adults. A curative treatment was sought urgently.

The Wolff-Parkinson-White syndrome had long fascinated Dr. Howard Burchell. Born in Athens, Ontario, a farming community south of Ottawa, Burchell received his medical degree from the University of Toronto and trained at Toronto General Hospital, the London Hospital Medical School and Heart Hospital, and the Mayo Clinic in Rochester, Minnesota. He remained at Mayo as a consultant cardiologist until 1968, when he became Chief of Cardiology at the University of Minnesota and served in that position until his retirement in 1975. From 1965 to 1970, he was the Editor-in-chief of *Circulation*, the scientific journal of the American Heart Association.

I have never met another man quite like him. Dr. Burchell, or "Dr. B" as many called him, was truly one of a kind. Whenever I spoke at a conference and saw Howard Burchell in the audience I immediately began to anticipate the inevitable, mind-bending question he would ask at the end of my talk. "Doctor Hauser," he would say in his soft, raspy voice, "have you ever thought about...." Then he would gently pounce. Usually I had never thought about this or that, but Dr. Burchell had, and often he challenged our minds to look at something familiar in a very different way. Dr. Burchell was a man of science, and in 1973 he wrote," ...to dismiss science as largely irrelevant in the education of the physician is to open the doors to another dark age of medicine."

In 1967, a 43-year-old Indiana mail carrier entered the Mayo Clinic for closure of an atrial septal defect—a hole between the two atria. He also had the WPW syndrome that caused him to faint once and nearly faint many other times. Dr. Burchell thought it might be possible to locate and cut the Bundle of Kent and cure the WPW that was distressing this patient more than the atrial septal defect.

On the day of the surgery, Dr. Dwight McGoon opened the patient's chest. Burchell and Dr. Robert Frye, a young cardiologist, were in the operating room with an EKG machine. Almost immediately, the patient spontaneously went into his rapid WPW rhythm. McGoon took a special electrode and placed it at different points on the surface of the patient's right ventricle, acquiring signals that Burchell recorded on the EKG machine

Later, Dr. Bruce Fye of the Mayo Clinic wrote, "Burchell was one of very few cardiologists in the world who knew how to piece the tracings [recordings]

together…" From this "electrical map" of the heart, Burchell identified the location of the Bundle of Kent, the accessory pathway that caused the patient's rapid heart beating. He asked McGoon to inject a local anesthetic in this area. Immediately the rapid heart beating stopped. However, an attempt to permanently severing the Bundle of Kent with a scalpel was unsuccessful.

Nevertheless, Burchell demonstrated the feasibility of mapping the electrical topography of the heart and treating WPW—and potentially other fast rhythms—surgically. This was the beginning of interventional electrophysiology—the physical elimination (ablation) of tachycardias—and the next leap forward occurred at Duke University in Durham, North Carolina.

Dr. Will Sealy was born and grew up in Reynolds, Georgia, a small agricultural town 40 miles west of Macon. His father was a banker. Will attended Emory University during the Depression and earned his way through medical school working for the largest undertaker in Atlanta. Early on, Sealy decided to become a surgeon and trained at Duke before entering the military in 1942, serving in England with the 65th General Hospital based in Suffolk. At the end of the war, he returned to Duke and became a thoracic surgeon, operating on many patients with advanced pulmonary tuberculosis.

By the mid-1950s, Sealy was doing open-heart surgery, using a combination of the DeWall-Lillehei bubble oxygenator and hypothermia. In the 1960s, he became interested in atrial arrhythmias that often occurred after the surgical repair of atrial septal defects. He worked with Dr. Andrew Wallace, a cardiologist who would become the Chief of Cardiology at Duke. Like Burchell at Mayo, they developed a system for mapping the heart's electrical system.

Sealy was aware of the WPW work at Mayo by Burchell and McGoon. In 1968, he saw a 32-year-old commercial fisherman from the Outer Banks of North Carolina who had bouts of rapid heart beating since he was four years old. At 28, the man began to experience shortness of breath with activity. He was treated for heart failure, with some improvement, but his episodes of tachycardia became more frequent and lasted longer. The EKG showed the slurred QRS pattern of Wolff-Parkinson-White. Attempts to slow his heart rate with drugs were unsuccessful.

After studying Albert Kent's original description, Sealy took the patient to the operating room and mapped his heart with a handheld electrode. He found the area where the electrical pulse from the atrium first appeared on the right ventricle. He thought this should be where the Bundle of Kent was located, and proceeded to cut the suspected tissue with a scalpel, severing the connection between the right ventricle and tricuspid valve. The incisions were more extensive than the one McGoon had tried at Mayo. It worked. Immediately the Wolff-Parkinson-White tachycardia stopped, and it never came back. This was the first successful ablation—physical elimination—of an abnormal heart rhythm, and it was the beginning of rapid, unprecedented advances in the diagnosis and treatment of abnormal heart rhythms.

Ansel Morgan was jolted out of a deep sleep by the noxious tones of his emergency pager. The alarm clock on the bedside table displayed the time: it was 3:22 a.m. He called the dispatcher at the county sheriff's office who told him there was a fire in a mobile home at the park on East River Road. Morgan had been a member of the volunteer fire department for three years. His gear was always ready to go in the back of his Ford pick-up. Within four minutes, he was backing out of his heated garage.

It had been five below zero when he went to bed. Now it was twenty below and his headlights reflected off the snow blowing across Highway 7 in western Minnesota. Twenty minutes later he saw the flashing red lights from the county's newest fire engine pulling into the trailer park. About 100 yards into the park, he saw a large mobile home engulfed in flames.

Morgan parked his truck next to the fire engine, strapped on his helmet over a fire-resistant hood, and stepped into his boots. He joined two other volunteers dragging a fire hose toward the flames. "Is anybody in there?" Morgan shouted.

"We don't know," one of them replied. Ansel Morgan grabbed a fire extinguisher and rushed to the front door. Suddenly his vision blurred; he thought he was looking into a tunnel. A wave of nausea brought a sour taste to his mouth. He felt warm and sweaty, despite the freezing cold. Then his legs buckled and he lost consciousness.

Morgan awoke as two firefighters dragged him by the arms, away from the burning mobile home. An ambulance had just arrived, and two paramedics lifted him onto a gurney and slid him into the back of the rig. They gave him oxygen through a facemask. A few minutes later, they recorded an EKG.

"What's happening?" Morgan groaned, not certain where he was.

"You blacked out," one of the paramedics replied. "No wonder. Your heart's going over 200 beats a minute. Have you had heart trouble before?"

"Once. I was sixteen," Morgan said. He tried to sit up but the paramedics had restrained him with safety straps across his chest and thighs. "I was having a fast pulse at times and saw a specialist at the University. He didn't think I needed anything. It never happened again—'til now, I guess. I was in high school." Ansel was 42.

"Well, whatever it was, it's back. We're going to take you into Rice Memorial," the paramedic said. "Do you want me to call someone?"

"Yeah, my wife." Morgan gave them his home phone number, and asked, "Were there any people in there—the mobile home?"

"No, the owners are in Texas for the winter. It all started with an explosion. The manager thinks something went wrong with the propane."

Twenty-five minutes later, the ambulance pulled into Rice Memorial hospital in Willmar, Minnesota. In the emergency room, an intravenous catheter was inserted into Morgan's vein in his right forearm and an EKG was done. Morgan told Dr. Enriquez, the emergency room physician, about the episode when he was a teenager.

"Ansel, you have a supraventricular tachycardia—an SVT," Enriquez said. "I'm going to give you a drug into your vein to stop it—or at least slow it down. You may feel a little funny for a minute or so. Your blood pressure is a little low, so we're giving you saline—salt solution—through your vein."

"Okay, doc, I'm feeling real crappy right now..." The tunnel vision came back and the ceiling lights faded. Morgan's chest felt like it was going to explode. Then he felt a rush and suddenly his body was quiet. He looked at the doctor who was watching the monitor. "What was that?"

"You're back in a normal rhythm. The drug worked," Enriquez said. "You felt the pause between the fast SVT and the normal rhythm. It was close to ten seconds. I gave you a drug called adenosine. It makes you feel weird."

"It sure did. Don't want to do that again," Morgan said.

"We'll keep you here for a few hours and monitor your rhythm," Dr. Enriquez said. "I need to do a few blood tests, make sure nothing else is going on. If everything checks out, you can go home. I don't want you to drive, though."

"Okay. I think my wife is coming. She may be here."

At that moment, Eleanor Morgan appeared in the doorway. She was a petite brunette with hazel eyes and her mouth was shaped in a smile. She always looked happy, and that was her nickname. No one, except her mother, called her Eleanor.

"Can I come in, doctor?" she asked. "I'm Happy Morgan, Ansel's wife."

"Yes, please come in. I'm Doctor Enriquez," he said, extending his hand. "Your husband is fine. He had a pretty fast SVT—fast heart rhythm—but we gave him a shot and it's gone now. I think he'll be able to go home in a few hours—as soon as we check a few blood tests. And assuming his heart behaves."

Happy took Ansel's hand and held it. She looked at the doctor and asked, "Why did he have it? It's never happened before…Is this a heart attack?"

"No, it's not a heart attack. Apparently your husband may have had rhythm problems as a teenager." Happy looked at Ansel, who nodded. "I think the stress of the fire emergency probably triggered it," Enriquez continued. "In any case he needs to see a heart specialist. What kind of work do you do, Mr. Morgan?"

"I work for the electric company, "Ansel replied. "I'm a lineman."

"Well, you can't get yourself into a situation where another spell could cause a serious injury. You shouldn't be on a ladder or roof, and you can't be responding to fires until this rhythm problem is sorted out. I'm going to start you on atenolol. It's a beta blocker, a drug that will slow your heart rate and hopefully prevent the SVT."

Three hours later Happy Morgan drove her husband home. The following day Ansel visited his primary care physician who told Ansel that he would be seeing Dr. Bill Katsiyiannis, an electrophysiologist at the Minneapolis Heart Institute. Katsiyiannis had trained at Washington University in St. Louis, Missouri, and specialized in the ablation of heart arrhythmias.

The most successful medical treatments have come about because a scientist or group of scientists figured out how a particular disease caused harm. Once the biologic mechanism(s) of a disease were known, therapies like drugs or surgical techniques could be devised to treat it. This was especially true for arrhythmias. I lived through an era when we tried multiple drugs and drug combinations to suppress rhythm disturbances before finding one or several that seemed to work reasonably well.

There was nothing scientific about this empiric practice: it was the dark age, as Burchell would call it, when unknowingly we gave antiarrhythmic drugs to patients that could kill them. Not until the late 1980s did we understand fully that certain antiarrhythmic drugs could also be *proarrhythmic*, meaning they could trigger lethal rhythms such as ventricular tachycardia and ventricular fibrillation. This revelation was one of the great wake-up calls for cardiologists during the last half of the 20th century.

For patients like Ansel Morgan, very fast rhythms meant they could not engage in professions where a blackout could place them and others in jeopardy. These were the patients who benefitted most from ablation, because they would be cured and return safely to their professions. For other patients, ablation was attractive because it relieved symptoms and eliminated the need for daily drug therapy.

The Global Positioning System (GPS) and Google Maps guide us from point to point and plot the fastest route from city to city. Electrophysiologists use mapping systems to locate the tissue in the heart that triggers or perpetuates a fast rhythm. Howard Burchell and Will Sealy used a simple electrode to identify the Bundle of Kent in the operating room. Modern mapping systems often employ dozens of electrodes on several catheters inserted into the heart through a vein or artery. These electrodes gather signals that are computer processed and displayed on a large monitor so that the electrophysiologist can locate the millimeters of tissue causing the arrhythmia.

Once the tissue is found, the electrophysiologist can ablate it -- physically eliminate it. Remarkably, it was not until the early 1980s that the first ablations by a catheter in the heart occurred. Electrophysiologists working independently at the University of California in San Francisco and Duke University in Durham, North Carolina announced their results in 1982.

In San Francisco, Dr. Melvin Scheinman had been perfecting his method for ablating the atrioventricular node in the animal laboratory. In April 1981, Scheinman saw a 60-year-old retired ironworker who had severe rheumatoid arthritis and bouts of very rapid atrial fibrillation that precipitated acute heart failure. When attempts to control the atrial fibrillation with drugs failed, Scheinman decided that the only treatment for this patient was to ablate—destroy—the atrioventricular node and create complete heart block. By ablating the atrioventricular node, no pulses from the atrium could be conducted to the ventricles. A pacemaker implanted in the ventricle would then control the heart rate.

Scheinman performed the experimental ablation by delivering a high-energy direct current (DC) shock from an external defibrillator through a catheter that he placed against the atrioventricular node in his patient's heart. The electrical energy burned the atrioventricular node, killing the tissue, disrupting its ability to transmit pulses from the atrium to the ventricle. Then he implanted a pacemaker and set it to 70 beats per minute. It was an elegantly simple solution and one that did not require open-heart surgery. The ironworker had a stable paced rhythm and his heart failure resolved.

But the high-energy DC shock was a problem. It caused a thermoelectric explosion that was traumatic and could damage more than the atrioventricular node. The explosion produced high pressures inside the heart and could form bubbles that traveled to the lungs and brain. How could electrophysiologists ablate the culprit tissue without damaging valves, coronary arteries, or healthy heart muscle?

Dr. Shoei K. Stephen Huang came to my office at Rush in 1983. Steve was one of our cardiology fellows at Rush-Presbyterian-St. Luke's Medical Center in Chicago. Born in Taiwan, Huang wanted to be a cardiac electrophysiologist. Steve told me he had an idea for ablation. Instead of high-energy DC shocks, he thought that radiofrequency energy would be safer and more effective.

For many years, we had used a radiofrequency cautery in the operating room to cut through tissue and coagulate bleeding vessels. Huang thought the radiofrequency current could be delivered through a catheter and burn only the tissue that the tiny metal electrode was touching inside the heart. It should not cause collateral damage.

Steve asked if I could help him test his idea in the animal laboratory. I was a bit skeptical, but intrigued. Besides, we wanted our cardiology fellows to pursue their research ideas. After preliminary animal work at Rush, Huang moved to the University of Arizona where he further investigated radiofrequency (RF) ablation, publishing his results in 1987. Soon RF ablation was being used in humans. Special steerable catheters and RF generators were produced and, in less than a decade, RF ablation was treating rapid rhythms in the AV node, atria, and ventricles.

By the time Ansel Morgan suffered his debilitating SVT, RF ablation was a safe and effective technique. It has cured tens of thousands of patients with a variety of abnormal rhythms. This technique did for heart arrhythmias what the heart-lung machine did for open-heart surgery: it was a tremendous enabler and allowed physicians to cure rhythm disorders that had once been unapproachable.

Shortly before I retired in 2015, Stephen Huang presented me with a signed copy of the third edition of his textbook, "Catheter Ablation of Cardiac Arrhythmias."

Three weeks after he blacked out fighting the fire in the trailer park, Ansel Morgan found himself lying on an X-ray table in an electrophysiology laboratory at the Minneapolis Heart Institute. He had seen Dr. Katsiyiannis in the clinic ten days before and he understood what was going to happen. Katsiyiannis thought Ansel had an atrioventricular nodal reentry tachycardia, a common arrhythmia that could be cured with ablation.

A technician applied EKG electrodes on Ansel's arms and legs. The nurse anesthetist gave him an injection of intravenous midazolam that made him sleepy. He could see a technician organizing instruments on a table covered with a light blue sterile cloth. Soft rock music played in the background from speakers in the ceiling. No one seemed to be in a particular hurry. It all appeared very routine, a comforting feeling.

"Good morning, Mr. Morgan," Katsiyiannis said as he positioned himself next to the X-ray table. Touching the skin over the femoral artery and vein in Ansel's right groin, he said, "You will feel a sting as I'm give you a local anesthetic—just as we talked about."

Ansel, groggy from the midazolam, whispered, "Okay."

Quickly Katsiyiannis numbed the tissue with lidocaine and placed a plastic vascular sheath into the femoral vein. Within minutes, he inserted four catheters into the right side of Ansel's heart.

First Katsiyiannis tested Ansel's conduction system, precisely measuring the milliseconds it took for the pulse produced by his sinus node to travel through the atria, atrioventricular node, His Bundle, and left and right bundle branches, to the Purkinje fibers of the left and right ventricles. As expected, all of the conduction intervals were normal, indicating that the tissue was healthy—no scar, no short-circuits, no surprises.

Next, he stimulated the heart with pacing pulses delivered via the catheter in the right atrium. The small electrical pacing pulses—each about 10 volts—stimulated the right atrium, causing the entire heart to beat, suppressing the normal biologic pulses from Ansel's sinus node. Katsiyiannis was now controlling the heart's rate and rhythm: he "captured" the heart by pacing it faster than Ansel's sinus rhythm.

Next Katsiyiannis would try to start-up Ansel's rapid heartbeat—the tachycardia—that had caused him to black out. To do this, he used a special stimulator—a computerized external pacemaker—delivering electrical pulses in a precise, timed sequence via the catheter in the right atrium.

He adjusted the stimulator to pace the atrium at 100 beats per minute. After the fifth beat, he delivered a stimulus that caused an early or premature beat. This premature beat produced a change in the electrical properties of Ansel's atrioventricular node. This precipitated Ansel's tachycardia which, as Katsiyiannis had predicted, was typical AV nodal reentry tachycardia. He knew it was the tachycardia that caused Ansel to blackout at the fire because it was identical to the one recorded in the ambulance.

The phenomenon called *re-entry* works like this: A beat from the sinus node may follow one of two pathways through the AV node to the ventricles. One pathway is faster than the other, so the beat that travels down the slow pathway is blocked by the faster beat. A premature beat, however, may alter the electrical properties of both pathways, so the beat traveling down the slow path not only goes to the ventricles but also travels *back up* the faster pathway—in the reverse direction—to the atrium. It does not stop there: the beat goes back down the slow pathway. It keeps going around and around, down the slow pathway and up the fast pathway, re-entering the circuit within the AV node. Consequently, beats are rapidly thrown off to the atria and ventricles, causing the fast AV node re-entry tachycardia.

Decades of research led to understanding this fundamental mechanism, called re-entry in which a beat, under certain conditions, re-enters a tissue pathway and endlessly loops around, generating a fast rhythm like AV nodal re-entry tachycardia. Re-entry can occur anywhere in the heart. Wolff-Parkinson-White tachycardia is a form of re-entry: the pulse loops around, using the AV node and the Bundle of Kent as pathways. Most ventricular tachycardias are caused by a re-entry phenomenon. In this case, the loop is often around a scar caused by a heart attack.

To treat these tachycardias with ablation, the electrophysiologist creates an electrical map of the heart, identifies the critical pathways necessary to start and maintain the re-entry tachycardia, and burns them with radiofrequency thermal energy or freezes the tissue with a cryoprobe.

Katsiyiannis located Ansel's slow pathway by recording signals from the catheter near the tricuspid valve. He gently manipulated the catheter while examining the electrical signals on the monitor. These signals, called electrograms, came from the atrium and the ventricle. The electrograms displayed a characteristic pattern when the catheter's electrode came in close contact with the slow pathway tissue. Burning this area would eliminate the slow pathway and prevent further episodes of AV nodal re-entry tachycardia.

The radiofrequency generator was on a stand next to the X-ray table. Katsiyiannis asked a technician to connect the catheter to the generator. He reconfirmed the position of the catheter in Ansel's heart by checking the electrograms. Then he applied the radiofrequency energy for 10 seconds; it traveled between the catheter electrode in the heart and a skin patch electrode that had been applied to Ansel's chest. The electrical energy delivered through the catheter was converted to thermal energy and the heat was transferred to the electrode. The heat fried the slow pathway tissue, creating a tiny burn, and eliminated the troublesome tachycardia.

Afterward Katsiyiannis tried to induce Ansel's AV nodal tachycardia with the same pacing sequence he used before the ablation. Nothing happened, demonstrating that the ablation was successful. Ansel Morgan was cured. He would need no medications, and he could return to his work as a lineman and volunteer firefighter.

The lives of many thousands of patients have been adversely affected, even threatened, by pathologic tachycardias. WPW and AV nodal re-entry tachycardia are two of a long list of heart rhythm disorders that originate above the ventricles. They can cause debilitating symptoms but they seldom kill or permanently disable their victims. The exception is atrial fibrillation, which can kill and disable people in many different ways, and I have observed all of them. One patient is the most memorable.

CHAPTER 21

My wife, Sally, and I checked into the Hotel Royal Riviera on a picturesque peninsula of rolling hills, landscaped terraces and a craggy coastline on the Mediterranean Sea. We had visited Cap Ferrat in France many times and we planned a relaxing three days before I spoke at a medical conference in Nice. Our hotel was six miles east of Nice on the Cote d'Azur, an ideal place to walk, jog or simply sit and watch the seagulls and sailboats.

We flew overnight from Minneapolis to Nice with a brief stop in Amsterdam. When we checked in at 5 p.m. on June 9, 2012, both of us eagerly anticipated an early dinner at the hotel followed by sleep. Our fourth floor room overlooked the pool with a splendid view of the beach. Sally wanted the shower first so I turned on CNN and began to unpack.

After hanging up my clothes in the closet opposite the bathroom, I turned and saw Sally standing at the sink, peering into the mirror. There was something odd about her posture and she was not moving. I stepped into the bathroom and asked, "Is something wrong?" She turned and tried to speak, but could not form the words. "I agh, I agh", she moaned, and collapsed into my arms.

I carried her to the bed. Her eyes were closed. Irrationally I thought how pretty she looked lying there. Sally opened her eyes, "I'm okay. I'm okay." Those were her last words. "Sally, squeeze my fingers," I told her. My mind raced: I struggled to remain objective. What could be happening? Her right hand was feeble, and she could not move her right foot. Then her eyes closed again, and she no longer responded to my voice or touch.

Sally was having a major stroke. She was right-handed. It involved the dominant side, the left side of her brain.

I called the front desk: "I need an ambulance. My wife is having a stroke. We have to get her to a hospital fast." Within minutes, the hotel manager arrived. Sally was lying motionless on the bed. "Do you need a doctor," he asked? I replied, "I am a doctor and we must have an ambulance quickly."

Where would the ambulance take her? What hospital? Should we go to Monaco or to Nice? I had no idea, nor did he. The manager said either way it would take an ambulance at least 30 minutes to get to the hotel along the congested coast road on a Saturday night.

Then he had an idea. "There's a fire station next door. I'll ask them!"

Ten minutes later, three large firefighters entered our room with a stretcher. Two of them gently picked Sally up and strapped her in. They did not speak English and my French was nil. The manager spoke to them for a few minutes and said, "They will take your wife into Nice—Hopital St Roch—I don't know it." I asked the manager to call the hospital and arrange for a neurologist to meet us in the emergency room.

The ride into Nice was swift. With its blue lights flashing and the characteristic French siren blaring, the large red fire ambulance deftly zigzagged its way around traffic on the boulevard Carnot and rue Delfy. The car traffic was bumper-to-bumper and opportunistic motorcyclists weaved between vehicles on the two-lane road. At one congested intersection near Vieux Port, the ambulance driver jumped the sidewalk, slalomed between trees and benches for half a block, and slipped back into traffic.

One of the oxygen tanks tore loose from its mounting and rolled about on the floor of the ambulance until the firefighter sitting next to me secured it. Sally, unconscious on the stretcher, was oblivious to the noise and jostling.

I could not take my eyes off her. We had eloped when she was nineteen and I was twenty-two. She had survived breast cancer. We had celebrated our fiftieth wedding anniversary the previous year in Paris. We had never been apart. She was my best friend. I could not fathom life without her.

We arrived at Hopital St. Roch on rue Pierre Dévoluy in 18 minutes rather than the 30 minutes I expected. I followed the stretcher into the emergency room. A young woman, no more than 5 feet 4 inches in height, stood in the hallway. She wore a white uniform with a stethoscope draped around her neck. The only thing I could think to say was, "Do you do lysis?" I repeated, "Do you do lysis?" She looked at me deliberately and replied, "Of course we do lysis—and I speak English."

Time lost is tissue lost when a major artery is blocked. It is especially true of the brain. Millions of brain cells begin to die within minutes when they are deprived of oxygen. These cells—neurons—consume 20 percent of the oxygen we take in even though they constitute only two percent of our body's tissue mass. Without blood flow, not only is the brain deprived of oxygen but also of glucose and other crucial nutrients.

The starved neurons begin to fail, abandoning critical functions, such as sending signals that enable speech and voluntary movements. The damage triggers an outpouring of chemical byproducts that poison vital metabolic pathways. The injury progresses with increasing rapidity. Fluid flows through pores, swelling the brain, ruthlessly forcing it against the rigid skull and deepening the coma. When this happens, all communication between the brain's complex nerve network and the rest of the body shuts down.

A large area on the dominant side of Sally's brain had no blood flow because her left middle cerebral artery was obstructed, most likely with a blood clot. Quickly opening the artery and restoring blood flow with a thrombolytic drug—lysis—could rescue Sally from a life of sensory isolation and immobility, unable to speak, visually impaired, and paralyzed. That is, assuming she survived the first 24 to 48 hours.

I remembered my days at Cincinnati General Hospital, first as a student and then as a medical resident. Stroke patients, like heart attack patients in that era, were put to bed with no active intervention. Treatment consisted of blood pressure control, and prevention of bedsores and bladder and bowel care. It was a grim disease, merciless in its capacity to destroy a person, and in those days we could only look on and hope this would never happen to someone we loved.

In 1958, two New Jersey neurologists, Bernard Sussman and Thomas Fitch, gave a thrombolytic drug—fibrinolysin—intravenously to a woman who was paralyzed for six hours. She had a history of atrial fibrillation due to rheumatic heart disease and an angiogram revealed that a clot, most likely from her heart, blocked her middle cerebral artery. The fibrinolysin seemed to work: her symptoms improved and a follow-up angiogram showed that blood flow was restored.

However, nearly 40 years elapsed before a thrombolytic agent, a clot buster, was approved by the FDA for use in patients with ischemic strokes—that is, strokes caused by the absence of blood flow to the brain. There are multiple reasons for this four-decade gap. Principal among them were concerns that available thrombolytic drugs could cause massive bleeding into that portion of the brain affected by the stroke. By 1991, a novel thrombolytic agent, tissue plasminogen activator (tPA), was available for clinical trials. Studies suggested that tPA was less likely to cause brain hemorrhage.

In 1995, two landmark clinical trials evaluating tPA in acute stroke patients were published. The first was a European study showing improved outcomes for a group of stroke patients who were treated with tPA. The second, a U.S. study, revealed that, when tPA was given within three hours of a stroke's onset, one-third of patients improved significantly and only three percent got worse. As important, one in eight patients had complete resolution of their stroke symptoms. The risk of bleeding into the brain, however, was increased by tPA: six percent of patients had this complication. Even so, by 2012, early thrombolytic therapy was considered beneficial for virtually all patients provided they received it *within three to four and a half hours of onset of their stroke symptoms.*

Within minutes of arriving at the hospital, Sally was carted off to radiology for a CT scan of the brain. She was still unconscious and I was reluctant to leave her in this unfamiliar place. The clock was ticking, and I wanted to be certain that she got tPA; provided, of course, that the CT scan showed no brain hemorrhage. Gesturing toward the cart carrying Sally down the hall I asked, "Can I go with her?" The nurse pointed to the waiting room and said something authoritatively in French. I did not understand her but got the idea. As I walked out, a distinguished woman in a long, white coat passed me in the hall. She was headed in the same direction as Sally, and she was in a hurry.

The waiting room was crowded. I sat next to a young woman holding a sleeping baby swathed in an indigo blue terrycloth blanket. I called neurologist Dr. Ron Taurel in Minneapolis from my cellphone. It was Saturday so I reached his answering service. The agent said she could not page Dr. Taurel unless I was an established patient. I explained that I was a doctor and my wife was having a stroke in a French hospital and I needed to speak with Dr. Taurel. She refused, repeatedly.

As my anger escalated, I drew stares from those around me, and woke the baby, who began to cry.

Finally, I gave up and dialed my own answering service and asked to speak to the on-call cardiologist. It was Dr. Chuen Tang. I asked him to find Taurel or one of his partners and arrange a call. Ten minutes later, my cellphone rang. It was Taurel. I explained what had happened and asked if he had any suggestions or knew of a neurologist in Nice. Taurel assured me that France had one of the best, if not the best, acute stroke care systems in the world. He recalled that a very prominent stroke neurologist practiced in Nice but did not remember her name.

At that moment, the emergency room clerk came into the waiting room and called my name, as the French pronounce it—"Misseur Hows-air." I raised my hand and stood up. In fragmented English the clerk instructed me to go to the neurology intensive care unit on the third floor.

My imagination took over as I followed the signs through the dark hallways of Hopital St. Roch. Is Sally alive? Is it hopeless? Does she need something they cannot provide here? Will she be transferred to another hospital? Where would that be?

At last, I found the elevator to the neurology unit.

St. Roch's neurology floor reminded me of the old Cincinnati General Hospital where I was a student and first year resident. The "waiting room" consisted of a few red plastic chairs in the hallway. The walls, often patched and painted, were white and the floor, doors, and chairs were blood red. There were several sparsely furnished double rooms near the elevator that were occupied by patients.

Further down the hallway a nurse sat at a desk in a large room where white curtains screened visitors from patients. This was the neurology intensive care unit. I introduced myself, expecting to hear the worst. Instead, the nurse called to someone in the doctor's work area. It was the distinguished woman in the long white coat who had passed me in the emergency room. She introduced herself, "I am Docteur Mahagne. Your wife is over here."

We stepped around the curtains and there was Sally, lying in bed, her head slightly elevated. Sally looked up at me, smiled, and said, "Hi." The relief I felt was so profound that I just wanted to kneel at the bed and thank God. I would do that later. For now, I took Sally's hand and returned her smile. "Where am I?" she asked.

"What happened?" Tears began to form in her gray-green eyes, and I squeezed her hand. "You had a small stroke," I said, "but you are going to be fine."

Docteur Mahagne explained what transpired after Sally arrived in radiology. The CT scan revealed a clot in Sally's left middle cerebral artery that blocked all blood flow. She showed me a copy of the scan. "You are a physician?" she asked. I said I was a cardiologist. Pointing to the clot, she said, "the thrombus was not very large and there was no evidence of hemorrhage, so we gave her tPA while she was in the scanner."

The tPA attacked the small clot, slashing the fibrin strands and releasing the clumps of cells and debris. Blood flow to the dominant, vital side of Sally's brain was restored. Within 30 minutes, she was awake, able to speak and move her previously paralyzed right side. It was a gift from God.

The clot was gone but questions remained: where had it come from and how could another one be prevented? Blockage in an artery supplying blood to the brain causes about 80 percent of acute strokes. Bleeding into the brain causes the other twenty percent. Thankfully Sally fell into the 80 percent group. Did a clot form within her artery (an atherosclerotic plaque that ruptured, the cause of most heart attacks) and block blood flow, or did a clot develop elsewhere in her body, break off, and travel to her brain? The latter is called an embolism, and atrial fibrillation is the most frequent cause of an embolism that ignites a major stroke.

Atrial fibrillation (AF) is a common rhythm disorder. It occurs more often as we age and in patients who have diabetes, high blood pressure, heart failure, or a heart valve problem. An overactive thyroid may cause AF and AF may be inherited, too. AF is a notorious cause of embolic strokes and accounts for 15 percent or more of all strokes. AF is also a cause of heart failure because it can result in very fast heart rates that, over time, overwhelm and fatigue the left ventricle. Too often, the first symptom of atrial fibrillation is a stroke or severe heart failure.

When the atria fibrillate, their electrical systems are no longer coordinated. Individual cells and groups of cells contract randomly and do not propel blood through the valves to the ventricles in one effective beat. Blood pools and tends to become sludge in a useless structure called the left atrial appendage. Like the appendix in the colon, the atrial appendage is an evolutionary remnant that has no known function.

The sludge may form clots that break off and enter the blood stream. These clots can travel to any artery in the body and create a blockage. When the clot embolizes the brain, it causes a stroke; if it embolizes in a coronary artery, it precipitates a heart attack; if it embolizes in a leg artery, it threatens loss of the limb.

Sally had never experienced atrial fibrillation. A year earlier, she had noticed heart palpitations, but several days of EKG monitoring revealed only a few premature beats and no sign of AF. However, while she was in the neurology intensive care unit, a nurse reported seeing a brief burst of atrial fibrillation on the EKG monitor. This episode was not recorded, so there was no way to confirm the observation. Nevertheless, it was a "smoking gun" that could not be ignored. Docteur Mahagne thought Sally should be anticoagulated as soon as a CT scan indicated that her brain tissue had healed sufficiently.

After three days, Sally moved out of intensive care to a double room down the hall. She began rehabilitation. Another CT scan of her brain showed that the area affected by the stroke was undergoing the changes expected following such a massive insult.

An echocardiogram was entirely normal. She also had a special echocardiogram, called a transesophageal echo, whereby an ultrasound probe is passed through the mouth into the esophagus. This places the ultrasound source very close to the left atrium and permits exquisite views of the interior of the heart. The test revealed no clots in her heart, including the left atrial appendage, and there was no evidence of a hole in her heart that could allow passage of a blood clot from elsewhere in her body to her brain.

Ten days after the rapid ambulance ride into Nice, Sally left Hopital St. Roch. I drove her to the Hotel Royal Riviera where she thanked the manager and his staff for their kindness. We did the same at the fire station next door. Then we drove along the coast to Monaco and checked into the Marriott. We would not fly back to Minneapolis until she could take a blood thinner. Sally would rehab on the Riviera.

A week later, we returned to Hopital St. Roch where Sally had a follow-up CT scan. Her brain had healed and the neurologist started injections of low molecular weight heparin, a blood thinner, which I gave her every 12 hours. I called Delta Airlines and scheduled our return flight to Minneapolis. Three days later, we were home. Except for very mild weakness and tingling in her right hand and occasional difficulty finding words, Sally was back to her usual self. Our three daughters were there to meet us. We celebrated the fourth of July together.

We have long underestimated the pernicious nature of atrial fibrillation. It is another disease that can remain silent until it incubates a blood clot that embolizes to the brain, heart, or leg. Clots are like stealth missiles: they may remain undetected until the acute event.

When I reflect on that night in June of 2012—those two critical hours surrounding Sally's stroke—I look to heaven and say, "Thank you, God." The seemingly serendipitous sequence of events began when I happened to be with Sally at the moment she had the stroke. It could have struck in the airplane over the Atlantic or during our flight to Nice. Then there was the extraordinarily helpful hotel manager, and the fire department ambulance that, very critically, was located next door to the hotel. Finally, it ended with the expert care provided by Docteur Marie-Helene Mahagne and her staff at the Hopital St. Roch.

Remarkably, Docteur Mahagne was not just any neurologist: she was one of the stroke neurologists who conducted the groundbreaking study, published in the *New England Journal of Medicine* in 1995, showing that tPA could be an effective drug for treating acute strokes like Sally's. Perhaps God did not arrange it, but we will be forever grateful that she was on call that Saturday night in Nice.

CHAPTER 22

The beach in front of the hotel on Grand Turk island was a welcome relief for Stanley Hildebrandt. He had flown in from Minneapolis the previous day, escaping the accumulated snow and ice and the below zero temperatures. His wife, Martha, and oldest daughter, Melissa, accompanied him. They looked forward to the sun and casual lifestyle of their favorite Caribbean island.

Stan was a venture capitalist, 57 years old, and already thinking about cutting back his business commitments. Martha was talking about a home on Grand Turk. It would be a third home, complementing the mini-mansion on Lake Minnetonka west of Minneapolis, and the cabin on the North Shore of Lake Superior. The "cabin" was a sprawling collection of cottages and a lodge that Martha had remodeled into a comfortable five-bedroom home. It was a wonderful place to hold the annual family reunion that included his two brothers and three sisters.

A graduate of Ohio State, where he majored in computer science, Stan had forsaken business school to start a financial software company that he and his roommate founded in 1980. Five years later they sold the company to a Japanese bank for $38 million. Stan took a year off, and met Martha while he was visiting his cousin in St. Paul, Minnesota. They were married eight months later when she was pregnant with Melissa. They bought the home on Lake Minnetonka and had three more children, another girl, followed by twin boys.

Stan rode the Internet wave in the 1990s, expanding his fortune to over $500 million, and exiting well before the bubble burst. He was shrewd but never greedy. He believed in Business Lesson #1: "pigs get fat and hogs get slaughtered."

Now in February of 2014, resting on the beach in a cushioned lounge chair, Stan was thinking of nothing more complicated than where they should have dinner that evening. Martha and Melissa were off somewhere diving for conch shells. Melissa had recently graduated from St. Catherine University—St. Kate's, as most knew it—where she obtained her bachelors in nursing. Good nursing jobs were scarce but she had secured a position at Abbott Northwestern Hospital on a cardiology floor. She would start in mid-March, four weeks away.

At 4:12 pm, still lying on the lounge chair, Stan felt his heart pounding, rapidly and somewhat irregularly. This had been happening on and off for several months. He had cut back his caffeine consumption with some improvement. Stan took a deep breath and coughed several times, but the pounding persisted. A few minutes later his chest felt very uncomfortable, and he sat up. He placed an index finger on his radial pulse: it would be fast for a few seconds then pause and slow down. "What the hell," he whispered. "I'll go back to the room."

Stan stood up. He was wobbly and unsure what was happening. He nearly fainted. Sitting back down, he stared at the surf, and waited. Several minutes passed. He felt better. Gradually, the discomfort in his chest waned, and then it was gone. The rapid beating stopped too, and his pulse was again steady and strong.

From behind him came a voice. It was Martha. "Stan, honey, you missed a wonderful dive." She sat next to him on the chaise lounge. "You look a little bedraggled. Are you okay?"

Ignoring the question, he asked, "Where's Melissa?"

"She's in her room. I came down here to keep you company." Martha paused then repeated, "Are you okay?"

Stan replied, "I don't know. I just had some skipped beats and a little heaviness in my chest. He paused, took a deep breath, as if to clear something in his lungs that was not there, and continued, "but it's gone now."

Martha studied her husband. He was a typical male minimizer: nothing ever caused him to panic or outwardly worry. The alpha male in him was always composed, never vulnerable. "I think you should tell Melissa. She's a nurse now, you know." Martha reached for her cell phone.

Stan gently grasped Martha's wrist. "No, I'm fine. Let's not start our vacation with a fuss over nothing. If it happens again, I'll tell her. Come on." He stood and motioned for Martha to get up and walk with him. But she sat there, looking up at him. Something did not seem right, but she could not define it. Sighing, Martha stood and followed him to the hotel. There was no point in pursuing the issue with this stubborn man.

They had dinner at a restaurant on the beach about 600 yards south of their hotel. It was bustling with a happy hour crowd when they arrived. Stan asked for the table closest to the surf, as far as possible from the bar. He was particularly delighted to be with these two beautiful women. Martha and Melissa were both blonde, blue eyed, and trim. It was not easy to know that they were mother and daughter; one would have to study Martha carefully to know that she was twenty years older.

Stan inherited his distinguished silver gray hair and deep brown eyes from his mother. He was just over six feet and weighed exactly eleven pounds more than he had at his college graduation. The exercise equipment he had in their home in Minnetonka was a good investment: the treadmill, stationary bike, and Bowflex™ gym allowed him to workout every morning. It was after one of these workouts during the Christmas holidays that he first experienced the burst of fast heartbeats and chest heaviness.

The three of them were walking back to the hotel along the beach when Stan felt lightheaded. He continued on for a few feet, and then reached out for Martha and Melissa on either side of him. Melissa said, "What's wrong, Dad?"

"I don't know…I need to sit down…" He started to squat, and then fell back onto the sand, unconscious.

"Mom, go get help! Dad, Daddy, can you hear me?" Melissa knelt by her father, feeling for his carotid pulse. Stan moaned. "Are you having pain, Dad?" He did not answer. Melissa felt a faint, rapid pulse.

Gradually the gray veil lifted and Stan was aware of his daughter kneeling in the sand next to him. He was cognizant of flashing lights and strong hands applying something cold to his chest. A fuzzy figure was taking his blood pressure. He could hear Melissa talking to a man, several men. Where was Martha? He was perplexed, trying to focus but his brain was muddled. He blacked out again.

Lightning struck him, an electric shock like none he had ever experienced before, stronger than the painful one he had received while trying to fix an electric outlet in the boathouse years ago. He grabbed at someone's arm and opened his eyes. Melissa's face filled his hazy vision: she was moving her lips, saying something, but he could barely hear her. "Dad, squeeze my fingers!" He felt them in his right hand and squeezed, weakly at first, then more firmly as the haziness lifted from his brain.

"Whaa, what, what happened," Stan asked his daughter. She was surrounded by people, three of whom wore the uniform of paramedics.

"You blacked out, Dad. We're taking you to the hospital."

Dr. Hein Wellens was born in The Hague, Netherlands, in 1935. He became a member of a storied group of Dutch physicians and scientists whose founding father was Dr. Dirk Durrer, one of the true giants of cardiology. Durrer was a big thinker, and his fertile mind and limitless enthusiasm generated more knowledge about the electrical properties of the heart than any of his predecessors.

Wellens was of the same ilk. Working together—Durrer encouraged teamwork—Wellens and Durrer and their colleagues sparked a revolution in cardiology by showing how rapid heart beats—tachycardias—could be started and stopped by tiny electrical pulses that were delivered to the heart in a precise sequence. The method of delivering these electrical pulses is called *programmed electrical stimulation* or PES.

Without PES, the modern understanding and treatment of heart rhythm disorders would not exist. Like coronary angiography, echocardiography, and the heart-lung machine, programmed electrical stimulation was a foundational methodology: it allowed investigators to study tachycardias and understand their mechanisms—how they work. Once mechanisms were understood, successful treatments followed. Dr. Katsiyiannis used PES to start and stop Ansel Morgan's tachycardia. PES allowed Katsiyiannis to locate the slow pathway and ablate it.

Around 1970 Wellens began to apply programmed electrical stimulation to patients who were suffering from ventricular tachycardia (VT), a rapid, dangerous, often lethal rhythm. Up to this time, no one had dared to deliberately initiate—start—ventricular tachycardia in a patient. Ventricular tachycardia was ominous, frightening, and nothing caused more anxiety than to see a patient in rapid ventricular tachycardia: it was like smelling thick acrid smoke in your home in the middle of the night, or watching your child standing in the center of a busy highway at rush hour.

Why in God's name would anyone ever want to start ventricular tachycardia in a patient? The answer is another question: how else are you going to understand it and figure out how to treat it? Ventricular tachycardia was killing or disabling thousands of patients every year—together with ventricular fibrillation, it was a major cause of sudden cardiac death. In 1970, drug therapy for ventricular tachycardia was hit or miss, and the implantable defibrillator existed only in the brain of Michel Mirowski and would not be available for another 15 years.

By 1971 Wellens and Durrer had studied five patients who had had multiple episodes of ventricular tachycardia. Each of these studies took place in the catheterization laboratory at the University of Amsterdam where Wellens inserted four catheters into the right side of their hearts. With three of the catheters he recorded signals from inside their hearts and the fourth catheter was used to stimulate the ventricles with small, 10-volt electrical pulses. First, he stimulated the ventricles, overriding the patient's sinus rhythm, at 100 beats per minute. This stimulus was called "S1". Then he introduced a second stimulus, called "S2". S2 would follow S1 by a shorter interval of time, in effect producing a premature or early ventricular beat. Wellens continued to shorten the interval between S1 and S2 until he triggered ventricular tachycardia. In effect, the S1-S2 stimuli found a vulnerable spot in the heart's electrical cycle and initiated—jump-started—the tachycardia.

After starting these ventricular tachycardias, Wellens stopped them by delivering another premature electrical stimulus. So stimulating the heart, with precisely timed pulses, both induced and then terminated ventricular tachycardia in all five patients. Importantly, none of the patients suffered a complication.

In 1971 Wellens and Durrer submitted a manuscript describing their findings to *Circulation*, the journal of the American Heart Association. The journal's reviewers were very critical, stating that the study was unethical, that deliberately causing ventricular tachycardia in patients was far too hazardous, and that the manuscript should not be published. Fortunately, Dr. Howard Burchell, who knew Durrer and Wellens, was the former editor of *Circulation*; he rescued the manuscript from rejection, and it was published in the journal in the summer of 1972.

The research published by Wellens and Durrer would prove to have momentous consequences. Dr. Mark Josephson, who in 1972 was a young cardiac electrophysiologist, later said, "This article had perhaps the greatest impact on my career than any article written before or after.... Despite the anxiety of others, I was reassured that programmed stimulation of the ventricles in patients with ventricular tachycardia, was not only safe, but a potent tool to understand the pathophysiologic basis for ventricular tachyarrhythmias, and develop successful therapy for them".

The doctor in the Grand Turk emergency room confirmed what Melissa suspected: it was ventricular tachycardia that caused her father's cardiac arrest. The EKG from the external defibrillator had recorded the fast rhythm before the paramedics shocked him. Each tachycardia beat was the same shape, i.e. monomorphic, meaning that the rapid heartbeats were most likely coming from a single spot in the ventricle.

The emergency room was equipped with a SonoSite™ handheld ultrasound instrument that the doctor used to perform an echocardiogram. Stan's left ventricle was enlarged, his ejection fraction was low—25 to 30 percent, and one region of muscle on the underside of his heart did not seem to move at all. Stanley Hildebrandt probably had an ischemic cardiomyopathy due to coronary artery disease. A heart attack in the past left him with scar tissue, a potentially fertile ground for ventricular tachycardia.

Martha Hildebrandt remained in the waiting room where she could use her cell phone. She succeeded in getting through to her internist in Minneapolis. Dr. Jason Reid listened to Martha's description of the event and asked to speak with the emergency room doctor. Reid had never seen Stan professionally but he had met him when Martha was hospitalized briefly with pneumonia the previous summer. The two physicians agreed that Stan should be evacuated to the United States as soon as his condition was stable.

Five days later I met the Hildebrandts on Station 5200, the cardiology floor at Abbott Northwestern Hospital where Melissa was scheduled to begin her nursing career in three weeks. Stan had spent two nights at the 10-bed National Hospital on Grand Turk. Then he was transported to Minneapolis in an air ambulance that refueled and passed through immigration in Fort Lauderdale. Martha and Melissa accompanied him.

Stan had had no further episodes of ventricular tachycardia. He was feeling "great" and wondered why he needed to be in the hospital. I had met Stan some years previously at a social event. He was distinguished, one of those men who looked the part he played in real life, and he had the intellect and personal appeal to go along with his appearance. He was the total package, and soon his private room on 5200 was filled with friends and business associates.

I knocked and entered. "Is there room in here for a doctor?" I joked. Stan smiled and extended his hand and introduced me to Martha and Melissa. One of the visitors said, "Stan, we'll get out of here and let the doctor do his thing." He hugged Martha and Melissa and ushered the others out.

I reviewed Stan's history and the details of the recent episode. Melissa was an astute observer and filled in details not present in the records that accompanied him from the hospital on Grand Turk. The most important document was the EKG taken at the time of Stan's cardiac arrest. It showed a monomorphic ventricular tachycardia at a rate just over 200 beats per minute. The EKGs and blood tests at Grand Turk showed no evidence of an acute heart attack.

"You are going to have a busy twenty-four hours," I said after examining Stan. "You will have an echocardiogram here in your room, and after that you will be seen be seen by one of our electrophysiologists…"

"What's an electrophysiologist?" he interrupted.

"A cardiologist who specializes in heart rhythms," I replied. Then I continued, "Tomorrow, we have you scheduled for a coronary angiogram. I explained the procedure, and said, "If we find a blockage or blockages that should be treated with a stent, we will go ahead and do it right away." I paused.

Stan Asked, "Doctor Hauser, what in your opinion is going on with me?"

"You may have had a heart attack in the past. We will know more after the echocardiogram, but your main pump—the left ventricle—appears to be weak based on the report from Grand Turk. Scar tissue could be responsible for the ventricular tachycardia—that is, the rapid rhythm. If you have coronary artery disease, a stent or bypass surgery may be the next step.

"Will he need to have an implantable defibrillator?" Melissa asked.

I replied, "I think so, but that will be up to the electrophysiologist."

The echocardiogram was completed that afternoon. I reviewed it with Dr. Dick Nelson. Stan's left ventricle was mildly enlarged but the left ventricular ejection fraction was lower than reported from Grand Turk. It was 20-25 percent. The lower portion and side of the left ventricle was not moving, indicating these areas could be scar, due to one or several heart attacks.

So Stan Hildebrandt did have a heart attack in the past. Of all heart attacks, about 25 percent are unrecognized at the time and therefore untreated; they are diagnosed only when the patient sees a doctor and has an EKG or echocardiogram that shows an old heart attack. Approximately half of these unrecognized heart attacks are truly silent, meaning that the patient has no suspicious symptoms. The other half of unrecognized heart attacks are heralded by symptoms that are not "typical" of a heart attack or heart pain; these may be heartburn or unusual fatigue, and they occur more often in women and older men. Stan was an outlier, a member of a group of patients who have coronary artery disease that remains silent until a catastrophic event like sudden cardiac arrest or acute heart failure and shock.

Dr. Adrian Almquist, an electrophysiologist, evaluated Stan late in the afternoon. Because Stan had suffered an out of hospital cardiac arrest due to ventricular tachycardia, he recommended that a defibrillator be implanted prior to discharge from the hospital. This was "secondary prevention," meaning that Stan had had an episode of sudden cardiac death, had been resuscitated, and was at high risk for another episode. The next time he may be alone, or asleep, or in a situation where he could not be saved. This is the essential benefit of having an implantable defibrillator: it monitors the heart rhythm 24 hours a day, and can terminate ventricular tachycardia or ventricular fibrillation promptly.

The coronary angiogram revealed that one of Stan's coronary arteries, the circumflex, which supplied blood to the left and underside of his heart, was totally blocked. This total blockage was not unexpected. We were somewhat surprised to find that the left anterior descending and right coronary arteries each had an 80-90 percent blockage—plaque build up—near their origins from the aorta. These were severe proximal narrowings—stenoses—that were limiting blood flow and depriving his heart muscle of oxygen, particularly during activity. Wes Pedersen placed drug eluting stents in both of them. When Pedersen was done, the arteries were wide open.

Stanley Hildebrandt had a common cardiac condition: ischemic cardiomyopathy, the consequence of coronary artery disease affecting all three of his principal arteries. The scar tissue, the myocardial infarction, was affecting his left ventricle in several ways. First, the scar had caused the ventricle to reshape, or remodel itself around the scar; this remodeling process adversely affected its pumping performance by increasing its size, reshaping it like a basketball, and reducing the ejection fraction. We would treat Stan with triple drug therapy in order to minimize—and hopefully reverse—some of this remodeling. These generic drugs would include an angiotensin converting enzyme inhibitor or ACE (lisinopril), a novel beta-blocker (carvedilol), and an aldosterone antagonist (spironolactone).

The other consequence of the scar was ventricular tachycardia, the rhythm that could have killed him on Grand Turk, and was a present danger. Stan had had no further episodes of ventricular tachycardia during the 10 days he had been hospitalized. This was reassuring, but he was still at high risk for sudden cardiac death.

Two days after his stents were inserted, he underwent implantation of a Medtronic dual chamber implantable cardioverter-defibrillator (ICD) by Dr. Chuck Gornick, a veteran electrophysiologist and head of the department. Gornick placed a pacing lead wire in Stan's right atrium and a high voltage wire in his right ventricle; both wires were inserted through the left subclavian vein. He connected them to a multi-function ICD that was placed under the skin, below the left collarbone.

The ICD consisted of a sophisticated electronic circuit and a lithium battery that were sealed in an oval titanium metal can. Unlike the original implantable defibrillator developed by Michel Mirowski, this ICD was a modern pacemaker as well as a defibrillator. It monitored Stan's rhythm and paced his heart if the rate was too slow, coordinating the beats in the atrium and ventricle. If ventricular fibrillation occurred, the ICD would deliver a defibrillating shock via the lead in the right ventricle.

For ventricular tachycardia, the ICD would first try to terminate it with rapid pacing pulses, also sent through the right ventricular lead. Hein Wellens had shown that critically timed pacing pulses could stop certain types of ventricular tachycardias. Unlike a shock, pacing pulses are painless because they are low energy, five to ten volts. If the pacing pulses failed to stop the ventricular tachycardia, the ICD would charge its capacitors and terminate the arrhythmia with a high-voltage shock.

Stan's ICD was a medical and technological marvel, evolved over decades of scientific research and engineering innovation, and requiring hundreds of millions of dollars of investment and multiple clinical trials. His ICD cost $40,000 and would last about six years, until the battery depleted, requiring replacement.

The morning after the surgery, Linda Retel, a specialist from the Minneapolis Heart Institute, came to Stan's hospital room with a Medtronic programmer. This was an instrument that could communicate with his ICD through the skin. She placed a circular wand over the ICD. The wand had a coil antenna that sent coded radiofrequency signals to the ICD that was encapsulated in tissue below Stan's left collarbone. These signals commanded the ICD to disclose the rhythms Stan had had during the previous 12 hours; they were stored in the ICDs electronic memory. A few seconds later the ICD sent signals back to the programmer, which printed a report containing the ICD's diagnostic data.

The report said that Stan had had a normal rhythm during the night, he had no episodes of ventricular tachycardia, and that he had not needed neither pacing nor a shock. The report also noted that the ICD's battery was at 100 percent capacity, and that the electrical resistances in the lead wires were normal. At the end of the report was an EKG recorded by the two leads inside Stan's heart: the P-wave and QRS were normal in size and shape.

When I entered Stan's room, Martha was sitting on the built-in sofa bed by the window where she had slept during the night. "Good morning," I said. "Hope you got some sleep last night."

Martha said, "It certainly is a busy place. There was some kind of emergency down the hall around three o'clock this morning."

"I didn't hear a thing," Stan remarked. "I slept through the night until they woke me up around seven to draw blood."

"I just saw Linda at the nurse's station," I said. Your ICD looks good. I think you are ready to go home."

"Thank God," Stan exclaimed. "I can sleep in my own bed tonight!" He gave me two thumbs up.

Martha stood and walked toward the bed. "Are you sure, Doctor Hauser. Isn't it too soon?"

"He'll recover faster at home. There is no reason why he needs to be in this place." I smiled and turned to Stan. "Anne Hendrickson will go over your medications. I want to see you next week in the clinic for a check-up and blood tests. Meanwhile, I want you to relax around home, stay away from the office, and don't drive the car. Dr. Gornick or Dr. Almquist will decide when you can drive again."

Martha looked at Stan and back to me. "He may get upset with this question, but my husband is quite amorous, if you know what I mean…"

"Sex is okay," I broke in, "Just take it easy at first. You understand." Martha nodded.

Stan acted as though he did not hear this exchange. He cleared his throat. "We sure have had good care here."

In 1980, Dr. Marc Josephson and a cardiac surgeon, Dr. Alden Harken, developed a procedure subsequently tagged the "Pennsylvania Peel," a graphic reference to the novel surgical technique they performed in Philadelphia. The goal was to remove—cut away—the scar tissue responsible for causing ventricular tachycardia. This was surgical ablation, akin to the one Will Sealy had done on his fisherman with WPW syndrome in 1968. Only the ventricular tachycardia ablation involved far more tissue, and therefore was more extensive. In addition, the patients were much sicker with weak hearts and multiple chronic medical problems. The Pennsylvania Peel, technically called endocardial resection, was often a last resort to silence debilitating ventricular tachycardias.

Radiofrequency ablation of ventricular tachycardia became feasible as electrophysiologists learned more about this elusive arrhythmia. Once again, understanding mechanisms—how the arrhythmia worked—was critical. Unlike most other tachycardias, ventricular tachycardias come in many sizes and shapes, and they behave differently from patient to patient and even in the same patient. Also ventricular tachycardia can cripple the heart's pumping function, resulting in circulatory collapse and shock. This limits the time available for the electrophysiologist to locate and ablate the tachycardia.

Despite these obstacles, electrophysiologists made steady progress, catalyzed by the development of sophisticated computerized mapping systems that created 3-D color pictures of ventricular tachycardias as their electrical waves passed around and through the heart. These maps could pinpoint the tissue producing the tachycardia, as well as the paths within the heart that the tachycardia used to maintain itself. Once the pathways in the heart were located, the electrophysiologist could guide a radiofrequency catheter to these spots and burn the tissue.

I saw Stan in clinic eight days after he was discharged from the hospital. He was regaining his strength after weeks of inactivity. His blood pressure was where I wanted it. The incision over his ICD was healing nicely. I listened to his lungs and heart: no concerns. I removed the stethoscope from my ears and sat down at the little desk in the exam room and began perusing his chart on the computer. I asked routine questions, as I clicked through his hospital records, reviewing his blood tests and EKGs.

"You haven't had any racing. But have you noticed any skipping, any irregularities?"

"Now that you mention it," Stan replied, "I had something after dinner yesterday. I felt a very brief pounding. It lasted only a few seconds, then it stopped. Happened again around 10 p.m. But not since. It was so trivial I didn't think to tell you."

"We'll find out what it was. We'll interrogate the defibrillator. Wait here. Linda

Retel—you met her in the hospital—will bring the Medtronic programmer in and upload the data."

About 20 minutes later Retel showed me a printout from the programmer. She had interrogated Stan's ICD, which had stored the two episodes he felt the previous day, and one additional episode from the past week that apparently did not cause symptoms. These episodes were brief runs of ventricular tachycardia that were correctly identified by the ICD, which appropriately stopped them with brief bursts of pacing pulses. This is called *antitachycardia pacing*, and it evolved out of the groundbreaking work by Wellens, Josephson and others, who in the 1970s showed that pacing could not only start ventricular tachycardia but also stop it. Antitachycardia pacing was a neat, painless way to terminate tachycardia without resorting to a shock.

I went to the exam room and explained the findings to Stan. "Your ICD is doing its job. What you felt last night after dinner was ventricular tachycardia—the same rhythm you had on Grand Turk. Only this time the ICD quickly recognized it and stopped it with pacing. It happened again, around 10 p.m. You also had one other episode last week that you must not have been aware of."

"Does this mean I'm getting worse?", Stan asked.

"No, you are not getting worse. This is the same rhythm you had on Grand Turk. I'm going to increase the dosage of your beta-blocker—that's the carvedilol, and also the lisinopril. I want you to see the electrophysiologist in the clinic soon. He will decide what, if anything, needs to be done about the tachycardia."

"What might be needed," Stan asked.

"The options, "I replied, "are to maximize the medications we are giving you and continue to monitor you closely." I paused. "So option number one may be to wait and watch and do nothing more, unless the tachycardia becomes more frequent or causes symptoms. The second option is to add a drug to suppress the ventricular tachycardia. These drugs are potent and they can cause side effects. Option number three is to go into your heart with a catheter, find the area causing the tachycardia and try to eliminate it with a technique called ablation. Basically, the tissue is burned, and hopefully the tachycardia is gone."

Stan touched his chin and said, "I like option three—you said ablation?" I nodded. "Why not get rid of it and be done?"

"It's great when it works, but there are risks, and it is possible to actually make the rhythm worse or create a new one. I'll defer to the electrophysiologist."

We gave Stan a monitor he could use at home to send data over the telephone to a Medtronic computer that, in turn, would send the information to our clinic. During the next month he had three episodes of ventricular tachycardia that the implantable defibrillator quickly terminated with pacing pulses. Two of the three episodes occurred while he was sleeping, and the third caused no symptoms. He saw Adrian Almquist in the clinic and it was decided to continue monitoring and not pursue ablation or any drug therapy as long as the tachycardia was infrequent and not troublesome.

Four months later, in late August, I was seeing patients in the hospital when my iPhone rang. It was our emergency room. Stan had been brought in by ambulance from his home after receiving a shock from his ICD. I took the service elevator down to the first floor and walked into exam room #14 where Linda Retel was already interrogating Stan's defibrillator with the Medtronic programmer.

When Stan saw me, he exclaimed "Holy Christ this thing hurts! It knocked me out of my chair!"

I frowned, remembering the time when I was accidentally shocked by an external defibrillator while resuscitating an elderly patient after heart surgery. I said, "I know. I'm sorry. We'll see in a minute what happened." I looked at Retel typing commands into the programmer, which printed out a long report, including EKGs showing Stan's rhythms before and after the shock.

The problem was immediately apparent: Stan had an episode of ventricular tachycardia that was correctly identified by the defibrillator. It tried to stop the tachycardia with a burst of rapid pacing pulses. This had worked multiple times before. But this morning, instead of stopping the tachycardia, the pacing pulses, for some reason, made it go faster. In other words, rapid pacing accelerated the tachycardia, to over 220 beats a minute. When the defibrillator detected this very fast and potentially lethal ventricular tachycardia, it charged up its capacitors and shocked Stan with over a thousand volts, restoring a normal rhythm and probably saving his life.

The defibrillator had performed perfectly. We had long known that pacing could accelerate ventricular tachycardia. This is why we had never been able to safely apply simple pacemakers for treating ventricular tachycardia. The hazard of acceleration had been made clear in clinical trials during the early 1980s. As a result, antitachycardia pacing was not used without the safety net of an ICD's high-energy shock.

I admitted Stan to the hospital. His blood tests were normal: no evidence of a heart attack or electrolyte abnormalities. A repeat echocardiogram revealed that his left ventricular function had improved and his ejection fraction was now 40 percent. This was good news: Stan was benefiting from the drugs, and the coronary stent implants that had restored blood flow to his pumping chambers.

Almquist saw Stan and reviewed the printouts from Stan's defibrillator. He had a lengthy discussion with Stan and his family. Ultimately it was agreed that he should undergo ventricular tachycardia ablation. Curing the tachycardia was the best option for several reasons. First, Stan was young and the improvement in left ventricular function suggested his prognosis for living many years was quite good. Second, shocks and rapid pacing may be life limiting, and painful shocks, however infrequent, cause anxiety and diminish a patient's sense of well being. Lastly, effective drugs, like amiodarone, have serious long-term side effects, some of which may be fatal.

However, ablation had its own set of complications. Patients had died or suffered a stroke during or after the procedure for a variety of reasons, some related to placing catheters in the heart, but also due to overly aggressive ablation, i.e. trying to do too much, burn too often, or too deeply. There is an aphorism attributed to Voltaire stating that "Perfect is the enemy of good." This wisdom applies to many procedures, including ventricular tachycardia ablation. The goal of the ablation should be to eliminate the tachycardia, the arrhythmia, that the patient has experienced, and avoid ablating tachycardias that may be seen incidentally during the procedure but have never been recorded outside the laboratory.

Always the executive, Stan asked, "Who will do this and when?"

Almquist replied, "Dr. Melby will do the ablation in the morning." Melby was a graduate of the University of Minnesota Medical School and an expert in complex catheter ablation.

At 8 a.m. the following morning Dr. Dan Melby inserted electrode catheters through the femoral vein into the right side of Stan Hildebrandt's heart. Stan had been deeply sedated and was unaware of his surroundings. The electrophysiology laboratory included high resolution X-ray equipment and large monitors displaying Stan's EKG and arterial blood pressure. Prior to the procedure Linda Retel had turned Stan's ICD off with the Medtronic programmer. Defibrillation electrodes had been applied to his chest and a Physio-Control external defibrillator would be used to deliver a rescue shock, if necessary.

Melby had studied the EKGs that had been recorded in Grand Turk while Stan was in ventricular tachycardia. They indicated that the tachycardia was originating from the left ventricle in the region of the scar tissue on the underside of his heart. This scar had been delineated by the cardiac MRI that been obtained prior to implantation of Stan's ICD. Melby had reviewed the MRI with Dr. John Lesser the previous afternoon.

Just as Wellens had done 40 years earlier, Melby started Stan's ventricular tachycardia (VT) by pacing the right ventricle and delivering extra, premature pacing pulses in deliberate, programmed sequences. Three premature pacing pulses were required to start the VT. Within a minute this fast VT—nearly 220 beats per minute—caused Stan's blood pressure to drop precipitously.

"Shock him", Melby commanded.

The nurse standing by the external defibrillator triggered a shock that converted the VT to normal sinus rhythm.

Stan had "unstable ventricular tachycardia", namely VT that promptly caused his blood pressure to plummet and, if untreated, would lead to death within minutes. This instability meant that Melby would not have time to map the left ventricle during VT and locate tissue that he could burn with the ablation catheter. Without a specific target, Melby could destroy good tissue, cause irreversible damage, and miss the area responsible for the tachycardia.

There was an alternative, a complex method that had been evolved during decades of research and technology development. It involved pacing the left ventricle and finding a spot where pacing produced a QRS—a heartbeat on the EKG—that looked like the QRS of Stan's ventricular tachycardia. If found, such a spot should be close to the tissue causing the tachycardia.

Melby could then use a sophisticated electrical mapping system, called Carto, that would create a topographical picture, a color map, of the spot in the left ventricle where the tachycardia lived. The colors would signify the amount of voltage produced by the tissue; very low voltages that were typical of scar tissue would produce hues of red, yellow, and green, while high voltages, characteristic of normal heart muscle, would be represented in blue and purple.

The map would be displayed on a high definition video screen so that Melby could identify the few millimeters that may be causing or propagating the ventricular tachycardia. This would be the target, and he could guide the catheter to this spot and burn it. It would be tedious and time-consuming and the success rate would be about 75 percent. But the overall risk was low, and the potential benefit was worth the effort.

Melby stood by the X-ray table where Stan was sedated and covered by light blue surgical drapes. The catheter he used to pace the inside of Stan's left ventricle was steerable, and the Carto 3-D mapping system allowed him to precisely navigate the catheter tip from one spot to another. It took 40 minutes but he found the location where the QRS he stimulated with the catheter looked just like the QRS of the ventricular tachycardia recorded by the paramedics on Grand Turk island. This was the "fingerprint" of Stan's ventricular tachycardia.

Very precisely, Melby began to pace and record signals. The goal was to find the longest time between the electrical stimulus and the QRS. This would identify the tissue that was sustaining the tachycardia. Electrophysiologists called this zone the "isthmus" because it was a narrow channel of living tissue surrounded by scar. Over the next hour and a half the meticulous process of moving the catheter, recording signals, and constructing the 3-D map evolved until the boundaries of the isthmus were clearly delineated. Using the radiofrequency catheter, Melby created two parallel burns in the tissue of the isthmus, interrupting it so that no signal could cross it and re-enter the tachycardia's circuit. The endless loop that was essential to maintaining the ventricular tachycardia was interrupted. It was like digging a deep ditch across the oval track of the Indianapolis 500: the tachycardia's beats, like the racecars, had nowhere to go and came to an abrupt halt when they encountered the charred tissue.

The procedure was not over. Melby had to show that he could no longer electrically induce—start—the tachycardia. Using the same sequence of three pacing pulses that had originally triggered Stan's VT, Melby was unable to start the tachycardia, despite multiple attempts. Satisfied, he removed the catheters from Stan's heart. The ablation was complete.

Stanley Hildebrandt was one of the last patients I cared for at Abbott Northwestern Hospital. He had no further episodes of ventricular tachycardia or shocks from his ICD. Instead of building a home on Grand Turk, Stan and Martha bought a condominium in Florida. Their daughter, Melissa, became a nurse practitioner, married, and lives with her husband on a cattle ranch in Wyoming.

It was 2014 and I was on the glide path to retirement. I decided to confine my practice to our clinics in Minneapolis and around the state. At the age of 75 I found great satisfaction in seeing patients and their families whom I had known for many years. There was one particular patient from Chicago who I had never expected to see again. His name was Harold Swanson.

CHAPTER 23

Early one morning in the late summer of 2014 I drove to Olivia, Minnesota, to see patients in the Renville County Hospital cardiology clinic. There was no road construction or detours, so I made good time on U.S Route 212 as it meandered west through lush farm country. The tall fields of corn promised a healthy harvest, and several farms were baling their second or third cuts of hay. Occasionally a massive green John Deere tractor would swing onto the road ahead of me as it darted from one field to another. Otherwise the only pause in my journey was the single traffic light in Bird Island, a quiet town just east of Olivia.

As I drove into the outskirts of Olivia I could see the construction site for the new hospital on the south side of 212. The old Renville County Hospital, which had been built after World War II, was an antique. But the doctors and nurses were top notch and dedicated. Many of them had grown up in Renville County, or nearby, and they shared a culture of kindness and compassion and loyalty to their community.

I parked my car and walked into the front entrance of the hospital. There on the wall was a picture of Dr. James Arthur Cosgriff, Jr. "Doctor Jim," as he was known to patients and friends, was a remarkable physician who dedicated his life and career to the sick. He was born near Olivia in 1924, and graduated with honors from the University of Minnesota Medical School in 1946. A scholar, Doctor Jim could have entered any field of medicine he chose. Instead, after serving in the Navy, he returned to Olivia where he practiced with his physician father who had moved to Olivia in 1929 from Mankato in southern Minnesota. They made house calls, delivered babies, and staffed both their clinic in Olivia and the then-new Renville County Hospital. The younger Cosgriff gained a reputation as an astute diagnostician.

Whenever Dr. Jim asked me to see one of his patients, he would always dictate a letter, describing the patient's medical history and specifying the problems he wanted me to address. He also anticipated the tests I might need, and those results were also available at the time I evaluated his patients. Every caregiver should aspire to such discipline and attention to detail.

A year before his death in 2009, Dr. Cosgriff was asked, "What do you see as the greatest change to health care since you became a doctor?" He replied, "The diminution of the private physician-patient relationship." He added, "Society has substituted third-party intervention and control [Medicare, private insurers] for the practice of medicine, so that it becomes more difficult for a doctor and his patient to decide what is best for the patient." My great uncle, Dr. Charles Hauser, who began his practice in 1899, would have agreed wholeheartedly with Dr. Jim.

I sat at the desk in the clinic and looked over the printed schedule. The first patient sounded familiar: his name was Harold Swanson. How many Swansons had I met in Minnesota during the past 27 years? Well, this is another one, I thought. So I opened the door to the exam room. Immediately an elderly gentleman stood and extended his hand, "Hello, Doctor Hauser," he said, "I'll bet you don't remember me."

I smiled but did not reply right away. The hand I held in mine was soft, unlike the calloused farmers' hands I was used to in this part of the country. He was bald with fair skin and green eyes behind bifocal lenses that were set in dark blue designer frames. His tan wool slacks were creased, and he wore an open collar pale yellow silk shirt, probably from Tommy Bahama. Sitting next to him was a thin woman with short thick silver hair. She was fashionably attired, and I guessed she had at least a four-carat diamond wedding ring on her left hand.

"You and Doctor Messer and Doctor Ruggie took care of me in Chicago in the mid-1980s," Harold exclaimed. "And you were the intern when Najafi did my bypass in 1969!"

I shook my head, "My goodness," I said, "what a coincidence, and this is your wife. How do you do, Mrs. Swanson." She took my hand. "I'm Jean," she said.

After I sat down in the large exam room, Harold asked, "Doctor Hauser, how did you come to Minnesota from Chicago?"

I replied, "In 1987 I was recruited by Eli Lilly to be an executive in their pacemaker division in St. Paul, and help them develop the implantable defibrillator.

I did that for six years and then joined the Minneapolis Heart Institute fulltime in 1992. Since then I've been coming to Olivia about once a month." I paused, looked over at Jean, turned back to Harold, and said, "I'll ask you the same question… Why are you in Olivia?"

Jean uncrossed her legs and leaned forward. "I grew up here. Our families have been farming south of Olivia since 1892. Over five hundred acres altogether. We come back every summer and stay in the old farm house my grandfather built." She beamed, "I don't really do any of the farming anymore, but I can still drive the tractor—and change the oil!"

Harold continued, "We spend most of our time in Lake Forest, in Illinois, and winter in Arizona. My son is running the Swanson businesses with one of our granddaughters. It's worked out just as we hoped it would…"

I wanted to learn more about the Swansons but, regrettably, I had a schedule to keep. A new patient every 30 minutes; that was the drill. I asked Harold, "What brings you into the clinic today?"

"We were having dinner at my cousin's farm last week when he mentioned that he has been seeing a cardiologist, a Dr. Hauser, at the Renville clinic. I checked, and found out it was you. I couldn't believe the coincidence." Harold shook his head, and continued, "Anyway, I have an abdominal aneurysm that my internist in Lake Forest has been following. I saw a vascular surgeon in Chicago last May. He said the aneurysm was approaching a size—I think it's about five centimeters—where it should be repaired. But it wasn't quite there yet. He warned me that if I had any pain in my back or abdomen that I should see a doctor right away. Well, last week I started to have some back pain and it's still there. So here I am."

I went through Harold's history, and reviewed his medications. He was taking aspirin, Prinivil® (ACE inhibitor), Lopressor® (beta-blocker), and Viagra® (more power to him). His very high cholesterol had responded well to the 40 milligrams of Crestor® he took daily. He was having no angina or shortness of breath. In fact, he had no heart symptoms since his angioplasty 20 years previously. A nuclear stress test earlier in the year was normal. It was quite remarkable, considering that he had symptomatic premature coronary artery disease when he was 38-years-old.

I examined Harold. His blood pressure was slightly elevated and his rhythm was regular. I heard a modest murmur over his aortic valve, but the valve's closure sound was crisp, suggesting that the valve was probably okay. His breath sounds were normal. Then I placed my hand lightly on his abdomen: the aorta was enlarged, no doubt due to an aneurysm. It was pointless and somewhat risky to probe further. I had all the information I needed.

Sitting next to Harold on the exam table, I said, "You're not going to be happy with what I am about to tell you…"

Jean jumped in, "He has to come into the hospital?"

I turned to Harold and said," I'm concerned your aneurysm could be leaking. In all likelihood you will need surgery, and soon. So my recommendation is that we send you by ambulance to Abbott Northwestern Hospital in Minneapolis. I'll call ahead and have a surgeon see you right away."

"Why an ambulance?" she asked

"It's safer and faster," I replied in a firm tone that discouraged discussion.

Harold said, "Whatever you say, Doctor Hauser. I want to hang around a while."

Before Harold left in the ambulance I called the vascular surgery office at the Minneapolis Heart Institute and asked for the on-call surgeon. It was Dr. Tim Sullivan. I summarized Harold's situation and heart history, and said we would send an EKG and blood test results along with the patient. Sullivan replied that he would get an emergency CT angiogram of Harold's aorta and leg arteries before deciding what procedure to perform.

There were two surgical options for Harold. One was the traditional open repair where the surgeon exposes the aortic aneurysm through an incision in the abdominal wall, cuts the aorta above and below the aneurysm, and sews in a graft made of Dacron™ or a similar woven material. This procedure, described in chapter one of this book, is often the choice when a patient is unstable or in shock. This was not the case with Harold.

The second option was an endovascular stent graft that the surgeon inserts into the aorta without opening the abdomen. The graft is mounted on a flexible metal frame and it is deployed in the aorta through two small skin incisions over the femoral arteries in the groin. This less invasive second option was the lowest risk, especially in elderly patients who had heart problems like Harold Swanson.

Tim Sullivan grew up in Ohio and trained in vascular surgery at the Cleveland Clinic before joining the Mayo Clinic, where he was the director of the endovascular surgery program. He became head of the vascular and endovascular surgery department at the Minneapolis Heart Institute in 2007. Given Harold's heart history, I was pleased that Sullivan, a pioneer and expert in endovascular repair, would be managing his care.

After Harold arrived at Abbott Northwestern Hospital, he underwent a high-resolution CT angiogram of his abdominal aorta and leg arteries. Sullivan reviewed the images with Dr. John Lesser. They revealed a large six-centimeter aortic aneurysm that was leaking blood, causing swelling and pressure against Harold's spine. The aneurysm began just below the arteries to the kidneys (renal arteries) and ended before the aorta branched into the two iliac and femoral arteries that supplied blood to his legs and pelvis. Except for the aneurysm, there was no other important vascular disease.

Harold was taken to the third floor of the Heart Hospital and placed on a table in the hybrid operating room. This large room was designed and equipped to serve as both an operating room and a catheterization laboratory, so that procedures requiring X-ray visualization and major surgery could be performed in one place under sterile conditions. Sullivan was one of the room's designers; it had advanced imaging devices that were particularly useful for endovascular surgery, the type of procedure Harold was about to undergo.

An anesthesiologist sedated Harold and inserted an endotracheal tube in his windpipe. Sullivan made a half-inch incision over each femoral artery. He then inserted a needle and guidewire through the right femoral artery and, using fluoroscopy, moved the guidewire up the aorta until its tip could be seen well above the renal arteries.

Next he took a Medtronic Endurant II™ endovascular stent graft from the scrub nurse and inserted it over the guidewire into the right femoral artery and up the aorta above the renal arteries. The endovascular stent graft had a tubular metal frame made of nitinol (nickel titanium) which had shape memory at different temperatures. This shape memory allowed the metal frame to expand in the aorta at body temperature. High-density polyester fabric covered the metal frame. The frame was wrapped around a plastic rod that served as an insertion tool. At the tip of the graft was an uncovered, bare metal stent with tiny barbs that would anchor the graft to the inner wall of the aorta.

Using fluoroscopy, Sullivan rotated the stent graft within the abdominal aorta, unfurling it from the rod of the insertion tool, and deploying it in the lumen of the aneurysm. The graft was shaped like an upside-down 'Y' so that the lower, larger limb was in the aorta, and the two smaller limbs were in the left and right iliac and femoral arteries. After precisely adjusting the graft to the aorta's anatomic landmarks, including the aneurysm, Sullivan inserted a large, radiopaque balloon and expanded it, driving the stent and nitinol frame into the walls of the aorta and the iliac and femoral arteries.

The procedure was complete. Blood flowed through the stent graft from the aorta in the chest and upper abdomen to the arteries in the legs and pelvis. Thus the aneurysm was excluded from the circulation and eventually, with time, it would collapse into a harmless mass of scar tissue. The procedure took exactly 93 minutes, and soon Harold was awake in the post-anesthesia recovery room.

The day after Harold's surgery I went to his room on Station 5200. The room was empty, so I asked his nurse where he might be. She said he and his wife were sitting in the solarium overlooking the front entrance of Abbott Northwestern Hospital.

I found them sitting on a couch, holding hands. It was a familiar, often poignant sight: elderly couples touching, sharing quiet moments in the hospital, not knowing if one of them may be alone soon. I filed these pictures in my subconscious, snapshots of everyday people savoring precious moments. Somehow it was comforting, a counterweight to a world continuously in turmoil.

Jean Swanson saw me first. "This is an excellent hospital," she said as I sat down next to Harold. "The nurses are just wonderful!"

I smiled, and said, "I couldn't agree more." Turning to Harold, I continued, "Doctor Sullivan told me the surgery went very well, and you should be ready to go home in the next few days. How do you feel?"

Harold could hardly control his enthusiasm. "I went online this morning and found a lot of information about the surgery I just had. Amazing. Fewer complications. Shorter hospitalizations. The other way must be hard on patients, especially for guys like me."

"It's a terrific technology," I said. "It took twenty years to get the stent graft to this point. Actually, Doctor Sullivan helped develop it. You're right, it is much less invasive and that fact usually means fewer complications, and fewer deaths related to the surgery. You were fortunate because your aneurysm and aorta were perfect for this kind of graft."

I changed subjects. "Harold, you have a heart murmur. It is probably coming from your aortic valve, the valve that leads out of you heart. You're not having any symptoms, but I think it would be a good idea if you had an echocardiogram. You can have it done here or back in Chicago."

Harold asked, "When do you think I'll be going home?"

"That's up to Doctor Sullivan," I replied," but probably in the next day or two."

"Then I might as well have it here," Howard said.

The echocardiogram was completed that afternoon. Harold's aortic valve was scarred and somewhat calcified, but the leaflets moved fairly well and there was only mild stenosis. The left ventricle was in pretty good shape, although the muscle supplied by the right coronary bypass graft did not move very well. The bypass had probably closed many years ago. Altogether I was happy with the result and said so to Harold and Jean. I thought he should have another echocardiogram in a year. I told them to stop by the clinic next summer if they were visiting Olivia.

Harold said, "I like seeing you but I hope I never have to see you professionally again." Having heard this many times before, my ready reply was, "Then let's make it a social visit."

I saw Harold in the summer of 2015. He and Jean stopped by my cardiology clinic in Renville County Hospital to say hello. They had just celebrated Harold's 85th birthday at the Novak's farm south of Olivia. Unlike his father and uncles, Harold Swanson had the good fortune to live in an era when the major advances in the treatment of coronary artery and vascular disease became available.

In fact, I too was a big beneficiary. It is time to tell my story

CHAPTER 24

In the summer of 2004 I was training hard for the Lifetime Fitness triathlon in Minneapolis. I had placed first in my age group in 2002 (the other old guy fell off his bike), but barely finished in 2003. I was determined to reclaim the top spot or at least equal my best time. Every day after working in the hospital I would swim or bike or run. On the weekends I would do all three, a "mini" triathlon, if you will.

On this day, I was running around Long Lake near my home west of Minneapolis when suddenly I felt a severe, sharp pain in the left side of my chest. I slowed to a walk. It went away after a few seconds, and I resumed running, only more slowly. After a block or so, I came to my senses and walked the remaining half-mile home. On the way, I did what doctors should never do: I analyzed my pain. What caused it? It was not typical. "Probably muscular," I assured myself. I was not short of breath, sweaty or nauseated. So I must be fine, right?

The next morning, while driving to the hospital, I remembered that a new CT scanner had been installed in our clinic in southwest Minneapolis. It was capable of imaging the coronary arteries. I called my partner, John Lesser, who was leading our CT imaging program. I told him about the brief chest pain and asked if he could scan my coronary arteries. He told me to come by that afternoon.

Around 5 p.m. that same day, I climbed into the CT scanner. The nurse inserted an intravenous catheter into a vein in my right arm. She connected it to a powered syringe that injected X-ray dye while the CT scanned my heart. I felt a warm rush as the dye circulated through my body. I could see Lesser and Bjorn Flygenring through the leaded glass window looking at the video screen while the CT whirled around my body.

Ten minutes later the nurse removed the catheter from my arm. After dressing I joined Lesser and Flygenring who were hunched over the computer screen where the CT images of my heart and aorta were displayed. Lesser looked up and said, "Your coronaries are okay but you have an ascending aortic aneurysm. There's no dissection but we should do an MRI. Also, your aortic valve may be bicuspid. Have you had an echo?"

Abruptly, unexpectedly, my life had become very complicated. At the age of 64 I had a serious genetic disease that was responsible for more deaths and complications than all other congenital heart defects combined. My aorta was deficient in fibrillin-1, a connective tissue protein, and this deficiency had gradually disrupted the muscular middle layer of my aorta, causing it to weaken and enlarge. It was like a tire with a soft spot on a hot summer day: it could rupture and blow. The only treatment was major surgery.

A few days later I had an MRI of my heart and aorta and an echocardiogram. The MRI confirmed what was found on the CT scan. The aneurysm measured 5.2 centimeters. There was no evidence of a dissection or tear on either the CT or MRI scans. The echocardiogram confirmed that I had a bicuspid aortic valve: instead of the normal three leaflets, my valve had only two. Luckily there was no evidence that the valve was narrow or leaking. The bottom line was I needed my aorta repaired. The aortic valve could wait.

I called Dr. Vib Kshettry and asked him to review my tests. A few hours later he paged me. "Bob," he said, "I reviewed the scans. We should do your surgery soon." I agreed, and said that I had a trip planned to take my two granddaughters, Hannah and Ella, to Disneyland. The surgery would be done the week after I returned. I had an ominous feeling about the surgery and wanted to spend this time with my family.

Disneyland was delightful. We stayed at one of the Disneyland hotels and did all the things that tourists do, sometimes twice, and the three days passed all too quickly. I drove my daughter, Jennifer, and the two girls from Anaheim to the Palm Springs airport. I dropped them off at the departure zone and watched them disappear into the cavernous lobby, thinking it could be the last time I would see them. How many times had I watched my patients bid good-bye to their loved ones as they disappeared into the operating room or catheterization laboratory? It was a sobering, throat-tightening moment. I took a deep breath, swallowed and exhaled slowly, erasing a flash of melancholy.

On the morning of the surgery, I drove myself to the hospital and parked in the doctors' garage. Thirty minutes later, at 7 a.m., I was in a hospital gown on a gurney. A nurse started an iv and placed EKG electrodes on my chest and abdomen, well away from the sternum where Kshettry would make the incision. Sally and my three daughters arrived and remained with me until I was carted off to the operating room. As I was being wheeled down the hall, Dr. Raj Dwarakaneth, my anesthesiologist, injected propofol into a vein. It was the last thing I remembered.

Sally and my daughters went to the crowded surgery waiting room in the basement of Abbott Northwestern Hospital where they signed in with the receptionist. Vib Kshettry appeared three hours later, still in his surgical scrubs. He took Sally and our daughters to a side room and closed the door. Sally later recalled that Kshettry looked very dour, a marked departure from his usual cheerfulness. "The blood was gone from his face," Sally said. "I knew right away that something had gone wrong."

In fact, what had happened during those three hours was brilliant surgery that saved my life. After opening my chest and exposing my heart, Kshettry placed me on the heart-lung machine to maintain my circulation while he repaired the aneurysm. When he cut through the aorta above the aortic valve, he was surprised to see a tear in the wall, a dissection that had not been visible on either the CT or MRI scans. The dissection extended upward, to the innominate artery, and was inches away from the arteries supplying blood to my brain. I was on the doorstep to a stroke, even death.

The location and extent of the damage to my aorta was such that Kshettry could not repair it while I was on the heart-lung machine. He looked a Dwarakaneth standing at the head of the operating table. "We'll repair it under circulatory arrest", he said. "Let's cool him." They gave me Solu-Medrol, a steroid, and packed me in ice, lowering my body temperature to 59 degrees Fahrenheit.

Then they stopped the heart-lung machine. My heart was not beating, so my circulation was shut down as completely as an automobile whose engine is turned off. No blood was flowing anywhere, and no oxygen was being delivered to my brain or body. I was suspended in cold hibernation, a passenger on a silent journey that could end in the hereafter or even worse, a permanent vegetative state.

The minutes ticked away as Kshettry severed the aorta on either side of the aneurysm and inserted a 32mm-Hemashield™ synthetic tube graft composed of a knitted material impregnated with collagen. He worked quickly, placing a double layer of sutures through the wall of the aorta and graft, until the graft was securely attached on either end of the aorta, and the dissected—torn—segment removed. Every second was precious if I were to have any chance of surviving with a reasonable chance of having a life worth living.

The repair was completed in 20 minutes, an eternity under the circumstances, but very short considering the complexity of the surgery that Kshettry had to perform. Minutes later I was back on the heart-lung machine and once again blood began to flow through my body. One of my young partners, Dr. Betty Grey, came into the operating room and inserted an ultrasound probe down my esophagus to assess the completeness of the repair. Everything looked good.

I was gradually rewarmed and my heart began to beat on its own. Unknowingly, I had flirted with death, and indeed had existed somewhere between the living and the departed for nearly half an hour. As Kshettry sutured my sternum back together with steel wires, he did not know if I would wake up and, if I did, walk out of the hospital. This was why he looked so distressed when he entered the waiting room to speak with my family.

I was taken from the operating room to Station 10, the surgical intensive care unit where I had spent so much time managing my own post-operative patients. Sally and my daughters were allowed to visit once my nurse was ready for them to see me. I was asleep, connected to the ventilator, and there were multiple i.v. pumps delivering fluids and drugs. Sally said I looked very peaceful, but she knew that the next 24 hours were critical.

Sometime during the night I woke up. The room was dark but I could make out the shadowy figure of my nurse as she injected something into my iv. Shortly afterward the anesthesiologist removed the tube from my trachea and I was breathing on my own. I could move my arms and legs. I knew who I was, where I was, and why I was in the hospital.

Then the drugs started playing games with my mind. I flipped out. In the morning I called my administrative assistant, Marsha Burmaster, and told her that I was going home and to bring my briefcase. I even tried to take out my iv. A neurologist was called. Perhaps I had had some kind of stroke. The neurologist, Dr.

Richard Shronts, thought it was the drugs and stopped them. Gradually I returned to my senses, aided greatly by my nurse, Edith, who closed the door to my room and refused to let any visitors in except my family. "I do not want anyone to see Dr. Hauser like this," she told Sally.

The crisis passed and I was transferred to Station 41, a regular cardiac floor. At 7 a.m. on the fourth day after surgery I attended the Monday morning cardiology conference. Later that day I convinced Kshettry that I was ready to be discharged from the hospital. Five weeks later I was back at work.

My triathlon days were over. Despite the repair, the remainder of my aorta suffered from the same inherited deficiency and it would be unwise for me to engage in sustained, vigorous exercise. The mechanical stresses were too great and the consequences—dissection and aneurysm formation—were too dire. I rebooted my exercise program, downgrading my physical activities to walking and moderate biking. Of course I also took medications to keep my blood pressure down and to blunt the forces applied to my aorta with every heartbeat.

Road biking became my leisure activity passion. I kept my speeds around 14 m.p.h. and took frequent breaks, which enhanced my enjoyment of the rich Minnesota countryside from late Spring to early Fall.

On a Sunday morning in 2010 I mounted my Trek bike and glided down the driveway of our home. I turned right onto County Road 6, heading west toward Baker Park three miles away. The first mile was uphill and, as usual, my legs began to burn with the effort. This morning, though, my chest tightened as I reached the steepest section next to the Wolsfeld Woods, a forest of rare giant maples.

I backed off my pedaling and coasted to a stop. The chest tightness quickly resolved. I knew what the discomfort was: it was classic angina pectoris, the symptom of heart disease that I heard countless patients describe. The following day I told my friend and colleague, Bjorn Flygenring. He knew my history well. He ordered a CT scan to check my aorta and an echocardiogram to assess my aortic valve. The echocardiogram showed that the aortic graft looked fine and the aortic valve, though calcified, was not so narrow that it could be the cause of my exercise induced angina pectoris.

Thus my angina was most likely due to a blockage in a coronary artery. "You need an angiogram," Flygenring said. "Let's do it tomorrow. I'll see who is in the lab."

The following morning Mike Mooney inserted a Judkins coronary catheter into my right femoral artery. I was awake, lying on the table in the catheterization laboratory. Flygenring was sitting at the monitoring console behind a leaded clear glass window. I watched the catheter on the x-ray screen as Mooney maneuvered its tip into the opening of my left coronary artery. Next Mooney injected a bolus of x-ray dye.

All of us watched as the dye flowed through the left main, and into the left anterior descending and large circumflex arteries. There, in the middle of the dominant circumflex, was a 90 percent blockage, a pile of plaque restricting blood flow to the left and underside of my heart. No wonder I had angina. At least there was no significant disease in the other arteries.

Prior to the procedure I had said to Mooney that I would like to discuss the treatment I should receive after he completed my angiogram. Mooney had smiled, saying nothing. He had dealt with doctors like me before.

Now I lay on the table, knowing that I had a severe blockage in a major coronary artery. Mooney and Flygenring were off to the side of the room talking, but I could not hear them. When Mooney returned to the table, I asked, "What do you think, Mike?" He replied that he was going to place a stent in the circumflex blockage. Before I could respond, Mooney turned to the nurse standing at the head of the table and nodded. She injected midazolam, a sedative, into my intravenous line. Immediately I was in la-la land. Mooney, completely focused and undisturbed, proceeded to insert a drug-eluting stent into my circumflex. A handy drug, that midazolam.

The stent Mooney implanted worked, my angina was relieved, and I resumed biking. I enjoyed the remainder of the summer, but the echocardiogram showed that my aortic valve was getting worse. At the moment I had no symptoms but I knew the day would come when the valve would have to be replaced, meaning another open heart surgery.

That day came sooner than I had expected.

The winter of 2010-2011 was the fourth snowiest in 100 years. In April, however, we had a few days with temperatures in the 70s. Most of the snow had melted and I took my Trek bike out of storage. At the bottom of my driveway I turned right and began pedaling up the hill. Midway up, before Trinity Lutheran Church, I felt pressure in my chest. It was centered over my breastbone and spread outward toward my shoulders. I felt a little breathless. Could this be? Was this actually happening to me?

My aortic valve disease had progressed. Now the valve area was only half a square centimeter (normal is 3-4 cm^2). The echocardiogram revealed that my valve's two leaflets were densely calcified and barely moved. Given my symptoms it was time to replace the valve. I had another angiogram several days before the surgery; the stent Mooney had inserted the previous year was wide open and my other coronary arteries had some plaque but no blockages.

It was May 2011 and once again I was taken to the operating room by Vib Kshettry. Once more Raj Dwarakaneth was my anesthesiologist. Sally and my daughters sat in the waiting room, just as they had in 2005. It was a haunted place for them, replete with ominous memories. They hoped never to be there again.

This time, however, Kshettry emerged from the operating room with a smile. While he encountered a lot of scar tissue from my first operation, he removed the aortic valve without difficulty and inserted a 23 mm St. Jude Trifecta™ bovine (cow) tissue aortic valve. I was on the heart-lung machine for one hour, 48 minutes. My heart started to beat on its own, without any need for temporary pacing.

Anyone who has had heart surgery knows the malaise that grips you for weeks after the operation. I had very little incisional discomfort and rarely took a pain pill. But for weeks I had no ambition and alternated between sleeping and watching the French Open, which Rafael Nadal won, defeating Roger Federer in the finals. My favorite foods were Graeter's chocolate chip ice cream and Sally's Cincinnati chili (these were not included in the discharge diet prescribed by the hospital).

Five weeks later I was back seeing patients part time. By summer's end, I was biking and keeping a full schedule.

One of my college English professors remarked that a good story should have some irony. I never quite understood that until now. How ironic it is that so much of what I witnessed during my career ultimately affected me. I have been a direct beneficiary of many of the pioneering efforts of men and women I have known. Thank you, Walt Lillehei, for open-heart surgery, and the heart-lung machine. Thank you, Albert Starr and Alain Carpentier, for the valves. Thank you Andreas Gruentzig and Julio Palmaz for coronary angioplasty and stents. Thank you, Harvey Feigenbaum, for inventing the echocardiogram that diagnosed my aortic valve disease. Thank you F. John Lewis and Norman Shumway who showed us that hypothermia could protect the brain during heart surgery. And thank you to all the Owen Wangensteens and Howard Burchells of the world whose devotion to research and teaching made all of this possible.

Lastly, I am grateful and forever indebted to my colleagues at the Minneapolis Heart Institute and Abbott Northwestern Hospital. It is very simple: without their expert care and professionalism, I would have been dead long ago.

EPILOGUE

On the last day of my medical career I drove the familiar 125 miles northwest on I-94 to Alexandria and saw a half dozen patients. It was September 30, 2015. The clinic staff had a nice farewell party for me and I had my picture taken with my last patient—an old guy, like me.

The drive home was nostalgic. The exit signs signaled my passage to retirement: Sauk Centre, Freeport, Avon, St. Cloud, Monticello. I thought of my first patient, a young woman who had heart block after mitral valve surgery. Then there was John Leonard's death, and Rose Fisher's near catastrophic tachycardia after receiving her Starr-Edwards valve. My mind fast-forwarded to Blanche Simpson and Jack Pearson, the first patients in whom I implanted a pacemaker and defibrillator with my good friend, Dr. Marshall Goldin. And young Libby Palmer who raised a family during the 28 years she did not need pacemaker replacement surgery. Some people I could not help: John Young, who suffered intractable heart failure, and Janet Parker, who died suddenly awaiting a heart transplant. There was Peggy Lindquist, a 93-year-old great-grandmother, whom I helped in a different way; she had severe aortic stenosis and simply wanted to be comfortable and spend time with her family.

Most painful for me was the death of Joshua Oukrup, whom I think of almost every day. It was not just that Joshua was so young, but also because his death was so preventable, if only Guidant Inc. had behaved responsibly. Unfortunately, drug and medical device safety is not what it should and can be, and the potential for deadly adverse events like Joshua's still exists.

As I made my way southeast on Interstate 94, I remembered the great pioneers I had known: Lillehei, Starr, Mirowski, Greatbatch, Hartzler, Wellens, Wenger, Burchell, and Scheinman. They were as personally different from each other as a fiction writer could make them. But all of them approached their work with three critical attributes: creativity, passion, and tenacity. The same could be said of the great pioneers I did not know well or at all: Braunwald, Kouwenhoven, Sones, Favaloro, Shumway, Feigenbaum, Gruentzig, Endo, Carpentier, and Palmaz. Creativity and passion are vital but tenacity marks the men and women who overcome skepticism and setbacks to *implement* their ideas.

Could Lillehei, Starr, Greatbatch, Gruentzig, or Mirowski do today what they accomplished during the golden decades of 1955-1985? Most definitely the answer is no. The United States Food and Drug Administration alone would have throttled their efforts. Add to the FDA the vagaries and vicissitudes of Institutional Review Boards (IRB), and it is likely that none of their innovations would have reached millions of patients in time to save their lives.

It is not that the regulation of drugs and devices is unimportant, or that human research subjects need no protection. Well designed and judiciously applied regulations are essential for ensuring that products are safe and effective. Human research subjects, particularly those most vulnerable, deserve every protection we can afford them. But year after year the agencies that are charged with applying the law are expanding the regulations, a burden that is drowning innovation and discouraging investment in new drugs and technology.

Of all the pioneers I have described in this book, Michel Mirowski was the most remarkable. His focus and tenacity were unmatched. Walt Lillehei and Andreas Gruentzig possessed the same fire, as did many others. Yet Mirowski had to overcome so many obstacles from the moment he escaped the Nazis in 1939 until that day in 1980 when he implanted the first defibrillator at Johns Hopkins Hospital in Baltimore. His quest for a device that could prevent sudden cardiac death was Homeric in its scope and duration. My favorite Mirowski quote is: "It's not that it can't be done; [we] haven't found a way to do it. It's a question of mind, not facts."

Many of the major advances were considered radical or unethical at the time. Consider what Lillehei did: he took a healthy father of twelve children to the operating room, and connected the man's artery and vein to his one-year-old son using plastic beer hoses and a dairy pump. Then he opened the boy's heart, and sutured close a ventricular septal defect. Andreas Gruentzig inflated a crude homemade high-pressure balloon in the left anterior descending coronary artery of an otherwise healthy 37-year-old businessman who could have been treated quite well with routine coronary artery bypass surgery. Hein Wellens and Dirk Durrer deliberately caused sustained ventricular tachycardia, a life threatening rhythm, so they could study it. Melvin Scheinman created a thermo-electric explosion in a patient's heart to stop an uncontrollable tachycardia. Nanette Wenger overcame dogmatism, baseless preconceptions, and inertia to focus our attention on women's cardiovascular health.

At first glance, many of these events were audacious, but almost without exception they were preceded by careful research, had the support of the pioneers' academic institutions, and the patients were informed of the risks. A prominent exception was Geoff Hartzler who, based on logic and intuition alone, performed emergency angioplasty on patients in the throes of an acute heart attack. What he did, and was criticized for, is now such a high standard of care that hospitals are graded on how fast they get a heart attack patient to the catheterization laboratory, and how quickly the angioplasty balloon is inflated!

I arrived at the junction of I-94 and I-494 where I turned south toward my home in Medina. I reflected on the people who were responsible for the prodigious medical advances that occurred during my career. They were men and women of many races, religions, and nationalities. Physicians and scientists set aside their political, religious, and cultural differences to defeat heart and vascular disease and end human suffering. If only the rest of the world could do the same for its many political, social, and environmental ills.

Indeed, it is difficult to think of any other human endeavor that has benefited as much from diversity as medical science. Human creative and intellectual capital is precious. As you read this, somewhere in the world are boys and girls who, as adults, could discover something important, and others who could apply these discoveries to help patients and populations. While we do not know who these boys and girls are, we do know that they may be anywhere—in the mountains of

Japan, a town in rural Georgia, a refugee camp in Jordan, a village in Argentina, or a school in south Minneapolis. The critical thing is that we find them, or at least let them find us, and give them the opportunity to display their talents and do great things.

After arriving home from Alexandria, I hung my stethoscope on a hook in the closet where it will remain until someone else removes it. Also in the closet was a white lab coat with my name and MHI logo stitched on the front; it too will hang there as a remembrance. It has been a wonderful life, and I commend a career in medicine to anyone who wants to take care of people or do things that will help people live better lives. There will always be challenges, some annoying and seemingly insurmountable, and nothing is guaranteed except hard work and long hours. But the reward is the knowledge that nearly every day you have provided succor for another human being. This is a privilege that very few professions can claim.

I paused for many minutes, staring at my stethoscope and white coat, and thought of my parents. My throat tightened. I wished they and my daughters could be here to celebrate this day. So too my great uncle and his sons, Drs. Jack and Charles Hauser, who gave me more than I realized at the time.

Sally called me to dinner. We sat in front of the television, watching the evening news. It was Wednesday evening, and I would not have to go to the hospital or clinic in the morning. On the morrow I could sleep-in, bike, walk in Baker Park, or just hang out. Sally looked at me, smiling, and asked, "Now that you are retired, what are you going to do with all that free time?" I paused, as if pondering her question, and replied, "I'm going to write a book. I have some stories that should be told."